Praise for *Spicebox Kitchen*

"In a time when wellness has taken over food writing as a new guise for the same old diet culture, Dr. Shiue's science-based take on eating well and healthfully is so refreshing. Even before you get to the wonderful recipes, it's worth reading the intro in which she patiently dismantles myths around nutrition and taste and truly teaches the fundamentals of cooking nearly every ingredient under the sun, with angles fit for both beginners and experts. The book is rich with ideas and, I think, achieves its goal of making good eating unintimidating and accessible to all kinds of eaters."

—**SOLEIL HO**, restaurant critic, *San Francisco Chronicle*

"Looking to spice up your home cooking? In *Spicebox Kitchen* Dr. Linda Shiue brings a world of delicious flavors with accessible recipes full of discoveries from far and wide to your table. Linda's easy instruction, creative mind, and sound nutritional sensibilities gained over years as a physician and passionate diner transform your cooking and you into shining stars of deliciousness. Recipes from around the world make it easy for both novice and professional to cook with hunger and pride. Get ready to stain these pages as you create new favorites from your kitchen and delight your family and friends."

—**SUVIR SARAN**, author of *Indian Home Cooking*, *Masala Farm*, *Instamatic* and owner of The House of Celeste in New Delhi, India

---

"Wow! This book will change your health. My friend, physician and Chef Linda Shiue, MD, has traveled the world researching these recipes and it shows. Incredible flavors you can't imagine are waiting for you inside, along with the sage advice of an experienced doctor on what to eat."

—**DREW RAMSEY, MD**, assistant clinical professor of psychiatry, Columbia University

---

SPICEBOX
KITCHEN

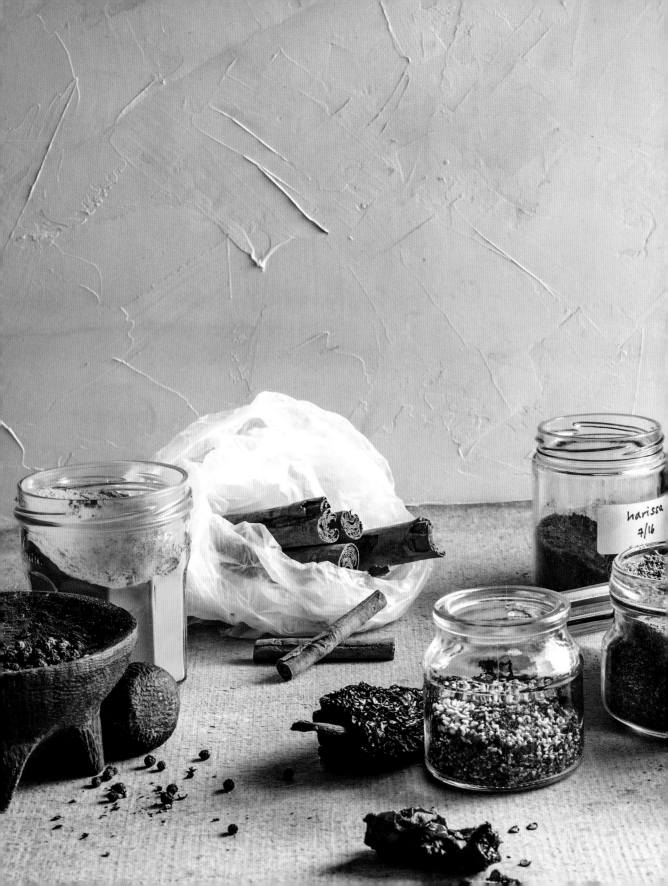

SPICEBOX
KITCHEN

Eat Well and Be Healthy
with Globally Inspired,
Vegetable-Forward Recipes

LINDA SHIUE, MD, CHEF
Foreword by Bryant Terry

Go
hachette
BOOKS
New York

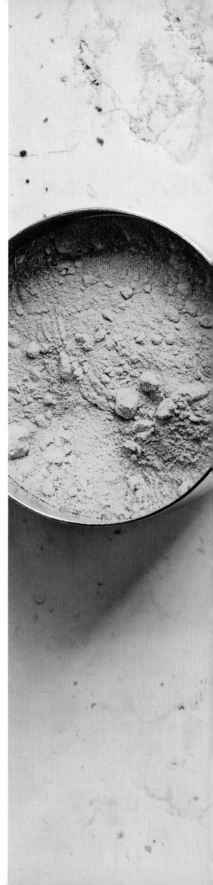

Copyright © 2021 by Linda Shiue
Cover design by Amanda Kain
Cover and interior photography by Michelle K. Min
Food and prop styling by Haley Hazell
Cover copyright © 2021 by Hachette Book Group, Inc.

Hachette Go,
an imprint of Hachette Books
Hachette Book Group
1290 Avenue of the Americas
New York, NY 10104
HachetteGo.com
Facebook.com/HachetteGo
Instagram.com/HachetteGo

First Edition: March 2021

Hachette Books is a division of Hachette Book Group, Inc.

The Hachette Go and Hachette Books name and logos are trademarks of Hachette Book Group, Inc.

The publisher is not responsible for websites (or their content) that are not owned by the publisher.

Print book interior design by Toni Tajima.

Library of Congress Cataloging-in-Publication Data

Names: Shiue, Linda, author.
Title: Spicebox kitchen: eat well and be healthy with globally inspired, vegetable-forward recipes / by Linda Shiue, MD.
Description: New York: Hachette Go, 2021. | Includes bibliographical references and index.
Identifiers: LCCN 2020028303 | ISBN 9780738286020 (hardcover) | ISBN 9780738286013 (ebook)
Subjects: LCSH: Cooking (Vegetables) | LCGFT: Cookbooks.
Classification: LCC TX801 .S558 2021 | DDC 641.6/5—dc23
LC record available at https://lccn.loc.gov/2020028303

ISBNs: 978-0-738-28602-0 (hardcover); 978-0-738-28601-3 (ebook)

Printed in China

IM

10 9 8 7 6 5 4 3 2 1

FOR MAMA.

When making a dish from far-off lands, perhaps
no ingredient is as important as curiosity.
Cooking, and eating, foods from places we've
never seen is as good a way as any (and
better than most!) to expand your horizons, to
remember that the world is a big, beautiful place
of endless magic and surprise.

—Samin Nosrat, *Salt, Fat, Acid, Heat*

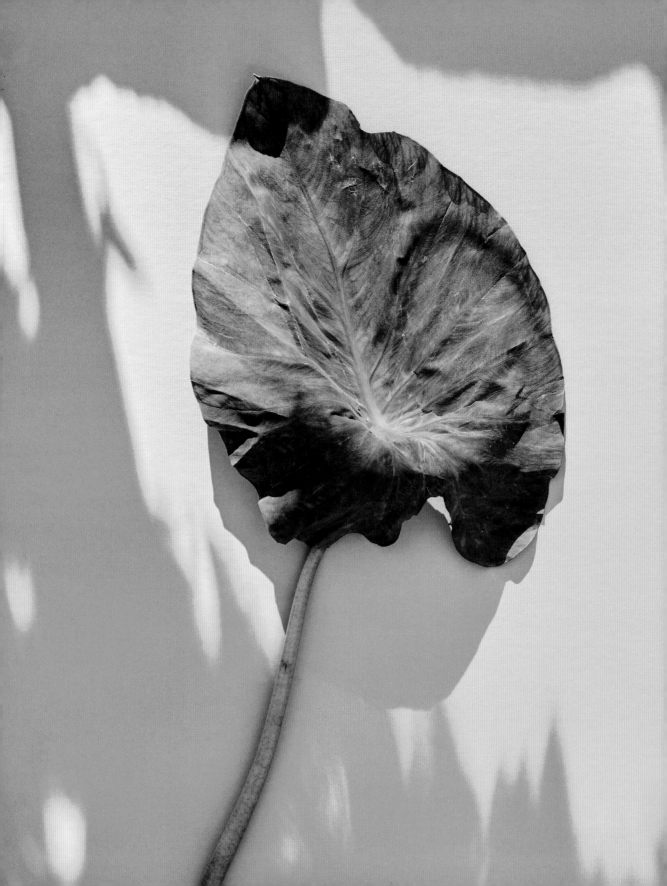

contents

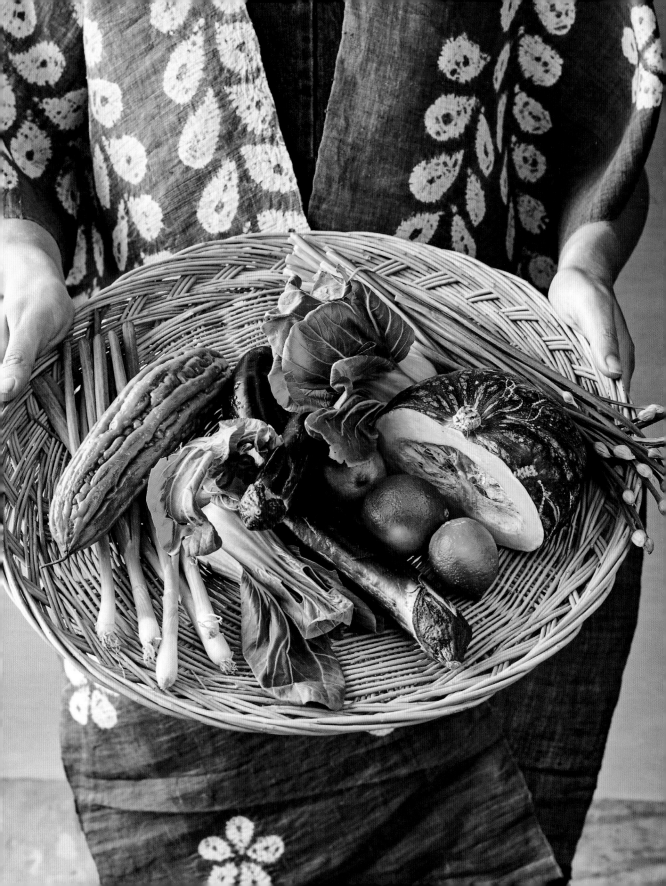

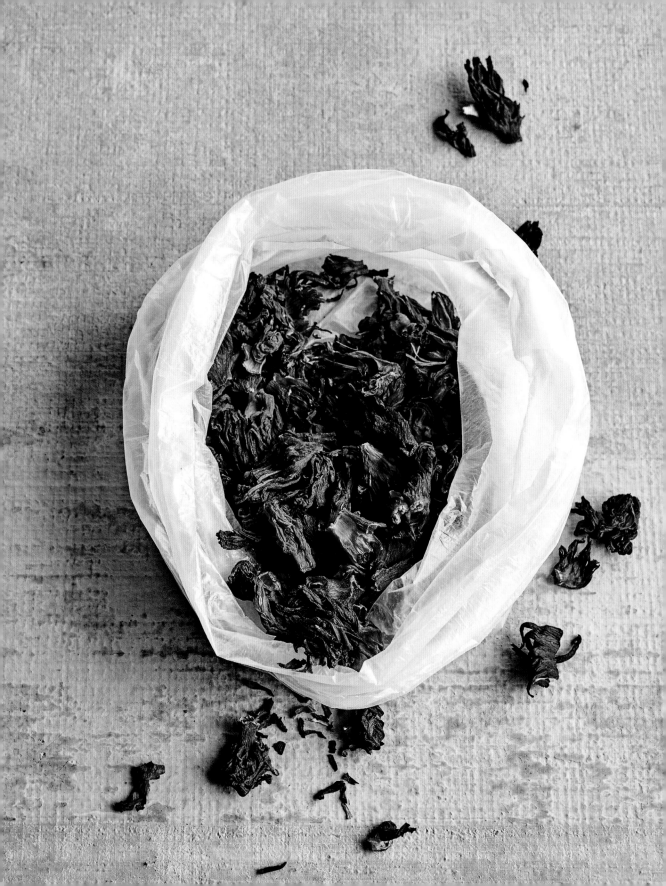

foreword

I FIRST MET LINDA SHIUE IN 2018 when she attended a dinner I organized in my role as Chef-in-Residence at the Museum of the African Diaspora (MoAD). Linda's colleagues with whom she was sitting introduced her as a "chef-doctor" or something like that, and I was immediately intrigued. I had no idea that one of the leaders in the field of culinary medicine came to my event that evening! During our brief conversation, I learned that Linda founded the groundbreaking Thrive Kitchen, a hands-on healthy cooking program aimed at empowering physicians and their patients with knowledge and fundamental culinary skills geared toward improving health and wellness, and inspiring people to get cooking at home.

When Linda and I met for tea several weeks later, we immediately hit it off. She and I discovered that we were both working to shift people's perception of "healthful" food being bland, boring, and brown to a vision of vegetable-centered dishes bursting with flavor, creativity, and vibrancy. I also learned that we both wanted to move eaters beyond simply using staple ingredients and spices from world cuisines and excite them to celebrate the varied dishes and patterns of eating from culinary traditions around the globe. We knew that dishes from these traditional diets could be another tool for improving public health, especially for those most impacted by diet-related chronic illnesses.

Since then, I've had the privilege of serving as guest chef a couple of times at Thrive Kitchen. It was such a joy connecting with patients and other community members in attendance. Linda's classes attract a crowd that's not unlike those who come to my programs—including not just patients, but culinary and medical students and people who grow or cook food for a living. The excitement and eagerness of the diverse crowds who attend Linda's classes are a testament to the effectiveness of her focus on flavor as a way to encourage people to make healthful eating a lifestyle and not a fad.

You'll be glad to know that this book brings the same joy, warmth, and delicious flavor profiles of Linda's classes right to your home kitchen. The recipes are simple enough for the novice or busy cook, and the dishes burst with complex flavors inspired by Linda's home base in California, the varied cuisines of Asian countries she's spent time in, the Mediterranean and Middle Eastern flavors she learned to cook during her restaurant externship while in culinary school, and the Caribbean flavors from her husband's home in Trinidad. Her recipes offer creative twists on traditional favorites, in some cases gently nudging them in a more vegetable-forward direction, which often actually means getting closer to their roots.

Linda also helps you stock your pantry with nourishing staples and spices, and she offers menu suggestions to point you in the right direction. I'm excited for you to begin cooking the wide-ranging recipes in this book, and I imagine you will learn a lot from the comprehensive and user-friendly overview of spices and healthy staple ingredients that form the basis of the dishes. We're all lucky we can experience Linda's words, recipes, and generosity of spirit in the pages that follow. Gather your family and friends around the table, and welcome to *Spicebox Kitchen*!

—**Bryant Terry**, Chef-in-Residence at the Museum of the African Diaspora (MoAD), James Beard Award Winner, author of *Vegetable Kingdom*

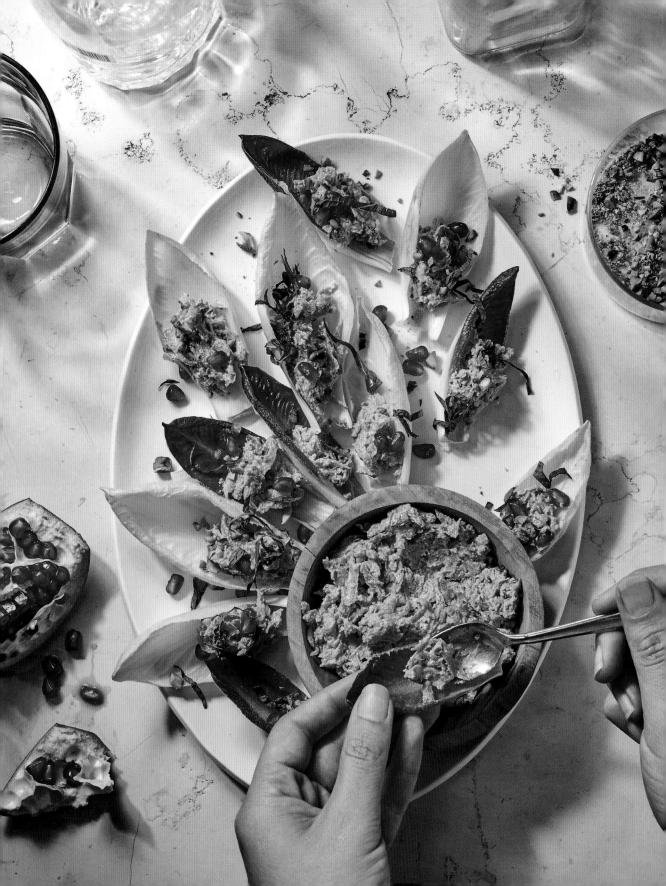

introduction

My Journey from the Clinic to the Kitchen

EATING WELL IS ABOUT FOOD AND HEALTH but equally also about celebration and community. There is a world of flavor, and the passport is spices. I connected my lifelong love of food and cooking to my work as a physician eight years ago, when I attended a medical conference that transformed the way I practice medicine, after a decade as a primary care physician. At that time, I was feeling burned out. I knew that I was helping my patients, but I didn't feel that I was making an impact in the way I really wanted. Despite my support and advice, my patients struggled to lose weight, to control their cholesterol and blood pressure and blood sugar, and they were tired, anxious, and depressed. I wrote many prescriptions, for cholesterol medications, for blood pressure medications, for diabetes medications, and for antidepressants and sleep aids. My patients didn't feel better, and I felt ineffectual.

Then, I went to that fateful medical conference, called Healthy Kitchens, Healthy Lives, cosponsored by Harvard School of Public Health and the Culinary Institute of America. We reviewed the latest updates in nutrition science, and how this knowledge could help patients. We were also taught to cook incredibly delicious food that was also health supportive, by the culinary school's chef-instructors.

That conference was my lightbulb moment. My practice changed immediately: Before, at the end of routine physical examinations, I would review my findings with the patient, discuss their weight, blood pressure, and lab results, and make some vague suggestions for modifying their diet and exercise routine. Typically, it might have ended there. But after my epiphany, with my next patient, I pulled out my prescription pad—and wrote a recipe for kale chips. A week after the conference ended, I taught my first cooking class to patients, and I was hooked. I began teaching cooking classes on a regular basis and felt as exhilarated as my students were. I shifted my practice to include culinary medicine, a new evidence-based field that blends the art of food and cooking with the science of medicine. I did this to address some dismal statistics: About 75 percent of visits are due to lifestyle-related conditions. Half of premature deaths are attributable to our overfed, yet malnourished, society. Only 10 percent of Americans meet dietary guidelines. Practicing culinary medicine is a low-cost, accessible, and culturally adaptable intervention.

A few years after I began to teach cooking, I attended culinary school and earned a certificate in plant-based nutrition, after which I founded a formal cooking program for patients. I also teach medical students and residents—doctors in training—because only a quarter of medical schools offer a course in nutrition, despite the fact that diet is the top cause of death and disability. While this path is nontraditional, it reinvigorated my joy in my career and, equally important, allowed me to help patients in a way I had previously been unable to do. Whether patients take a hands-on cooking class with me or simply accept my offer of a recipe, they are surprised, grateful, and inspired. They tell me that I have changed their life. It might mean reversing diabetes, going off blood pressure medications, or avoiding weight-loss surgery. At the least, eating better makes people feel better. Helping people find their way on this path is my mission, and a joy.

The best way I have found to make transitioning to eating more healthfully a joy is to bring in flavors from around the world. My food influences have always been global and wide-ranging, and I love the adventures you can have in your own kitchen just by exploring different spices. I believe that the best way to get to know a culture is to sit down and break bread (or roti, or a bowl of rice or noodles) with the locals. What I cook and what I teach in my cooking classes are recipes inspired by the people I have met from around the world. I grew up with parents from Taiwan, lived in Singapore for a year in college, and married a man from Trinidad. No matter where I am cooking, I rely on spices to capture the flavors of a particular cuisine. And I am never without my own spicebox. Known as a *masala dabba*, the spicebox found in the kitchen of Indian homes is a large, flat-bottomed, round steel container in which nest several smaller steel bowls for the cook to fill with a personal VIP list of spices. I like to think of a spicebox as the cook's equivalent of a doctor's bag—containing the essential tools to use in the art of cooking. Learning to use spices is the best way to add interest and vibrancy to simple home cooking. As our first medicine, spices also play a role in our health and wellness.

This cookbook shares my love for flavors from around the world from my unique perspective and nutrition knowledge as a physician and professionally trained chef. Whereas most "healthy

cookbooks" focus on nutrition over flavor, these recipes celebrate eating for pleasure. At my table, food is meant to be savored. I won't prescribe you a diet, advise you to count calories, or tell you what to eat. I believe that our food choices should be personal; the best diet for one person may not be the best for another. I do recommend that everyone eat "mostly plants," for many reasons, including taste, variety, the environment, ethical concerns, and, yes, health. My goal as a physician is to improve patients' health by inspiring them to cook more and eat more vegetables. My goal as a cooking instructor and recipe developer is to get people to love and crave vegetables by showing them the many ways to prepare them, deliciously. While this book celebrates vegetables and the recipes that follow are mostly plant based, I have also included recipes with seafood, eggs, or dairy when those ingredients are essential to the recipe. This approach reflects the "mostly plants" omnivorous diet I follow and that I recommend to my patients and students. Cooking these recipes, I think you'll realize that the measure of a cook is not how they cook a piece of meat, but how they are able to coax a variety of flavors and textures from vegetables, legumes, whole grains, seeds, and nuts. I am confident that eaters of all types will find much to enjoy in these recipes. In fact, I can't tell you the number of times a self-declared carnivorous student finishes their meal with gusto and surprise and says, "I don't miss the meat at all!"

While I teach people to eat more healthfully and deliciously, really, it's a party, and a means of building community. After all, a great way to spread happiness and build bridges is to cook for others. Even if you can't join me in person for one of my cooking classes, you can re-create the experience in your own kitchen with this cookbook.

HOW TO USE THIS BOOK

I've organized the recipes into four geographical regions to which I have a personal connection: California, Asia, Mediterranean/Middle East, and Trinidad. I chose these broad areas not only because I enjoy eating and cooking their cuisines, but also

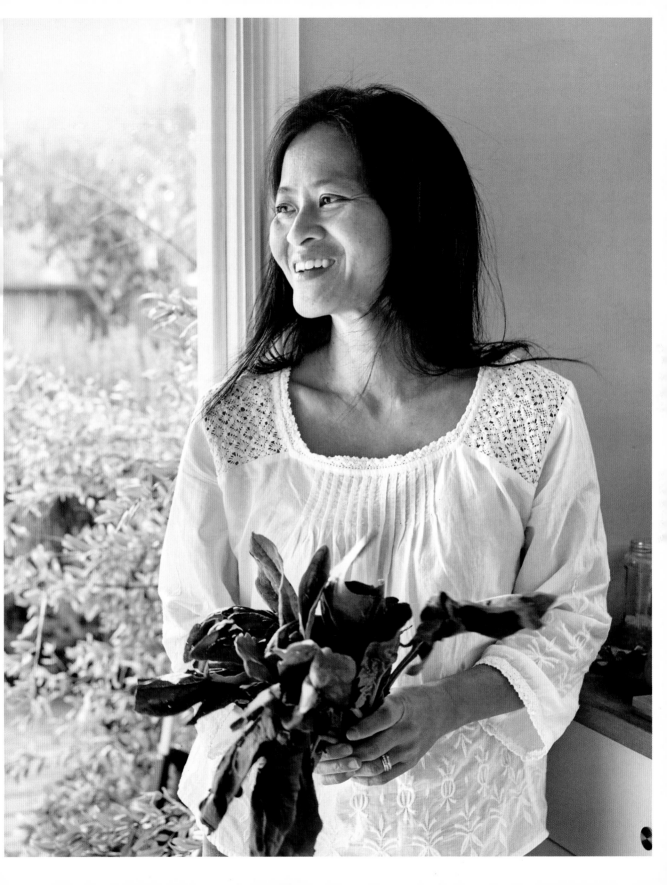

because they represent the diversity of our country and are all cultures with rich traditions of spice-filled, health-supportive cuisine. Each culture has its own way of cooking for health, with distinct uses of spices, herbs, and other flavoring agents. There are also commonalities shared among these diverse cuisines, all of which feature health-promoting ingredients, such as whole grains, vegetables, nuts, and seeds, and such techniques as fermentation.

Most of these recipes are designed for weeknight cooking. Organizing geographically makes it easy to assemble a menu by a cultural theme. For many of these recipes, side dishes can be mixed and matched to make a meal, meze style, whereas others are more traditional main dishes that can be served with one or more side dishes. This opens up the possibility of other ways of creating a menu. For example, you can assemble a menu by theme—choose several dishes from one section of this book. You can also combine recipes from different sections of this book with similar spices, as several of these cross over into different regions. Seasonality is another way to set a menu. Or you can go the more traditional route, with an appetizer, soup and/or salad, and main dish, and finish with fruit or a dessert. But no matter how you choose to assemble a meal, it is good to have a balance and contrast of flavors and textures, just as you would have in an individual dish. Although mixing it up is encouraged, I've also included sample dinner menus for each section.

I designed this book for the home cook of all levels of experience—so, no matter whether you've never boiled water or you're a wiz at sous vide,

there's something here for you. Part One functions as a how-to and reference guide. If you're a novice cook, you may want to spend more time here, to get stocked on cooking equipment and build your healthy pantry, as well as to learn fundamental knife skills and cooking techniques, with special attention on how to make vegetables the star of the show. If you already know your way around the kitchen stove but are seeking to make healthier food, you'll learn about healthy ingredients and how to select and store them. And everyone can benefit from some tips that chefs use to transform food from good to fabulous, including a primer to acquaint you with spices typical for each region. If you want to cook more often, but find it challenging to work it into your schedule, check out the meal planning and meal prep section. And I hope everyone will read the section on reducing food waste, which I consider as important as all these other topics.

Part Two takes you on a culinary tour; you'll discover recipes spanning breakfast, appetizers, soups and salads, side dishes, entrées, desserts and other sweet treats, and pantry items, including spice blends, sauces, snacks, and fermented foods. Please have fun exploring and consider these recipes to be templates. Once you get familiar with the ingredients, you can swap in similar ingredients depending on what is in season, what you have in your kitchen, or simply what flavors you prefer. For recipes that include non-plant-based ingredients, I've included substitutions whenever appropriate. Each recipe highlights key spices marked with → and key healthy ingredients marked with → that you can learn more about in Part One.

Information presented in this book is not intended as medical advice. If you are making a change in your diet, I encourage you to first discuss your individual needs with your doctor or dietitian. In particular, if you will be eating a completely plant-based diet, you will need to take supplemental vitamin B12 and may also need iron, zinc, vitamin D, and omega-3 fatty acids.

PART ONE

HEALTHY COOKING 101

A RECIPE FOR HEALTH

What should you eat? I don't prescribe a one-size-fits-all diet. I encourage you to eat the foods that connect you to your culture, using whole, minimally processed ingredients, and, for both flavor and health, to incorporate a wide variety of spices. That said, I have some basic recommendations on how to eat a balanced and varied diet. The two eating patterns for which we have the most scientific evidence are the Mediterranean diet and the whole food, plant-based diet (WFPBD). Both of these emphasize a wide variety of vegetables and fruits, whole grains, seeds and nuts, and healthy fats, while the Mediterranean diet also can include small amounts of fish, poultry, meat, and dairy products. These diets are both associated with lower rates of chronic diseases, including diabetes, heart disease, and cancer, as well as lower risk of early death. My approach to healthy eating takes into account both of these diets, with spices and a few other ingredients thrown in for flavor and variety:

Eat whole, real food, not processed, and emphasize vegetables and fruits as much as possible. This is better for your health and the environment, and also more delicious. If you do purchase processed food, always read the label, and avoid foods that have sugar in the top three ingredients, or more than five ingredients. (Keep it simple!) Think more about quality, not only the quantity, of your food.

Make small changes. Don't let perfection be the enemy of progress. Every bite counts! This can mean having one plant-based meal per week (e.g., Meatless Monday), and going from there. It's your overall diet that matters, what you eat most of the time. Think in terms of "treat days" as opposed to "cheat days."

Try to achieve a balance of foods. This isn't necessary at every meal, but overall in a given day. Following the "MyPlate" method and filling each plate with 50 percent vegetables and fruits, 25 percent carbohydrates, and 25 percent protein will get you on the right track, with ample room for customization.

Eat as wide a variety of colors and types of fruits and vegetables as possible, which will cover different nutrients and antioxidants. Aim for five or more servings a day. In the Mediterranean diet studies, people who ate ½ cup of fruit and 2 to 3 cups per day of vegetables had health benefits. If I'm going to recommend any one category of vegetables to eat more of, it would be leafy greens (see guide beginning on page 19). One very specific tip that I follow to make sure I get enough leafy greens is to buy baby greens—which are already prewashed—and eat them three times a day. This can be raw (green smoothies and salads) or cooked (they will wilt immediately when thrown into anything that you cook, whether that is a sauté, soup, or stew).

Get your carbohydrates mainly from vegetables and fruits. When you eat grains, aim for whole grains. There is such a variety of flavors and textures, and they offer much more in the way of nutrition than processed grains. (For more info on whole grains, see ingredient spotlight on page 22.) Studies of the Mediterranean diet recommend eating 1½ cups of whole grains daily.

Expand your protein horizons. Minimize red meat, especially processed meat, for both health and environmental reasons. Think of meat as a condiment rather than as the main event. Leaner and more sustainable sources of protein are plant-based sources, of which there is a wide variety, including legumes, tofu, nuts, and vegetables. The amount of legumes that showed benefits in studies was a mere 2 to 3 ounces per day, or about ¼ cup per day.

Make simple swaps. Find a whole-grain bread you like to replace your current bread; if you love white rice, try replacing half with brown rice with a similarly sized grain (e.g., short-grain with short, long-grain with long).

Try something new. When you visit the farmers' market, grab a vegetable or herb you haven't tried before. Ask the farmer how to cook it—they'll usually have some ideas. Experiment with new-to-you spices, and learn how to use them in your cooking (see page 9).

Don't fear fat! When using fats for cooking or flavor, try to choose healthier, unsaturated fat sources, including olive and vegetable oils, such as grapeseed or canola oil, rather than saturated fats, such as butter, coconut oil, and lard. Nuts are a whole food source of fat that can add flavor and texture, and in the Mediterranean diet studies, the recommendation is ¼ cup per day. Walnuts might offer the most benefit—a great source of omega-3 fatty acids, they were shown to reduce death from cancer risk by 50 percent.

Explore fermented foods. We are learning more and more about the gut microbiome and its relationship to healthy digestion, inflammation, and chronic disease, and fermented foods promote a healthier gut. Beyond that, fermented foods are part of every traditional cuisine, a delicious way to add flavor and texture to food while also reducing food waste.

When eating sweets, make it worth it! In many cultures, fruit is served for dessert, whereas baked goods are more of an occasional treat. Frequently eating processed, packaged cookies, for example, will take a toll on your health, and also may not be as satisfying as the occasional well-made dessert or pastry. Amount and frequency make a difference here—why not share your dessert, or do what the Culinary Institute of America's Menus of Change calls the "dessert flip"—instead of fruit as a garnish, serve lots of fruit with a small amount of indulgent favorites. If you want a daily treat besides fruit, dark chocolate (at least 70% cacao) is a good choice, full of antioxidants and low in sugar.

Make it easy. Keeping your pantry stocked with healthy essentials will make it easy for you to eat well. (See page 33 for suggestions.)

DELICIOUSLY HEALTHY INGREDIENTS GUIDE

Flavor First

The best way to make healthier food choices is to start with flavor. Learning to spice, salt, and season your food will make all the difference from something you eat because it's good for you to something you eat because it's irresistibly good.

A Full Spicebox

Spices have been used for millennia for flavor, for trade, and as medicine. *Spices* refers to any part of a plant that can be dried to flavor food, except the leaf (which is called an *herb*). Spices might come from flower buds (cloves) and flowers (lavender and rose), bark (cinnamon), roots and rhizomes (ginger and turmeric), berries, seeds (cumin and coriander), arils (mace), fruit (chile pepper, vanilla beans, peppercorns), stigma (saffron), pods (cardamom), and gums or resins (asafetida/hing). All food, but perhaps vegetable dishes in particular, can be enhanced by thoughtful seasoning with spices. In addition, using spices can be a way of traveling to another culture through flavor.

Spices have also been used for their medicinal properties. Before we had pharmaceuticals, we had spices. Spices offer antioxidant and anti-inflammatory effects from their bioactive constituents, including sulfur-containing compounds, flavonoids, and polyphenols. Researchers are looking at effects of various spices on cancer, cognition, blood sugar, cholesterol, arthritis, and many other conditions. Beyond these effects at the molecular level, learning to use spices to flavor food can improve the nutritional profile of food by adding flavor without needing to use as much salt, sugar, and saturated fat. Here are some of the spices in my masala dabba:

Allspice, the dried berries of a Jamaican pepper plant, combines the flavors of nutmeg, cloves, cinnamon, and black pepper.

HOW TO USE: Allspice complements both sweet and savory dishes well, and is featured in the Spicebox Supperclub Flourless Chocolate Beet Cake

(page 99) and the Jamaican Jerk Tempeh Kebabs (page 294).

NUTRITION AND HEALTH BENEFITS: Allspice has been shown to have antibacterial and pain-relieving properties, and can lower blood pressure.

Amchar masala is a Trinidadian Indian spice blend that combines black mustard seeds, coriander, cumin, fennel, and fenugreek.

HOW TO USE: Amchar masala is used to make the condiment Kuchela (page 319) and other pickles.

NUTRITION AND HEALTH BENEFITS: See individual spices.

Amchur is a tart powder made from dried green mango.

HOW TO USE: Amchur is used as a souring agent and can be used in chutneys (try Nalin's Mint-Cilantro Chutney, page 182). Another use is to tenderize proteins.

NUTRITION AND HEALTH BENEFITS: Made from dried mangoes, amchur contains powerful antioxidants thought to prevent heart disease and cancer. It is also used to treat stomach upset.

Angostura bitters are a proprietary and secret blend of the herb gentian root and other herbs.

HOW TO USE: You'll find Angostura added as the classic bitters in many cocktails. In Trinidad, it's added liberally to lime juice (see Peter's Lime Juice with Angostura Bitters, page 317) and other beverages, and also finds its way into desserts, such as Pone (page 315).

NUTRITION AND HEALTH BENEFITS: Angostura bitters are promoted as improving digestion, in addition to relieving heartburn, nausea, cramping, bloating, and gas.

Asafetida, also known as hing, is a pungent plant resin that adds umami and an oniony flavor.

HOW TO USE: Asafetida is added to many Indian dishes to add a savory note. Try it in the Magical Mango-Tamarind Rasam (page 138).

NUTRITION AND HEALTH BENEFITS: Asafetida is best known for helping digestion, especially with legume dishes. It also helps respiratory conditions.

Black pepper enhances most types of food.

HOW TO USE: Use a pepper mill and always freshly grind your black pepper.

NUTRITION AND HEALTH BENEFITS: Black pepper's active compound, piperine, has antioxidant and anti-inflammatory properties. Black pepper has been thought to help with pain, asthma, and digestion.

Caraway. These seeds have a fennel-like aroma and taste.

HOW TO USE: Caraway seeds are most familiar to many in rye bread. They are also a component of harissa (see page 249 to make your own).

NUTRITION AND HEALTH BENEFITS: Caraway seeds contain magnesium, which supports a healthy heart and brain health. They also aid digestion and contain compounds with anti-inflammatory and antioxidant activity.

Cardamom, a sweet, floral, fragrant, and slightly spicy spice, comes in green and black varieties.

HOW TO USE: Cardamom is commonly used in Indian curries, rice dishes, and chai; Ethiopian coffee; Scandinavian baking; and more, which is a testament to its special appeal. I like to grind a few pods of green cardamom with my coffee beans to get the day off to an excellent start. Try it in the Spiced Granola (page 54), Spiced Green Smoothie with Arugula and Mango (page 55), and Khoresh Fesenjan (page 237).

NUTRITION AND HEALTH BENEFITS: Cardamom has been used in Indian medicine and Chinese Traditional Medicine for mouth and throat problems, lung disease, and digestive problems. It is a rich source of vitamins and minerals, such as potassium, calcium, magnesium, phosphorus, and vitamin C. Cardamom contains antioxidants and also has been shown to have antibacterial effects. One study showed that it has blood pressure–lowering effects, as well as lowers stroke risk, at a dose of ½ teaspoon of ground cardamom daily for three months.

Cayenne: See peppers.

Cinnamon comes in two types: true or Ceylon cinnamon, whose sticks are softer, paler, and layered; and Saigon cinnamon or cassia, which is the more vibrantly colored, reddish brown cinnamon with harder, more tightly rolled sticks that is widely available in North America.

HOW TO USE: Cinnamon is used primarily for desserts in Western cooking, but much of the world uses it to add a touch of sweetness to savory dishes, such as Indian curries, Moroccan tagines, Vietnamese pho, and more. Try it in the Tepache (page 100), Zaalouk (page 208), and many other recipes in this book.

NUTRITION AND HEALTH BENEFITS: Cinnamon, which has both essential oils and polyphenols, has been shown to reduce blood pressure and blood sugar. It is protective both against heart attacks and diabetes. A note of caution: Cassia contains high levels of coumarin, which can cause liver damage at a high dose. Ceylon cinnamon has much lower levels.

Cloves are the dried flower buds of a tree native to Indonesia and have an aromatic, warm, and sweet scent and flavor.

HOW TO USE: Cloves are a component of pumpkin pie spice and spiced apple cider, and Trinidadian Sorrel (page 312). They are also one of the spices included in curry powder and garam masala.

NUTRITION AND HEALTH BENEFITS: Cloves are rich in the mineral manganese, which plays a role in bone health and blood sugar control. They also contain an anti-inflammatory compound called eugenol, which can be used as a mild anesthetic and antibacterial agent when applied topically.

Coriander refers to the seeds of the cilantro plant. It has a floral and pungent flavor with a citrusy taste.

HOW TO USE: This is a component of Indian curry and garam masala blends as well as Middle Eastern spice blends, including dukkah, harissa, and za'atar (see pages 252, 249, and 253 to make your own).

NUTRITION AND HEALTH BENEFITS: Coriander has been used since ancient times—it was included in

King Tut's tomb; Hippocrates prescribed coriander for heartburn; and it has been used in folk medicine as a seizure medication. It is currently being studied for antibacterial and anti-inflammatory effects, which are from its high concentration of antioxidants. Coriander seeds are a very good source of dietary fiber, copper, manganese, iron, magnesium, and calcium, and are thought to help manage diabetes and cholesterol.

Cumin. These earthy seeds are common in Mexican, Indian, and Middle Eastern cuisines.

HOW TO USE: Either whole or ground, cumin is used alone or as a component of spice blends in many savory dishes. Toasting the seeds or infusing them in oil enhances their flavor. You'll find it used throughout this book, including in the Pozole Verde (page 73), Shakshuka (page 197), and Salade Marocaine (page 209).

NUTRITION AND HEALTH BENEFITS: Cumin aids digestion and is a good source of iron, important for making red blood cells and avoiding anemia, as well as energy metabolism and immune function.

Curry powder. A blend of Indian spices with endless variations; Trinidad curry powder (page 325) often contains cayenne, cumin, coriander, fennel, fenugreek, and turmeric.

HOW TO USE: Curry powder needs to be cooked, either dry, or in oil or water, for best flavor. Try it in the Chana and Aloo (page 310) and the Trinidadian Curry Shrimp (page 300).

NUTRITION AND HEALTH BENEFITS: See individual spices.

Dukkah is an Egyptian spice blend that contains various seeds, nuts, herbs, and spices, commonly including sesame seeds, cumin, and coriander. (See page 252 to make your own.)

HOW TO USE: Use it with olive oil as a dip with bread and crudités, or try it as a rub or crust on proteins.

NUTRITION AND HEALTH BENEFITS: See individual spices.

Five-spice powder is a Chinese spice blend that combines cinnamon, cloves, fennel, Sichuan peppercorn, and star anise.

HOW TO USE: This adds a sweet and aromatic note to many Chinese and Vietnamese dishes. Try it in Mama's Chhá Bí-hún (page 165).

NUTRITION AND HEALTH BENEFITS: See individual spices.

Furikake is a Japanese rice seasoning made of seaweed, sesame seeds, and other flavorings. This is similar to gomasio, another Japanese seasoning, made of toasted sesame seeds and salt.

HOW TO USE: Furikake is often sprinkled on steamed rice as a seasoning. It is also used to make musubi in Hawaii, such as the Teriyaki Tofu Musubi (page 159), and as a seasoning for poke. Try the Hawaiian-Style Tomato Poke (page 139).

NUTRITION AND HEALTH BENEFITS: The seaweed in furikake is a vegan source of iodine, which is essential for thyroid function, as well as many other minerals that have cardiovascular benefits.

Garam masala, which means "hot spice," is an Indian spice blend that often includes fennel, black pepper, cloves, cinnamon, cardamom, cumin, coriander, and mace.

HOW TO USE: This is a key component of many curry dishes. Try it in the Trinidadian Curry Shrimp (page 300).

NUTRITION AND HEALTH BENEFITS: See individual spices.

Garlic is the pungent aromatic that flavors foods around the world.

HOW TO USE: To maximize its benefits, chop garlic and let it sit for ten minutes before using.

NUTRITION AND HEALTH BENEFITS: Garlic's sulfur compounds, including allicin, have been shown to lower cholesterol as well as blood pressure. Garlic is also thought to have antimicrobial effects, as well as anti-inflammatory properties, can help regulate blood sugar, and is being studied for cancer-fighting properties.

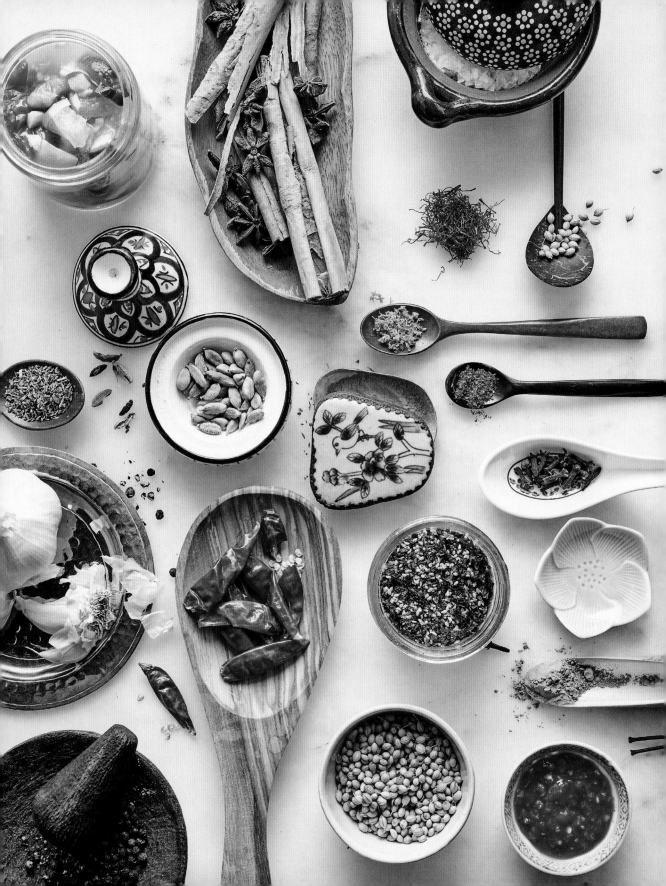

Ginger is a rhizome and is used in both sweet and savory dishes around the world, the latter particularly in Asian cuisine.

NUTRITION AND HEALTH BENEFITS: Ginger has been proven to be an effective antinausea treatment, with as little as 1 gram. At higher doses, it is thought to have benefits for cardiovascular health and possibly for joint and muscle health (it also contains gingerols, anti-inflammatory compounds that can reduce arthritis symptoms). In addition, ginger can help with pain. In one study, just ⅛ teaspoon of ground ginger was as effective as the migraine medication sumatriptan (Imitrex). The same amount was shown to be equally as effective as 400 mg of ibuprofen for menstrual cramps.

Harissa is a spice paste or powder native to Tunisia and popular in neighboring North African countries, including Morocco. It combines chile peppers with red bell peppers, garlic, and spices, including caraway seeds, cumin, and coriander (see page 249 to make your own).

HOW TO USE: Try it as a spice rub for proteins, or enjoy as a condiment. It's featured in the Summer Peach Burrata Caprese with Harissa (page 64) and Shakshuka (page 197).

NUTRITION AND HEALTH BENEFITS: See individual spices.

Mustard seeds come in several varieties: white or yellow, brown, and black, which have slightly different flavors.

HOW TO USE: In Western cuisine, mustard seeds are most often ground and combined with vinegar to make prepared mustard. You can also quick pickle them for a grainier condiment. In Indian cuisine, these seeds add both crunch and pungency to Indian vegetable dishes and pickles. To use, toast in warm oil until they pop. Try them in the Magical Mango-Tamarind Rasam (page 138).

NUTRITION AND HEALTH BENEFITS: Mustard seeds provide phytonutrients, anti-inflammatory selenium, and magnesium, in addition to heart-healthy omega-3 fatty acids.

Orange flower (blossom) water is made from the essential oils of bitter orange blossoms.

HOW TO USE: Use like vanilla extract to add a delicate, floral note to beverages and baked goods, such as the Lemonade with Orange Flower Water and Mint (page 241) and Orange Flower Water–Scented Almond Cake (page 240).

NUTRITION AND HEALTH BENEFITS: Like oranges, orange flowers contain vitamin C. This extract has been used as a folk remedy for anxiety, headaches, and menstrual cramps, and used topically for skin care.

Peppers, or capsicums, include both sweet and hot (chile) peppers. Chiles, such as Scotch bonnet, are known for capsaicin, which gives them their heat. They come in many levels of heat and can be used whole, crushed, or ground, depending on the dish. Almost all cultures use chile peppers in different ways. Some sweet varieties are dried and ground into paprika.

HOW TO USE: Chile peppers can be added to both savory and sweet dishes, if spicy is your thing. One trick for people who like the flavor of smoked and cured meats in greens and soups is to use smoked paprika, a.k.a. pimentón, instead, for a meatless substitute. Try this in the Spanish Spinach and Chickpeas (page 228), Sancoche (page 278), and Trinidadian Black-Eyed Peas for Old Year's and New Beginnings (page 289).

NUTRITION AND HEALTH BENEFITS: Some studies showed that eating spicy food can lower risk for mortality, in addition to lowering cholesterol and improving blood sugar control. In addition, chiles are thought to reduce the risk of heart disease by reducing cholesterol levels and having protecting antioxidants, including beta-carotene. Some studies have also shown benefits in weight and blood pressure control.

Pimentón (smoked paprika): See peppers.

Saffron, the world's most expensive spice, is the highly pigmented and fragrant stamen of crocuses, with a grassy or haylike flavor.

HOW TO USE: A little goes a long way! Make sure to bloom saffron in warm water to bring out its flavor before adding to sweet or savory dishes. Saffron is used to flavor rice dishes from many cuisines, including in the Middle East and the Mediterranean, and is also used in Scandinavian baked goods and Mediterranean seafood dishes, such as the Saffron-Scented Mediterranean Fish and Fennel Stew (page 225).

NUTRITION AND HEALTH BENEFITS: Saffron is a source of heart-healthy and mood-boosting B vitamins, including thiamine and riboflavin. Its pigments come from antioxidant anthocyanins and carotenoids, which are thought to protect against cancer, diabetes, and heart disease.

Sichuan peppercorns are the outer husk of the seeds from the berries of the prickly ash plant, a member of the citrus family. They have a numbing sensation and a flavor combining lemon and anise.

HOW TO USE: Most common in food from China's southwestern Sichuan province and combined with chile peppers for hot pot. They make a nice addition to Whole Wheat Scallion Pancakes (page 120) and Sichuanese Shredded Potatoes (page 124). Ground, they are a component of five-spice powder. They are also used in some Korean dishes and in the cuisines of Nepal, Tibet, and Bhutan.

NUTRITION AND HEALTH BENEFITS: Sichuan peppercorns are a source of vitamin A, important for eye health; vitamin K, which supports blood clotting; heart-healthy potassium; and immunity-boosting zinc and selenium, an antioxidant that additionally protects against thyroid and heart disease. The peppercorns also contain anti-inflammatory compounds called terpenes.

Sorrel, also called roselle or hibiscus, is a flower that is most often used dried to make an herbal tea.

HOW TO USE: This flower is brewed into an herbal tea, known as *agua de Jamaica* in Mexico, or sorrel in the Caribbean, where it is often infused with sweet spices (see page 312 to make your own).

NUTRITION AND HEALTH BENEFITS: Rich in antioxidants (more than green tea) and vitamin C,

sorrel is thought to lower cholesterol, blood sugar, and blood pressure. It also has laxative and diuretic effects.

Star anise. This beautiful star-shaped spice has a flavor similar to anise but also with notes of clove and cinnamon.

HOW TO USE: This is a component of five-spice powder and is used in stews in many Asian cuisines. Try it in the Taiwanese Tea Eggs (page 125).

NUTRITION AND HEALTH BENEFITS: Star anise has been used traditionally for digestion and respiratory illnesses, and is used to make the antiviral medication known as oseltamivir (Tamiflu).

Sumac is a tart, lemony-tasting powder used in Middle Eastern cuisine, made from the dried berries of the sumac bush.

HOW TO USE: Use a sprinkle of sumac as a beautifully red garnish on any savory Middle Eastern dish, where you might otherwise use a squeeze of lemon. Terrific in spice blends, such as za'atar (see page 253 to make your own), or as a garnish on hummus.

NUTRITION AND HEALTH BENEFITS: Sumac is rich in antioxidants and has been shown to help lower blood sugar.

Turmeric is a vibrant, yellow-orange spice with a peppery and earthy flavor. A key component of curries, it is also one of the best known spices for its medicinal properties.

HOW TO USE: To greatly increase the absorption and bioavailability of turmeric, use it together with black pepper and a source of fat. Try it in the Curry Mango (page 290).

NUTRITION AND HEALTH BENEFITS: The active ingredient in this rhizome is curcumin, which is the most potent naturally occurring anti-inflammatory substance. It has been shown to be beneficial against arthritis, heart disease, Alzheimer's disease; autoimmune diseases, including inflammatory bowel disease and lupus; as well as prostate and colon cancer. Turmeric also lowers cholesterol, helps control blood sugar, and has a high concentration of antioxidants. In an eight-week study, a dose of 500 to 1,000 mg of curcumin per day, equivalent to 3 to 5 teaspoons of ground turmeric, was shown to produce anti-inflammatory effects. In another study, patients with primary knee osteoarthritis who consumed a dose of 2 grams per day of turmeric extract for six weeks had similar pain relief as the patients who consumed 800 mg per day of ibuprofen.

White pepper is from the same peppercorn as black pepper but dried after the outer skin has been removed. It has an herbaceous, pinelike taste and is less spicy than black pepper.

HOW TO USE: Use when you might use black pepper but with less spiciness. It is commonly used in Chinese cuisine. Try it in the Roasted Sweet Potato and Corn Salad (page 66) and Mama's Chhá Bí-hún (page 165).

NUTRITION AND HEALTH BENEFITS: See black pepper.

Za'atar is a Middle Eastern herb and spice blend combining an herb of the same name as well as thyme, sesame seeds, sumac, and salt (see page 253 to make your own).

HOW TO USE: Use as a condiment with flatbread and olive oil, as a rub for proteins, or as a garnish for hummus or labneh.

NUTRITION AND HEALTH BENEFITS: See individual ingredients.

Herbs

In addition to adding vibrancy, fragrance, and fresh flavor to food, herbs are loaded with health benefits. Herbs contain vitamins, minerals, and antioxidants and count toward your recommended intake of vegetables. They have been used for millennia for medicinal purposes, as with spices.

Basil, a member of the mint family, adds a fragrant and bright note to Mediterranean cuisine and is also used in Asian cooking. It has many variants, including sweet basil, Thai basil, cinnamon basil, chocolate basil, and tulsi (a.k.a. holy basil).

HOW TO USE: Basil is a delicate herb and is best used fresh. Try freshly picked leaves with summer vegetables and fruits, including tomatoes, zucchini and yellow squash, eggplant, stone fruit, and watermelon. To prevent discoloration, it can be blended with olive oil in a pesto or herb oil. Try the Chinese Eggplant with Black Vinegar and Thai Basil (page 148).

NUTRITION AND HEALTH BENEFITS: Basil contains antioxidants called flavonoids, and also volatile oils that are thought to reduce cortisol levels. It also contains vitamins A, C, K, and folate; minerals, including calcium, iron, and magnesium; and omega-3 fatty acids; and it is thought to have antibacterial and anti-inflammatory properties.

Bay leaf, also known as bay laurel, is full of essential oils.

HOW TO USE: Bay leaf can be used either fresh or dried, and works best when it can be simmered slowly for a long time, as in stews and soups, such as the Mexican-Spiced Roasted Butternut Squash Soup (page 70). It also scents the Spiced Coconut Rice (page 80).

NUTRITION AND HEALTH BENEFITS: Bay leaf has been used medicinally to soothe gastrointestinal conditions and ease digestion. Preliminary studies have found that bay leaf can also help with blood sugar regulation and cholesterol levels.

Cilantro is a bright-tasting herb from the same family as parsley and carrots. Cilantro is also known as coriander or Chinese parsley, and in Chinese as *xiang cai*, which translates as "fragrant vegetable."

HOW TO USE: Cilantro leaves make a terrific garnish for many dishes, especially in Mexican and Asian cuisines. It can also be used as a substitute for culantro, a related herb used in Trinidadian and other Caribbean dishes.

NUTRITION AND HEALTH BENEFITS: Cilantro is a good source of vitamin K, which supports blood clotting. It also contains many phytonutrients and antioxidant flavonoids.

Culantro, an herb with long, sawtooth leaves, is in the same family as parsley and cilantro but distinctive from the latter. It has a unique flavor that is used in the Caribbean, where it is known as *shado beni* or *bhandhania* in Trinidad, Guyana, and Suriname, and *recao* in Cuba, the Dominican Republic, and Puerto Rico.

HOW TO USE: Most of the recipes in the Trinidad section feature culantro, including the Green Seasoning (page 324).

NUTRITION AND HEALTH BENEFITS: Culantro has been used in folk medicine for many purposes, including burns, earache, fevers, hypertension, constipation, fits, asthma, stomachache, worms, infertility complications, snake bites, diarrhea, and malaria.

Garlic chives combine the taste of garlic and onion.

HOW TO USE: Try in Stir-Fried Squid with Chinese Chives (page 153), or cook them in a Chinese-style omelet.

NUTRITION AND HEALTH BENEFITS: Garlic chives contain both allicin, a sulfurous compound known to be good for heart health, and quercetin, helpful in lowering cholesterol and blood pressure. They also contain many antioxidants; B vitamins; vitamins A and C; and minerals including potassium, iron, and calcium, good for heart and brain health, strong bones, and more.

Mint comes in many varieties, the most commonly available being peppermint and spearmint.

HOW TO USE: Sweet, cooling, and refreshing, mint can be used on its own to make a tisane (herbal tea), or paired with green tea to make Moroccan mint tea. Equally appropriate for savory and sweet dishes, mint is used widely in Middle Eastern and Mediterranean cooking. It's great in salads, with summer produce, and pairs well with green peas. Mint is featured in the recipe for Eat the Rainbow Fresh Spring Rolls (page 128) and Chilled Minted Pea Soup with Indian Spices (page 136). Mint garnishes the Roasted Acorn Squash Salad (page 210), brightens the Lemonade with Orange Flower Water and Mint (page 241), and is essential to Moroccan Mint Tea (page 242).

NUTRITION AND HEALTH BENEFITS: Mint oil is refreshing and also has antibacterial properties. It helps with digestion, and is a source of fiber, and vitamin A, for eye health, as well as many antioxidants.

Parsley is widely used in European, Mediterranean, and Middle Eastern cooking, most commonly as a garnish.

HOW TO USE: Parsley adds a bright, fresh flavor and bright green color to food. My preference is for flat-leaf (a.k.a. Italian) parsley, which has a more delicate flavor and leaves than the curly variety, which is a common garnish. Recently, parsley is commonly included in green juices, where it maintains a bright green color. Try the recipe for Grilled Asparagus with Gremolata (page 215).

NUTRITION AND HEALTH BENEFITS: Parsley is a great source of vitamin K, which supports healthy blood clotting, and antioxidant flavonoids. It is also a source of immunity-boosting vitamin C as well as fiber.

Rosemary is a hardy member of the mint family, with a pungent pinelike scent and appearance.

HOW TO USE: Rosemary is great with potatoes and other root vegetables. Because it grows on thick stems, it can be also used as a skewer for grilling while it also gently scents the food. Try the Rustic Grape, Feta, and Caramelized Onion Galette (page 232) or Oranges in Rosemary and Orange Flower Water Syrup (page 238).

NUTRITION AND HEALTH BENEFITS: Rosemary contains substances that are useful for stimulating the immune system, increasing circulation, and improving digestion; it also contains anti-inflammatory compounds. It has been studied for positive effects on memory and also for upset stomachs. In addition, rosemary has been demonstrated to have antibacterial properties as well as to reduce the negative health effects of grilling or charring meat.

Tarragon is a delicate herb with a flavor reminiscent of anise, fennel, and licorice.

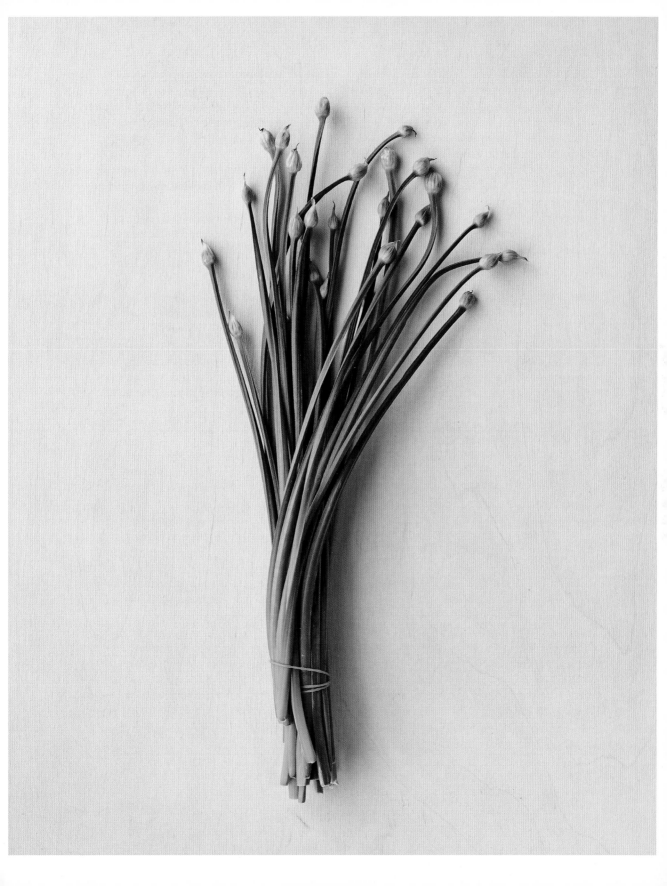

HOW TO USE: This herb is featured in French cuisine, such as the Salade Niçoise (page 231), and is also one of the herbs in *sabzi khordan*, a side dish of fresh herbs served with lavash and cheese as an accompaniment to Persian meals.

NUTRITION AND HEALTH BENEFITS: Tarragon has numerous medicinal properties, including fighting infections, and also improves digestion, heart health, and insomnia.

Thyme, another member of the mint family, is fragrant with a delicate and savory flavor.

HOW TO USE: For culinary purposes, thyme is used in European and Middle Eastern cuisines, including the Middle Eastern spice blend za'atar (see page 253 to make your own). Thyme is also used widely in Caribbean cooking, as a component of green seasoning and as one of the essential ingredients in Jamaican jerk seasoning (see pages 323 and 324 to make your own).

NUTRITION AND HEALTH BENEFITS: Thyme has been used as a natural remedy since ancient times for respiratory conditions, probably because of its many volatile oils, including the eponymous thymol, which has antioxidant and antimicrobial effects. It's also a source of vitamins A and C as well as fiber and minerals, all of which support heart health and prevent chronic diseases.

Salt

You may be wondering why I am recommending salt in a healthy cookbook. Salting food properly brings out all its other flavors and can make or break the difference between bland and incredible-tasting food. Sweet tastes sweeter, creamy tastes creamier—everything tastes more like itself, not salty. It is true that many Americans have an excessive intake of sodium in their diet, but most of that comes from processed/packaged or restaurant foods. Cooking most of your food at home is your best way to avoid excess sodium. When you cook, a little salt goes a long way, if used at the right time (during cooking, as opposed to at the table).

Varieties of salt. As the child of two chemists, I was dubious when I first learned that different types of salt could have different amounts of sodium and therefore different levels of saltiness—it is all sodium chloride, after all. But depending on how it is harvested—rapidly evaporated in a closed container (table salt), in an open container (kosher salt), or gradually (*fleur de sel*), it will form into different shapes of crystals with different densities and amounts of sodium. And depending on the source, salt may take on different colors and flavors, from other minerals and trace elements.

- *Table salt:* The kind in salt shakers and packets, typically iodized, sometimes with anticaking agents added.

- *Fine kosher salt:* A less dense crystal gives this about 50 percent of the sodium content and saltiness of table salt. Used by restaurants due to its pure flavor and ease of sprinkling. Measurements in this book refer to Diamond Crystal kosher salt.

- *Coarse kosher salt:* Larger crystals, dissolves slowly, often used for salting meat. Salty tasting—cannot substitute for fine kosher salt.

- *Sea salt, such as fleur de sel, Maldon:* Formed from gradual evaporation from seawater. These are finishing salts that are used for texture, crunch, and sparkle. I like Maldon salt from Britain; and Jacobsen Salt Co. in Portland, Oregon.

Salt should be stored in a saltcellar—a small, lidded jar designed just for salt, or any container with a lid. This will allow you to pick up a pinch, or use a measuring spoon, neither of which a shaker will permit.

BUILDING BLOCKS:
GREENS, GRAINS, AND MORE

Get to Know Your Greens

When people ask my advice on the one ingredient to eat more of to improve their health (though just one is a hard pick), I always say to eat more greens. What does that mean? There are dozens of varieties of leafy green vegetables, and some that I include in this category aren't leafy while others are not green. Most of these greens are members of the *Brassica*, or cruciferous vegetable genus, which is a varied and highly nutritious group of vegetables.

NUTRITION AND HEALTH BENEFITS: *Brassica* vegetables provide high amounts of nutrients important for preventing heart disease and diabetes, strengthening the immune system, and maintaining strong bones: vitamins C and K, manganese, and soluble fiber, as well as potentially cancer-fighting phytochemicals. To get the most nutrition from your greens, make sure to dress or cook them with a fat source, to be able to absorb the fat-soluble vitamins A, D, E, and K.

LETTUCE

This category of leafy greens contains mainly water and does not offer much in the way of fiber or nutrients. In general, to get adequate nutrition when eating lettuces, consider 2 cups per serving size, as opposed to 1 cup for darker leafy greens. Of the lettuce varieties, romaine lettuce is the most nutrient dense, with twice as much vitamins A and K as iceberg.

To increase nutrition, combine lettuce with other greens and vegetables. Lettuce can also be used as a cup or wrap for other fillings. Try cooking lettuce, too—romaine is also delicious stir-fried, braised, or grilled.

DARK LEAFY GREENS

Arugula is a beautiful, peppery-tasting green.

HOW TO USE: Excellent as a simple salad dressed with olive oil and lemon juice, arugula can also be quickly sautéed. Try it in the Spiced Green Smoothie with Arugula and Mango (page 55),

the San Francisco Summer Arugula Salad with Blackberries, Avocado, and Cucumber (page 62), or the Miso-Glazed Maitake Mushroom Burgers (page 169).

NUTRITION AND HEALTH BENEFITS: Arugula is rich in fiber; vitamins A, C, K, and folate; and calcium. Consuming 2 cups of arugula will provide 20 percent of vitamin A; over 50 percent of vitamin K; and 8 percent of vitamin C, folate, and calcium needs for the day. Arugula is excellent for gut, heart, and bone health and preventing diabetes; it is full of fiber and heart-healthy minerals, including magnesium and potassium, as well as cancer-fighting phytonutrients, which support gut, heart, and bone health and diabetes prevention.

Kale is inexpensive, in season year-round, and a nutrition powerhouse!

HOW TO USE: Kale can be eaten raw, massaged, baked into chips, stir-fried, thrown into soups, made into pesto, added to smoothies, or juiced. I use it anywhere I might use spinach. It's one of my favorite greens, so you'll see it throughout this cookbook. Start with the Thanksgiving Kale Salad with Roasted Root Vegetables (page 69), Pozole Verde (page 73), Kale-Walnut Pesto (page 244), Eat Your Greens! Fried Rice (page 140), or Indian Spiced Kale with Coconut and Turmeric (page 146). **Baby kale** is the young, tender leaves of greens that are often sold triple-washed and packaged, so are ready to go without additional preparation. Throw a cupful into whatever you're eating, raw or cooked. Baby kale leaves will wilt on contact with heat, so no additional cooking is needed when you add them to soups, stews, or stir-fries. Try baby kale in the Piña Kaleada (page 55).

NUTRITION AND HEALTH BENEFITS: Each serving contains 100 percent of the Recommended Daily Allowance (RDA) for vitamin K, for blood clotting; and lutein, for vision. Kale is also an excellent source of vitamins B_6 and C, beta-carotene, calcium, magnesium, copper, potassium, and fiber, helping prevent diabetes and heart disease. In addition, kale contains iron and is great for blood sugar control and digestive health.

Collards are dark, hearty greens with large leaves.

HOW TO USE: The large and sturdy leaves of collard greens are most often braised until very tender, but they can also be used raw, stir-fried, or blanched to use as a wrap. Try them in the Eat Your Greens! Fried Rice (page 140) or as a substitute for chard in the Eat the Rainbow Chard Polenta Rounds (page 202).

NUTRITION AND HEALTH BENEFITS: Very high in fiber and vitamins C and K, collards are also a member of the *Brassica* genus, all of which are a good source of potassium, calcium, and B vitamins. Supportive of heart, neurological and mental health, and bone health, collards also contain potentially anticancer phytochemicals called glucosinolates.

Microgreens are the underdeveloped greens of vegetables, such as kale, arugula, and broccoli, which are harvested just one to two weeks after planting. They range in flavors from peppery to tangy and are full of vital nutrients. Try adding a handful of microgreens to sandwiches and salads, or use as a garnish for soups.

ASIAN GREENS

Asian greens also fall into the *Brassica* genus as very nutritious vegetables in the mustard family. These are a good source of fiber, as well as potassium, calcium, vitamin C, and B vitamins, supportive of heart, neurological and mental health, and bone health. They also contain potentially anticancer phytochemicals called glucosinolates.

Napa cabbage, also known as Chinese cabbage, has a mild, slightly sweet taste.

HOW TO USE: In Chinese cuisine, napa cabbage is often stir-fried with ginger and garlic or added to soups, and in Korea, it is fermented to make kimchi. Shredded, raw napa cabbage can also be used in salads. Learn to make Quick Kimchi on page 177.

NUTRITION AND HEALTH BENEFITS: This cruciferous vegetable contains almost twenty different antioxidants beneficial for heart health. All cabbage is a great source of vitamins K (for blood clotting), C, mood- and nerve-supportive B_6, and folate; copper, potassium, and many other minerals; as well as fiber. Research is also looking into its benefits for type 2 diabetes and cancer prevention.

Bok choy comes in many shapes, shades of green, and sizes. From delicate baby bok choy to bloom-shaped tatsoi, all have tender, juicy stems with more delicate leaves, and some have edible yellow flowers. Their flavor is slightly sweet, with a touch of bitterness.

HOW TO USE: A natural for stir-fries and soups, bok choy can also be thinly sliced and eaten raw in salads, or sliced in half and grilled. See page 147 for a recipe for classic Chinese Stir-Fried Greens.

NUTRITION AND HEALTH BENEFITS: As a member of the *Brassica* genus, bok choy is a good source of fiber, as well as potassium, calcium, vitamin C, and B vitamins, supportive of heart, neurological and mental health, and bone health.

BEET FAMILY

Beets are related to spinach, chard, and quinoa.

HOW TO USE: Roast or boil, or slice thinly or grate raw to use in salads. Try them in the Roasted Beet Hummus (page 214) or the Beet Risotto (page 220). Sauté, braise, or add the greens to soup (beet greens are a great swap for spinach in cooked dishes).

NUTRITION AND HEALTH BENEFITS: Beets contain many nutrients beneficial for heart health, including vitamin C and folate, manganese, potassium, magnesium, and fiber. Their colorful pigments have antioxidant and anti-inflammatory properties. Beet greens are a source of vitamins A and K.

Chard, or Swiss chard, is also a member of the beet family. Its stalks can be white, yellow, orange, or red, supporting glossy dark green leaves.

HOW TO USE: Chard stems can be sliced thinly and sautéed or braised; the leaves are delicate and can be eaten raw, including as a wrap.

NUTRITION AND HEALTH BENEFITS: Chard is a great source of vitamin A and B vitamins; many minerals, including magnesium, iron, manganese, copper, potassium, calcium, phosphorus, and zinc; and many phytonutrients. These properties make chard beneficial for heart health, as well as blood sugar regulation.

Spinach is a dark leafy green familiar to most. Unlike many other leafy green vegetables, it has a tender stalk that is delicate enough to be eaten raw.

HOW TO USE: Baby spinach (often sold triple-washed and packaged, so ready to go without additional preparation) is ideal for salads, whereas whole leaf spinach is delicious sautéed. Try eating the bottoms of the stems, trimming off just at the roots—this is the sweetest tasting part, and high in nutrients. Throw a cupful into whatever you're eating, raw or cooked. They'll wilt on contact with heat, so no additional cooking is needed when you add them to soups, stews, or stir-fries.

NUTRITION AND HEALTH BENEFITS: Spinach is a great source of iron, fiber, protein, and other nutrients that protect against cancer and heart disease, and promote skin and hair health. In both mature and baby forms, spinach contains the highest concentration of folate and potassium among greens and is a great source of iron.

NONLEAFY GREENS:
OTHER CRUCIFEROUS VEGETABLES
Broccoli and romanesco. Broccoli is a vibrant green vegetable featuring a crown of florets arising from a thick stem. Romanesco is another bulbous green vegetable that looks like spiked broccoli.

HOW TO USE: These are excellent eaten raw, broken into florets, or cooked in stir-fries or soups, or roasted. And don't waste the stems—just peel and slice them. You can julienne stems for a slaw or slice into coins to add to your stir-fry, or add to your soup.

NUTRITION AND HEALTH BENEFITS: These are a good source of fiber, as well as potassium, calcium, vitamin C, and B vitamins, and supportive of heart, neurological and mental health, and bone health. They also contain potentially anticancer phytochemicals called glucosinolates.

Brussels sprouts look like tiny cabbages.

HOW TO USE: Like cabbage, these should not be overcooked—definitely not boiled. Use dry heat methods, such as pan or oven roasting, as the best way to bring out their sweet flavor without turning them mushy and sulfurous. They can also be thinly sliced and eaten raw in a slaw or salad, where they taste surprisingly delicate. Try the Gateway Brussels Sprouts (page 74).

NUTRITION AND HEALTH BENEFITS: Brussels sprouts are a good source of fiber, as well as potassium, vitamin C, and B vitamins, and supportive of heart and neurological and mental health.

Cabbage (green, red, or savoy) is a practical, unglamorous vegetable: available year-round, inexpensive, and long-lasting.

HOW TO USE: It's great raw (shredded, as a slaw) and equally delicious braised or charred in wedges, or fermented into sauerkraut. Red cabbage is one of the colorful garnishes for the Pozole Verde (page 73), and green cabbage gets fermented in the Taiwanese Pickled Cabbage (page 174).

NUTRITION AND HEALTH BENEFITS: This cruciferous vegetable contains almost twenty different antioxidants beneficial for heart health. All cabbage is a great source of vitamins K (for blood clotting), C, mood- and nerve-supportive B_6, and folate; copper, potassium, and many other minerals; as well as fiber. Research is also looking into benefits for type 2 diabetes and cancer prevention. On top of that, **red cabbage** contains anthocyanin antioxidants, which provide even more support for heart health.

Cauliflower. Like broccoli, cauliflower consists of florets on a central stem. While it is most commonly available in white, it also comes in vibrant shades of orange, green, and purple.

HOW TO USE: Cauliflower can be eaten raw as a crudité but reveals other dimensions when cooked. Roasting brings out its succulence and sweetness, and boiling or pureeing brings out its creaminess, making it an excellent mash or soup. It can also be grated and eaten either raw or cooked as a rice substitute. Try the Smoky Cauliflower Steak with Romesco (page 226).

NUTRITION AND HEALTH BENEFITS: High in vitamins C and K and many phytonutrients, cauliflower benefits the cardiovascular, digestive, immune, and inflammatory systems. Whereas raw cauliflower preserves the vitamin C content, cooked cauliflower has other benefits. In particular, cooked cauliflower can help lower cholesterol and also has more bioavailable lutein, for eye health. The more colorful varieties are higher in antioxidants, including anthocyanins in the purple variety.

Kohlrabi is a bulbous globe with leaves attached; it looks a little bit like something from outer space but is an underrated and very nutritious vegetable.

HOW TO USE: Kohlrabi can be eaten raw, when it is best thinly shaved, or cooked, when it develops an oniony flavor. To prep, snap off the stems and peel off the skin. Try kohlrabi in the Eat Your Greens! Fried Rice (page 140).

NUTRITION AND HEALTH BENEFITS: Kohlrabi is high in fiber and provides heart-healthy potassium and immunity-boosting vitamin C. Although it looks like a root vegetable, it has a low glycemic index, important if you're watching your blood sugar.

Whole Grains

Whole grains, which contain three components— the bran, germ, and endosperm—are full of nutrients. Refined grains, which contain only the endosperm, have been stripped of a quarter of the protein and up to two-thirds of other nutrients. When you eat this stripped-down grain, your body responds to it as it does to sugar, leading to a rapid blood sugar rise.

NUTRITION AND HEALTH BENEFITS: Whole grains provide fiber, iron, B vitamins, and many other nutrients that benefit digestion, blood sugar regulation, heart health and mood, as well as weight maintenance and decreased risk of colon cancer. They also contain protein, minerals, and healthy fats, as well as carbohydrate. They are more slowly digested into sugars and have been shown to reduce the risk of obesity, inflammation, and chronic diseases, including diabetes and heart disease, as well as colon cancer.

What about gluten? Of the dozens of whole grains, only four contain gluten: wheat (and its many variants), barley, rye, and triticale.

Beyond nutrition, whole grains also have great variety and are delicious! Once you learn to cook with them, I think you will prefer them to refined grains. Here are whole grains you'll find in the recipes in this book.

Corn is a whole grain that provides energy-providing carbohydrate, available as whole-grain **hominy** (try it in the Pozole Verde, page 73), **polenta**, and **arepa flour**, which is partially cooked (try the Arepas "el Diablo," page 93, and Auntie Doll's Baked Pastelles, page 307).

HOW TO USE: Whole-grain cornmeal makes delicious polenta or grits. Corn tortillas and popcorn are easy ways to incorporate whole grains into your routine.

NUTRITION AND HEALTH BENEFITS: Corn provides fiber and heart-health-boosting vitamin C, B vitamins, magnesium, and carotenoids.

Millet is a tiny grain that has many varieties, including recently repopularized fonio, cooks very quickly, and is a great swap for couscous. It can also be made into a porridge.

NUTRITION AND HEALTH BENEFITS: Like all whole grains, millet is rich in protein, fiber, B vitamins, and minerals, especially manganese, important for bone health and diabetes control.

Oats. Whether steel-cut, rolled, or Scottish porridge oats, or otherwise, all oats are whole grain. Oats are naturally gluten-free, but if you need to avoid gluten, check labeling to ensure they have been certified as such. Try the Sophisticated Ginger-Orange Oatmeal (page 50) or the Vegan Chocolate Banana Oatmeal with Hazelnuts, Jaggery, and Fleur de Sel (page 53).

NUTRITION AND HEALTH BENEFITS: Oats deserve their heart-healthy reputation—they contain a special kind of fiber called beta-glucan, which has been found to be especially effective in lowering cholesterol, and also have a unique antioxidant, avenanthramides, which helps protect blood vessels from the damaging effects of LDL cholesterol.

Quinoa is a good beginner whole grain because it is inexpensive and cooks very quickly. It comes in many colors, most commonly available in white, red, and black varieties.

NUTRITION AND HEALTH BENEFITS: Quinoa is a source of complete protein, as well as carbohydrates, fiber, B vitamins, and minerals, including calcium, iron, and magnesium. Quinoa also has antioxidants, especially in the darker-colored varieties.

Rice is a staple around the world because it is inexpensive, easy to cook, versatile, and comes in many varieties. It is also the most easily digested grain.

NUTRITION AND HEALTH BENEFITS: Whole-grain brown, black, or red rice benefits digestion, blood sugar regulation, heart health, and mood. **Haiga rice** is an intermediary between brown and white short-grain rice, with some of the nutritional benefits of whole grain, but a softer texture, similar to that of white rice. **Parboiled (converted) rice** has almost as many nutrients as brown rice and a similar glycemic index, though less fiber, and thereby a softer texture. Try it in the Okra Rice (page 283) and Pelau with Roasted Pumpkin (page 296).

Wheat. Bulgur and **freekeh** are cracked whole wheat grains that cook very quickly and are a good introduction to eating whole grains. **Farro**, which takes longer to cook, is another popular wheat variety. Try it in the Lemony Farro Salad with Avocado and Pistachios (page 65). **White whole wheat flour** is 100 percent whole grain and a good way to add fiber, B vitamins, and iron to your diet when eating baked goods. In most recipes calling for all-purpose flour, try replacing half with white whole wheat, as I do in the Whole Wheat Scallion Pancakes (page 120).

Semolina is a coarse flour made from durum wheat and, compared to standard wheat flour, has more fiber, protein, B vitamins, and minerals, including iron and magnesium. It's featured in Baghrir (page 191).

MAKING THE SWITCH TO WHOLE GRAINS
You probably already eat some whole grains (corn tortillas, oats, popcorn, and polenta made with whole-grain cornmeal are some common examples), but if you're used to eating only refined grains (white bread, pasta, and rice), whole grains might take getting used to. Here are some suggestions on helping you learn to enjoy them:

- **Switch your rice.** To get used to the texture of brown rice, I recommend trying softer brown rice varieties, such as brown jasmine or haiga rice. Or start with 50:50: replace half the white rice with brown, red, or black rice. Just try to match the grain size, for similar cooking time. You could even use other quick-cooking grains, such as quinoa, instead of half your rice. Get creative. In your rice bowl, fried rice, or risotto, substitute other whole grains, such as farro, bulgur, quinoa, and millet (these last two make a great swap for couscous). Any whole grain, not just oats, can be cooked into a sweet or savory porridge.

- **Buy whole-grain pasta**, or a blend that's part whole grain, part white.

- **Try different whole grains.** Good recipes to sample whole grains include Spiced Granola (page 54), Lemony Farro Salad with Avocado and Pistachios (page 65), Arepas "el Diablo" (page 93), Whole Wheat Scallion Pancakes (page 120), Kimchi Fried Rice (page 143), Turkish Bulgur Pilaf (page 218), Mujadara (page 234), Buss Up Shut (page 270), Auntie Doll's Multigrain Roti (page 275), and Rice Cooker Jamaican Rice and Peas (page 293).

Legumes

Legumes, which include beans, lentils, and peas, have been eaten as a varied and inexpensive source of protein since ancient times, in cultures around the world. They have a small carbon footprint and are highly sustainable, and they also benefit the environment because their roots fix nitrogen in the soil, reducing the need for fertilizers. Dozens of varieties of legumes are commonly eaten.

HOW TO USE: Legumes are an ideal pantry staple, whether dried or canned, making it easy to cook a meal. The same bean, prepared with different seasonings and spices, can fit into the cuisine of nearly any culture.

NUTRITION AND HEALTH BENEFITS: In addition to being a plant-based source of protein, low-calorie, and fat-free, legumes provide both soluble and insoluble fiber; complex carbohydrates; minerals, including iron; B vitamins; and antioxidants. Legumes aid in blood sugar regulation more than almost any other food group and can also reduce cholesterol.

BASIC LEGUMES

Lentils. Unlike other dried legumes, lentils do not need to be soaked and cook within thirty minutes or less. Eaten in many parts of the world, including Asia, the Mediterranean, and the Middle East, they come in many different colored varieties: brown, green, red, yellow, and black.

HOW TO USE: Brown lentils are the most common and work well in soups and stews, where they will maintain their shape. Green lentils are similar to brown lentils. Red and yellow lentils are sold split, so they cook quickly and completely, making them an excellent choice for dips and Indian dal (see page 287 for recipe). Black lentils are the firmest variety and hold their shape well, so are the best choice in salads. Lentils also make a surprisingly convincing textural substitute for ground meat in sauces, taco fillings, and shepherd's pie. Try the recipes for Lentil Soup for a Small Planet (page 82) and Mujadara (page 234).

NUTRITION AND HEALTH BENEFITS: Lentils are high in fiber, folate, molybdenum, iron, magnesium, and protein.

Chickpeas, also known as garbanzo beans, are a creamy, neutral-tasting bean.

HOW TO USE: Use chickpeas in soups, stews, curries, salads, or pureed into hummus. Try the Pumpkin Hummus (page 104), Spanish Spinach and Chickpeas (page 228), and Chana and Aloo (page 310).

NUTRITION AND HEALTH BENEFITS: Chickpeas are a great source of protein, as well as fiber—just 2 cups a day is enough to meet daily fiber requirements. They're also rich in folate, iron, and zinc.

Black beans are enjoyed in Latin American cuisine.

HOW TO USE: Use black beans as a side dish, taco or burrito filling, with rice, or in soup. Try them in the Arepas "el Diablo" (page 93).

NUTRITION AND HEALTH BENEFITS: Black beans are a great source of protein and fiber; they also contain resistant starch, which makes them low glycemic, as well as antioxidant anthocyanins.

Black-eyed peas are a distinctive-looking bean with a firm texture.

HOW TO USE: Eat them simply cooked, with rice—try the Trinidadian Black-Eyed Peas for Old Year's and New Beginnings (page 289).

NUTRITION AND HEALTH BENEFITS: These are a good source of fiber and protein, as well as folate and numerous minerals that help lower risk of chronic diseases, including type 2 diabetes, high blood pressure, coronary heart disease, and metabolic syndrome.

Cannellini beans have a creamy and delicate taste.

HOW TO USE: These beans taste great in salads, on their own, or in soup, such as minestrone. You'll find them in the Maltese Bread and Tomato Sandwich (page 200), Pantry Pasta with Cherry Tomatoes, White Beans, and Sardines (page 223), and other recipes in the Mediterranean section (pages 187–257).

NUTRITION AND HEALTH BENEFITS: High in protein, fiber, and calcium.

Edamame are green soybeans, which are widely available precooked and frozen.

HOW TO USE: Edamame can be simply defrosted and eaten as a snack, added to salads, or cooked in a stir-fry. Try them in the Taiwanese "Picadillo" (page 151) and Edamame Hummus (page 183).

NUTRITION AND HEALTH BENEFITS: Edamame are a great source of protein and fiber.

Kidney beans are a commonly used bean in salads, chili, soups, and more.

HOW TO USE: Try them in the Rice Cooker Jamaican Rice and Peas (page 293).

NUTRITION AND HEALTH BENEFITS: Like all beans, kidney beans are a good source of protein and fiber.

Peas. Fresh or frozen, green peas are a sweet and delicate legume.

HOW TO USE: If fresh, enjoy them raw! Otherwise, peas can be added to salads, stir-fries, and fried rice. Their sweetness is highlighted in the Chilled Minted Pea Soup with Indian Spices (page 136).

NUTRITION AND HEALTH BENEFITS: In addition to many vitamins and minerals, green peas provide the carotenoid phytonutrients, lutein and zeaxanthin, which are known to promote vision and eye health. They're also a source of heart health–supportive omega-3 fats in the form of alpha-linolenic acid (ALA) and, like all legumes, fiber and protein.

Pigeon peas are beans with a similar taste and texture as black-eyed peas. They are popular in India, Africa, and the Caribbean.

HOW TO USE: These beans are enjoyed with rice and in stews. Try them in the Pelau with Roasted Pumpkin (page 296) and Stew Pigeon Peas and Pumpkin (page 303).

NUTRITION AND HEALTH BENEFITS: A source of plant-based protein and fiber, as well as numerous vitamins and minerals.

Pinto beans are a creamy and soft bean popular in Mexican dishes and in Tex-Mex chili.

HOW TO USE: Try them in the Smokin' Hot Vegan Vaquero Chili (page 84) and Pozole Verde (page 73).

NUTRITION AND HEALTH BENEFITS: Pinto beans are a good source of sustainable protein and fiber, and are an excellent source of folate.

Split peas are dried and split preparations of a variety of peas, and come in yellow or green varieties.

HOW TO USE: These are most often cooked into soup or dal (see page 287 for a dal recipe).

NUTRITION AND HEALTH BENEFITS: Split peas are one of the best sources of fiber and are also a good protein source.

Other Ingredients

A great recipe starts with the building blocks of healthy ingredients and creating delicious flavors with spices and herbs. To expand on that base, I hope to get you comfortable with adding other produce, proteins, nuts and seeds, fermented foods, and more, for endless possibilities. This section gives a brief overview of the nutrition and health benefits of some of these other ingredients you'll find in the recipes in this book.

NONLEAFY VEGETABLES

Acorn squash. See winter squash.

Asparagus is an excellent source of heart-healthy quercetin, folate, potassium, and vitamin E, as well as B vitamins for brain and heart health, vitamin K for blood clotting, immunity-supportive vitamin C, as well as fiber, iron, protein, and many antioxidants and anti-inflammatory compounds.

Bell peppers are a great source of vitamin C, important for wound healing and immunity, and the antioxidant beta-carotene, beneficial for heart health.

Bitter melon is used in many cultures for diabetes/blood sugar regulation. It has three compounds that are thought to lower blood sugar and also improve fat metabolism. It is also rich in vitamin C, which supports immunity, as well as anti-inflammatory compounds.

Carrots provide heart-protective beta-carotenes, which were named after them, as well as vitamin A, important for vision.

Cassava, also known as manioc and yuca, is a tuber from which tapioca starch is produced. It must be cooked, to decrease naturally occurring cyanide. Aside from carbohydrate, cassava is also a source of immunity-supportive vitamin C.

Celery is low in calories, high in fiber, important for both digestive and heart health, and has many antioxidants, including immunity-boosting vitamin C.

Corn. See whole grains (page 32).

Cucumbers are a good source of vitamin K, for blood clotting, and silica, for healthy skin, hair, and nails. Leave in the seeds, which are rich in phytonutrients, including carotenoids and flavonoids, and beneficial for cholesterol, heart health, and chronic inflammation.

Daikon radish contains high amounts of potassium, vitamin C, and phosphorus—nutrients that are essential for heart health and immune function. In addition, it contains a digestive enzyme called diastase, which helps relieve indigestion and heartburn.

Eggplant provides fiber, vitamin C, potassium, and magnesium and also contains anthocyanin phytonutrients, which give it its purple color. These nutrients are supportive of heart and brain health.

Fennel contains heart-healthy potassium and folate, as well as fiber and vitamin C.

Jicama is high in fiber and low in calories, and is an excellent source of vitamin C, potassium, and iron, with benefits for heart health. The type of fiber it contains, inulin, is a prebiotic, which promotes good gut health and blood sugar control.

Kabocha squash. See winter squash.

Mushrooms are low in calories and fat and are cholesterol-free. They also contain a modest amount of fiber and over a dozen minerals and vitamins, including copper, potassium, magnesium, zinc, and a number of B vitamins, such as folate, in addition to antioxidants that can reduce chronic disease and inflammation. If grown in sunlight, they are also a source of vitamin D.

Okra is high in vitamin C and zinc, which support the immune system; vitamin K, for blood clotting; and B vitamins for heart and brain health; and is also a source of protein and dietary fiber. As an antioxidant-rich food, okra may support improvement in cardiovascular and coronary heart disease, type 2 diabetes, digestive diseases, eye health, and digestion.

Onions provide prebiotic fiber and contain higher levels of anti-inflammatory and antioxidant polyphenols than many vegetables, including tomatoes and carrots. They are one of the best sources of heart-healthy quercetin and also provide vitamins B_1, C, and folate, plus phosphorus and potassium. In addition, red onion contains the antioxidant anthocyanin.

Potato. See root vegetables.

Pumpkin. See winter squash.

Radicchio is high in the heart-healthy antioxidants known as anthocyanins.

Root vegetables are good sources of fiber, especially if their skin is left on.

Potatoes are a great source of many nutrients, including potassium, vitamin C, and B vitamins, as well as many antioxidant phytonutrients, all important for heart health and cancer prevention.

Sweet potatoes have the same heart-healthy nutrients as potatoes and are an excellent source of vitamin A, for eye health.

Taro also has a significant amount of the heart-healthy antioxidants vitamin E, potassium, and magnesium.

Seaweed, or sea vegetables, provide a great source of sustainable nutrition, in particular thyroid-supportive iodine, which can be deficient in vegan diets, as well as vitamins A, B, and C; iron; calcium; and magnesium, important for heart health. Sea vegetables also provide protein and fiber, in addition to having anti-inflammatory properties.

Sweet potato. See root vegetables.

Taro. See root vegetables. Also, taro leaves are a great source of vitamins A and C, various B vitamins, minerals, and fiber. They have benefits for the immune system, vision, cholesterol, and blood pressure. *Note:* Raw taro leaves can irritate the skin, so wear gloves when preparing raw leaves.

Tomatillos provide vitamin C, as well as vitamin K, for immune function and healthy blood clotting, in addition to lutein and zeaxanthin—carotenoids that may boost eye health.

Tomatoes provide lycopene, the heart-healthy antioxidant that is found in higher amounts in cooked rather than raw tomatoes, as well as immunity-boosting vitamin C. The antioxidant and anti-inflammatory benefits of tomatoes extend to many different body systems, including the cardiovascular system, musculoskeletal system, kidneys, liver, and skin.

Winter squash (e.g., acorn, butternut, delicata, kabocha, pumpkin). The orange-colored flesh of these squash attests to the high levels of carotenoids they contain, providing benefit against heart disease and other chronic diseases. While rich in carbohydrate, squash has a low glycemic index due to its fiber content. A 1-cup serving of squash offers one-quarter of the daily recommended intake of fiber.

Zucchini and other summer squash are very high in fiber, protein, B vitamins, and heart-healthy carotenoids and minerals, including copper, manganese, magnesium, phosphorus, potassium, calcium, and iron.

FRUIT

Apples provide immunity-boosting vitamin C, digestion-enhancing fiber, and blood sugar–regulating polyphenols.

Asian pears are rich in many antioxidants, anti-inflammatory compounds, and fiber. The phytonutrients found in pears have been shown to decrease risk of type 2 diabetes by improving insulin sensitivity.

Avocados, also known as "nature's butter," provide heart health benefits from their high amount of monounsaturated fat, similar to that in olives, and smaller amounts of omega-3 fatty acids. They're also a source of all B vitamins (except vitamin B_{12}), vitamin C, and several minerals.

Bananas are known as a good source of heart-healthy potassium, but also provide fiber, immunity-boosting vitamin C, and B_6, important for brain health and prevention of one type of anemia.

Blackberries, supportive of heart and brain health, are high in fiber as well as antioxidants, such as anthocyanins.

Cherries, a good source of fiber, are full of antioxidants and phytochemicals thought to fight inflammation and possibly help lower blood pressure.

Dates are a good source of essential minerals potassium, iron, and magnesium and B vitamins, and are also full of antioxidants.

Grapes are rich in numerous antioxidants, including resveratrol, which has been linked to decreased risk of heart disease and death. Grapes help with blood sugar regulation and also have beneficial effects on inflammation, immunity, and cancer prevention.

Lemons and their peels contain high amounts of vitamin C and other antioxidants associated with lower risk of death from all causes, including heart disease, stroke, and cancer, and, of course, protect against scurvy! Also a source of limonins, which are thought to be protective against cancer, the peel, which is what you eat from a preserved lemon, adds calcium, potassium, and fiber.

Lime juice adds a dose of vitamin C, to prevent infections, and protect against cancer and other chronic diseases.

Mangoes are high in fiber, potassium, many antioxidants, and pectin, which is a starch that can reduce cholesterol.

Olives, source of the **olive oil** shown to be so beneficial in the Mediterranean diet studies, are rich in heart-healthy monounsaturated fats and also boast phytonutrients, which have anti-inflammatory properties.

Oranges are high in fiber and vitamin C, a potent antioxidant and supporter of immunity. Citrus fruits have been shown to protect against cardiovascular disease and several cancers.

Papayas contain the digestive enzyme papain, which can help with constipation and other IBS symptoms. It is also a good source of fiber and antioxidants, in particular vitamins A and C and the carotenoid lycopene, reducing inflammation and possibly beneficial for heart health and fighting cancer.

Peaches are a good source of fiber, vitamin A, niacin, potassium, and vitamin C, all beneficial for heart health.

Persimmons are sources of vitamin A, beneficial for vision and immune function, immunity-supportive vitamin C, and antioxidants and fiber, which guard against heart disease and diabetes.

Pineapple contains the immunity-supportive antioxidant vitamin C, manganese, which plays a role in bone health and blood sugar control, and bromelain, which aids in digestion, as well as fiber.

Plantains. Also see bananas. Plantains have a higher starch and lower sugar content than bananas, and are eaten cooked, like a root vegetable.

Plums are a good source of fiber and vitamin C.

Pomegranates are rich in antioxidants beneficial for heart health.

Tamarind has a high fiber content, B vitamins, and several minerals, including iron. It is thought to have antibacterial properties, lower cholesterol, and help regulate blood sugar.

PROTEINS
Legumes. See pages 24–25.

Eggs are an inexpensive and quick source of protein with many other nutritional benefits. Egg whites provide the protein and egg yolks are a source of vitamin B12 and heart-healthy omega-3 fats, choline, vitamin D, and many other nutrients, which can support liver, heart, and neurological health. They're also a good source of iodine, for thyroid health, and the antioxidants lutein and zeaxanthin, which support eye health. Current guidelines recommend an egg up to once a day, but no more than three a week if you have diabetes, are at high risk for heart disease from other causes, such as smoking, or already have heart disease, given possible concerns about dietary cholesterol.

Fish. Just two 3- to 4-ounce servings of fish per week were shown to reduce risk of heart disease and death in the studies of the Mediterranean diet. Fish provide low-fat, high-quality protein and a good source of heart and brain healthy omega-3 fatty acids and vitamins, such as D and B2 (riboflavin), as well as minerals that include calcium, phosphorus, iron, zinc, iodine, magnesium, and potassium. Fish are also a source of selenium, a mineral with antioxidant properties that is important for many bodily processes, including cognitive function, a healthy immune system, fertility, and thyroid hormone metabolism. **Salmon, sardines, anchovies,** and other oily fish are particularly good sources of omega-3 fatty acids. Canned salmon, sardines, and anchovies are also good calcium sources because the bones are soft enough to eat.

Shrimp are a good source of low-calorie protein, very sustainable for the environment, and also rich in a variety of nutrients, including vitamins B_{12} and D, and selenium, making them good for bone health, the nervous system, preventing anemia, and supporting immune and thyroid function. They are also rich in omega-3 fatty acids, which is heart healthy.

Squid is a low-fat source of protein and a great source of minerals, such as phosphorus, zinc, copper, and selenium, important for bone and heart health, a strong immune system, and thyroid function.

Tempeh is a fermented soybean cake that originated in Indonesia and is now available in many super-markets. It can be eaten as is, or browned in a skillet or the oven for a little crispness. It is a good source of protein, probiotics, and soy isoflavones, which can help with menopausal symptoms, and calcium, for bone health.

Tofu is an excellent source of nutrients beneficial for bone health, heart health, diabetes, and menopausal symptoms, including calcium, manganese, copper, selenium, protein, phosphorus, omega-3 fatty acids, iron, magnesium, zinc, and vitamin B_1.

Yogurt is a source of probiotics and calcium, beneficial for gut and bone health, as well as protein. Strained forms, including **Greek yogurt** and **labneh**, have even higher concentrations of calcium and protein.

NUTS AND SEEDS

As a group, nuts and seeds provide flavor, texture, and common nutritional benefits of protein, minerals, and heart-healthy fats, including monounsaturated fats and omega-3 fatty acids.

Almonds provide monounsaturated fats, magnesium, and potassium, as well as fiber and

many antioxidants, especially when consumed in whole form with the skin. **Almond milk** does not have much nutritional value, unless fortified with calcium, vitamin D, or other nutrients, but is a good alternative to dairy milk.

Cashews have a lower fat content than most other nuts, and mostly unsaturated fatty acids, much of them monounsaturated fats. They're also a source of copper and other antioxidants.

Chia seeds are a source of omega-3 fatty acids, antioxidants, fiber, iron, and calcium.

Flaxseeds provide fiber and heart-healthy omega-3 fatty acids.

Hazelnuts, also known as filberts, contain many vitamins, minerals, antioxidant compounds, and healthy fats. They have benefits for cholesterol, regulating blood pressure, reducing inflammation, and improving blood sugar levels.

Pistachios, in addition to providing healthy fats and protein, contain fiber, antioxidants, and various nutrients, including vitamin B_6, and thiamine. They have been shown to have benefits for weight, cholesterol, and blood sugar regulation, and promote gut, eye, and blood vessel health.

Peanuts are a great source of monounsaturated fats, vitamin E, niacin, and folate, as well as resveratrol, the antioxidant found in red wine. **Pure peanut butter**, ground from peanuts without added emulsifiers, stabilizers, sugar, or salt, retains the nutritional benefits of peanuts.

Pumpkin seeds (pepitas) are a source of fiber, protein, and zinc, which is important for immune function, as well as manganese and other antioxidants. They are also a source of mood-enhancing magnesium, and iron.

Sesame seeds and **tahini** (sesame paste) are a good source of calcium (for bone health), magnesium (for heart health, asthma, migraines, and sleep), iron, phosphorus, vitamin B₁, zinc (for bone health), molybdenum, selenium, dietary fiber, and monounsaturated fats. Sesame seeds also contain lignans, a special type of fiber that can lower cholesterol and blood pressure.

Walnuts are an excellent source of omega-3 fatty acids.

OTHER

Chocolate and cocoa powder have heart-healthy antioxidants called flavanols. For the most benefit and lowest sugar, choose dark chocolate, at least 70% cacao.

Coconut milk, made from grated flesh of mature coconuts, is rich in many minerals that boost heart health, including manganese, phosphorus, iron, and magnesium. While it does contain saturated fat, this includes a medium-chain fatty acid called lauric acid that may have benefits for cholesterol and reduce inflammation.

Coffee is mainly a source of caffeine, but some studies have shown that its high levels of antioxidants may decrease risk of type 2 diabetes, dementia, and Parkinson's disease.

Fermented foods, such as **pickles, yogurt, kefir** and **labneh, kimchi**, and **miso**, provide probiotics, which support a healthy gut microbiome; these bacteria also influence our immune system and help with chronic inflammation, obesity, blood sugar metabolism, mental health, and cancer.

Kimchi, a fermented food, contains beneficial probiotics that support a healthy gut microbiome, the trillions of bacteria that live in our gastrointestinal tract. These bacteria also influence our immune systems and chronic inflammation, with effects on obesity, blood sugar metabolism, mental health, and cancer.

Matcha (green tea) contains L-theanine, an amino acid that occurs naturally in the tea plant and has both calming and stimulating properties. It also boasts many antioxidants that protect against heart disease, cancer, and diabetes. Because matcha is finely milled, it has higher concentrations of these compounds than does regular green tea.

Miso, fermented soybean paste, in addition to providing the benefits of all **fermented foods**, provides B vitamins, for brain health, and antioxidants, for preventing chronic disease.

Olive oil, an important component of the Mediterranean diet, is a source of healthy unsaturated fats as well as antioxidants called polyphenols, which may offer protection from cardiovascular disease, stroke, brain dysfunction, and cancer.

LET'S GO SHOPPING!

Now that you know all about the amazing ingredients that will add flavor and health to your plate, it's time to shop for them. You probably have your usual routine when you go grocery shopping and it may seem overwhelming to try a new way. I'll walk you through ways to approach this; these are the tips my students and patients also find most helpful.

First up, here are some resources to help you make the best choices when buying ingredients and storing them.

Spices. Spices lose both flavor and health benefits as they age. Whole spices will preserve flavor longest and can remain fresh if tightly sealed for a year or two, whereas ground spices will lose their flavor after six months.

- It's best to buy spices in small quantities, unless it is something you use very often.

- Grind whole spices using a mortar and pestle or a small electric coffee/spice grinder. Tip: To clean the grinder between spices, grind some uncooked rice, which will pick up the spices, and then brush it out.

- To make sure your spices are fresh, label your spices with the date of purchase. Alternatively, if their color has faded, or if they are no longer fragrant, it's time to replace them.

- Store spices in your own masala dabba or tightly sealed in glass jars, away from sunlight, in a cool, dry place. You can also store tightly sealed whole spices in the freezer.

Produce. Your food is only as good as your ingredients, and this is especially important for produce. If you are able to grow some of your own, even in a small container, that's ideal. Otherwise, whether you get your produce from a supermarket, local market, farmers' market, or farm stand, try to select produce that is in season. (The difference in flavor between a tomato in winter and one plucked off the vine in summer is the perfect example of what a difference seasonality makes.) If there's one nearby, try visiting your local farmers' market or farm stand. Buying locally and seasonally not only reduces the carbon footprint of your food, but the shorter distance also means more nutrient-dense food because produce begins to lose nutrients as soon as it's picked. This is usually the least expensive option as well, in addition to supporting your local economy. When you can't get seasonal produce, don't overlook frozen fruits and vegetables, which are typically flash-frozen soon after being picked, and are an inexpensive and convenient option.

    To find out what's in season in your area: https://www.seasonalfoodguide.org

    To find local farmers' markets, search by zip code: https://www.ams.usda.gov/services/local-regional/food-directories/

    To find a CSA: https://www.ams.usda.gov/local-food-directories/csas

    A question that frequently comes up is: "Do I need to buy organic?" My answer is a qualified, "Mostly, when possible, but it depends." The nonprofit Environmental Working Group provides annually updated lists of the "Clean 15" and the "Dirty Dozen," which guides you in which types of produce are least and most likely to carry pesticide residue, at www.ewg.org/.

Use Your Senses

Here are some tips on how to pick the best of the bunch. Use all of your senses to choose:

Look. Look for vibrant colors; inspect for obvious damage, such as bruising or discoloration as well as for insects. The skin of fruits and vegetables should be smooth and taut, not wrinkled. Greens should look fresh and perky, not limp, and the leaves should keep their form when you pick up a bunch. When choosing root vegetables, such as potatoes, avoid those with sprouts and wrinkled skin, which are signs that they are well past their prime. Check the bottom of a container of berries for any soft/moldy specimens, and remove them immediately to prevent spoiling others.

Feel. Check for soft spots or dents, which will quickly turn to rotting. Citrus fruits should not feel too firm or light, which indicates that they are dry inside. In general, when choosing citrus or melons, choose one that feels heavy for its size (this is obviously a matter of experience). Except for greens, vegetables should feel firm.

Smell. Fruit should smell like itself when it is ripe.

Taste. Another advantage of going to the farmers' market or a smaller market is that you'll be able to ask for a sample.

Storing produce. Storing your produce properly will prevent it from going to waste.

- Don't wash fruits and vegetables until you're ready to use or prep them.

- Store fruits and vegetables separately from each other.

- If you are using bags for storage, keep bags loose or puncture holes for some air circulation, whether in or out of the refrigerator.

- Keep the following produce in a cool, dark place. Note that tomatoes and the following items release ethylene, which can accelerate ripening, so it is best to keep those separate from other produce. Once avocados, stone fruit, and tomatoes have ripened, they should be kept refrigerated.

  - Avocados
  - Bananas
  - Eggplant
  - Garlic
  - Onions
  - Pears
  - Potatoes
  - Stone fruit
  - Sweet potatoes
  - Tomatoes
  - Winter squash

- Keep the following produce in the refrigerator in the crisper drawers. Before storing root vegetables with green tops, such as carrots, radishes, and beets, remove their greens and save them for use in pestos or other dishes.

  - Apples
  - Broccoli and cauliflower
  - Brussels sprouts
  - Celery
  - Citrus: lemons, limes, oranges, and grapefruit
  - Greens
  - Melons
  - Mushrooms
  - Peppers
  - Root vegetables, except potatoes and sweet potatoes: carrots, parsnips, radishes, and beets
  - Scallions, with the bulb wrapped in a damp paper towel
  - Zucchini and summer squash

- Herbs can be stored like cut flowers. Cut off the bottom of the stem on the diagonal, then store them in water, with the leaves loosely covered in plastic, in the refrigerator. (Basil is an exception, which should be kept at room temperature.) You can wrap delicate herbs, such as cilantro and dill, in a barely damp paper towel, and then keep them loosely covered in a plastic bag in the refrigerator.

Whole grains. If you are new to whole grains, you might be thinking about mushy brown rice. But in fact, there are dozens of whole grains, and only four of them contain gluten, for anyone who needs to avoid gluten. My favorite resource for learning about whole grains is the nonprofit www.wholegrainscouncil.org/. And my favorite way to try out whole grains without breaking the bank are the bulk bins of your local supermarket, where you can buy as much or as little as you want. Try different varieties. Some are quick cooking, such as **amaranth, bulgur, whole-grain cornmeal, freekeh, millet, oats, quinoa,** and many varieties of rice, including Japanese partially milled **haiga, brown jasmine,** and **parboiled (converted),** popular in the Caribbean. Longer cooking grains include **short-grain brown rice, black rice, farro,** and **wheat berries.** When purchasing products made from whole grains, such as bread, it can be confusing if it is truly whole grain versus containing some whole grains. Don't be confused by the words *multigrain* or *wheat*—if it isn't labeled "100% whole grain," then take a look at the nutrition label, do a quick calculation, and make sure the ratio of carbohydrate to fiber is 5:1 or less.

Protein. You might be surprised to learn that plants also offer complete protein (as well as fiber and a wide variety of vitamins, minerals, and antioxidants that are not found in animal products). So, explore plant-based proteins: beans and lentils; whole soy products, including edamame, tofu, and tempeh; nuts and seeds, including hemp and chia seeds; whole grains, especially quinoa; and green vegetables, including peas, broccoli, Brussels sprouts, kale, and cauliflower.

Fish and seafood. These provide excellent nutrition: they are a source of omega-3 fatty acids, which are important for heart and brain health, as well as vitamin D, selenium, and protein, and are low in saturated fats. Like vegetarian diets, pescatarian diets are associated with lower rates of obesity and risk of diabetes. However, many species of fish are endangered due to overfishing, and eating excess amounts of certain types of seafood can lead to excess levels of heavy metals, including mercury. For best choices regarding sustainability, Monterey Bay Aquarium's annually updated Seafood Watch (www.seafoodwatch.org/) is an excellent guide, with specific recommendations for different locations. Regarding heavy metal exposure, a good guideline is to restrict seafood to no more than twice a week and to avoid larger fish, which are more likely to contain heavy metals; this is especially important for pregnant or nursing women and young children under the age of six. These include king mackerel, marlin, orange roughy, shark, swordfish, tilefish, ahi tuna, and bigeye tuna but may vary by location, so check the EPA's website for current details: https://www.epa.gov/fish-tech/. For the best sources of omega-3 fatty acids, eat fatty fish, which include salmon, herring, mackerel, anchovies, and sardines. Wild fish and seafood are overall the best choice. Farmed fish and seafood are a less expensive source, but there are some environmental, toxic, and ethical concerns about this popular practice. If buying farmed fish, buy from domestic sources, which have a better chance of adhering to environmental regulations. No matter the source, just two 4-ounce servings per week showed health benefits in the Mediterranean diet studies.

Meat alternatives. "Fake meat" is becoming wildly popular, but for both flavor and nutrition, I prefer the centuries-old meat alternatives, which contain fewer ingredients and are less processed. These include tofu in all its textures, and tempeh. Made from wheat gluten, seitan has also been used for thousands of years as a chewy substitute for meat.

Meat, including beef, pork, lamb, and poultry. I don't include recipes for meat in this book, but if you do eat meat, it's important to consider the source. These animal-based proteins have different effects on the environment and health depending on whether they come from animals raised conventionally versus organic, grass-fed, and pasture-raised meat from animals raised by small producers. Meat from more readily available and inexpensive, conventionally raised animals generally contains hormones and antibiotics, and because of their lifestyles, more saturated fat than organic, grass-fed, pasture-raised meat. For your health, it is better to eat smaller amounts of more expensive, locally sourced meat less frequently than conventionally raised meat more often.

STOCKING A HEALTHY PANTRY

You're one step closer to a delicious, healthier meal if you build and maintain a well-stocked pantry and keep some basics in the fridge. Use this list as a jumping-off point for stocking your own.

PANTRY BASICS

- **Whole Grains**
  - Bulgur wheat
  - Cornmeal, coarse-ground
  - Farro
  - Oats, rolled and steel-cut
  - Quinoa
  - Rice: black, brown, haiga (partially milled), mixed, red
  - White whole wheat flour

- **Dried pasta and noodles: whole grain or legume based**

- **Dried or canned beans and pulses: black, chickpea, pinto, white, lentils, yellow split peas**

- **Sardines and anchovies**

- **Seasonings**
  - Diamond Crystal kosher salt
  - Black peppercorns with grinder
  - Spices: cardamom, cayenne, cinnamon, cumin, curry powder, dried chiles, garlic powder, ground ginger, nutmeg, smoked paprika, turmeric
  - Dried herbs: bay leaf, oregano, rosemary, thyme

- ☐ Low-sodium soy sauce or tamari
- ☐ Asian fish sauce (vegetarian versions are available)
- ☐ Unsalted vegetable broth
- ☐ No- or low-sodium diced tomatoes
- ☐ Aromatics: garlic, ginger, onions, shallots
- ☐ Acids: lemons, limes; vinegars: apple cider, balsamic, rice, red wine, sherry

- ○ Cooking fats: olive oil, neutral oil, such as canola or grapeseed
- ○ Flavoring oil: coconut oil, toasted sesame oil, walnut oil
- ○ Nuts (almonds, cashews, walnuts), seeds (pumpkin seeds, sesame seeds), nut butters (almond or peanut butter)
- ○ Sweeteners: agave nectar, honey, pure maple syrup, sugar
- ○ Root vegetables: potatoes, sweet potatoes, winter squash

Note: Canned food can be high in sodium, so whenever possible, choose versions that have no salt added. Draining and rinsing canned beans will reduce sodium significantly. Also look for cans labeled BPA-free, as there are health concerns with this chemical, which is commonly contained in can linings. Alternatively, look for Tetra Paks, which are always BPA-free.

IN THE FRIDGE AND FREEZER: THESE ARE THE ITEMS I MAKE SURE I REPLENISH EVERY WEEK; PRODUCE VARIES BY SEASON

- ○ Butter or vegan butter
- ○ Eggs
- ○ Milk or plant-based milk
- ○ Tofu, tempeh
- ○ Seasonings: chili sauce, Thai curry paste, miso, Dijon mustard
- ○ Fresh herbs: basil, cilantro, mint, flat-leaf parsley, thyme

- ○ Leafy greens: arugula, baby greens, chard, kale, lettuces, spinach
- ○ Cabbage
- ○ Carrots
- ○ Cucumbers
- ○ Mushrooms
- ○ Tomatoes or cherry tomatoes
- ○ Frozen fruit, corn, peas

EQUIPMENT AND TECHNIQUES

Equipment

Cooking equipment doesn't need to be fancy or expensive. Inexpensive, good-quality cookware can be purchased online or from discount retailers; a restaurant supply store open to the public is another great resource. Try to purchase pots and pans with oven-safe (metal) handles, for maximum flexibility. And even if you already have a stocked kitchen, here are some key pieces that make healthy cooking easier.

JUST THE BASICS

- ○ Cutting board (wood is best, followed by plastic. Glass cutting boards will dull your knife.)
- ○ Chef's knife and honing steel, to keep your knife edge sharp
- ○ Paring knife
- ○ Serrated knife
- ○ 2-quart saucepan
- ○ 10- or 12-inch skillet or sauté pan (best choices: stainless steel, cast iron, and if you want nonstick, ceramic preferred)
- ○ Set of three to five mixing bowls
- ○ Colander

- ○ Set of dry measuring cups
- ○ 2-cup glass liquid measuring cup
- ○ Set of measuring spoons
- ○ Vegetable peeler
- ○ Box grater
- ○ Can opener
- ○ Several wooden spoons
- ○ Spatulas
- ○ Tongs
- ○ Scissors
- ○ Pot holders
- ○ Dish towels

NEXT LEVEL

- ○ 4-quart saucepan with lid
- ○ 6-quart saucepan with lid
- ○ Dutch oven
- ○ 8-inch nonstick skillet or omelet pan
- ○ Baking sheets—get heavy-duty aluminum professional-grade sheets, so they won't warp. These sheet pans can be used for everything from cookies to full-on sheet pan dinners
- ○ Ladle
- ○ Whisk
- ○ Zester/rasp-type grater—can be used to zest citrus, grate ginger, garlic, chocolate, cheese, etc.
- ○ Collapsible metal steamer basket

OPTIONAL BUT VERY USEFUL

- ○ Salad spinner
- ○ Citrus squeezer

- ○ Mortar and pestle or electric spice/coffee grinder
- ○ Electric mixer
- ○ High-speed blender for smoothies, nut milks, cashew cream, purees, and sauces
- ○ Food processor—the mini type, with 4-cup capacity, which is great for chopping nuts and bread crumbs and making pesto
- ○ Immersion blender—for pureeing hot liquids
- ○ Electric rice cooker—not just for rice, for any whole grains
- ○ Slow cooker and/or electric pressure cooker
- ○ Digital scale—for the most accurate measurements

Healthy Cooking Techniques

Healthy cooking techniques allow you to coax the best flavor and texture from vegetables. I've started with knife skills because how you cut a vegetable can make a very big difference in texture and taste, as well as determine the best cooking method to use.

KNIFE SKILLS
Knowing the basics of choosing and maintaining knives and learning how to use them will make you a more efficient, safer, and better cook. Buy the best chef's knife you can because it will become a kitchen workhorse that can last a lifetime.

TYPES OF KNIVES—THE ESSENTIALS

Chef's knife: This is the knife you'll use most of the time. A classic chef's knife has a broad, tapering blade, sharp tip, and hefty handle. Choose one that feels comfortable in your hand.

Utility or paring knife: This small knife has a short blade, 3 to 4 inches long, which makes it easy to control. Best for small, soft ingredients, such as apples and potatoes.

Serrated knife: A large serrated knife, with its sawtooth edge, is useful for slicing bread, as well as slicing soft-skinned ingredients, such as tomatoes, and also hard ingredients, such as butternut squash, watermelon, and pineapples.

Knife (honing) steel: This is not a knife, but an essential accessory. A steel is a ribbed rod attached to a handle, used to maintain the edge of a knife's blade so that it stays sharp longer.

HOLDING, USING, AND MAINTAINING A KNIFE

- Here is the knife grip used by most chefs: The palm of the hand chokes up on the handle while the thumb and index finger grip the top of the blade. This allows for better control of the blade and is also more ergonomic. But the best way to hold a knife is the way that feels safest to you.

- The ideal position for your other hand, the "helping hand," is called the claw or C grip, with the fingertips curled under and knuckles pressing down on the ingredient to keep it from rolling or sliding.

- Use your arm and upper body, not just your hand and wrist, to put downward pressure on the knife.

- Move the knife in a rocking motion, from front to back, as well as up and down. It should glide smoothly and quietly rather than chopping straight up and down.

- Make sure your cutting board stays firmly in place on the counter by laying a wet kitchen towel underneath.

- After use, hand wash your knife, and dry with a towel immediately.

- Honing makes the blade of a knife straight and is done with a knife (honing) steel by drawing the blade over and over along an abrasive rod of metal, ceramic, or stone. Do this at least once a week. Keeping your knives sharp will allow for clean cuts, as opposed to mashing or crushing vegetables.

- Keep your knives sharp. Manual whetstones are best, but tricky to use. Bring your knives to a knife shop or hardware store to have them professionally sharpened once a year, more often as needed.

BASIC CUTS

Onion

SLICE. Cut the onion in half, in the direction of the lines on the skin. Cut off the root. Remove the skin. Place the cut edge on a cutting board, then slice into your desired thickness on a slight angle, following the lines of the onion.

DICE. Cut the onion in half, in the direction of the lines on the skin. Do *not* remove the root. Remove the skin. Place the cut edge on the cutting board and make one or more horizontal cuts; the size depends on how large you want your final pieces to be. Next, make vertical cuts, to your desired size, stopping short of the root by about ¼ inch. Then, make perpendicular cuts to make evenly sized cubes.

Other Vegetables

DICE. First slice off a thin slice of your vegetable to make a stable, flat cutting surface. Lay it on its flat side, then cut slices of the desired final thickness of your dice. Then, cut slices into batons/sticks of the same thickness. Finally, gather the batons into a flat bundle and cut across into equal-size cubes.

JULIENNE. This is the method to create matchsticks or batons, which are thicker. Start with clean, peeled vegetables. If it is a long vegetable, first cut crosswise into 2-inch-long pieces, and then cut one thin slice off each of those pieces lengthwise to get a flat, stable surface to place on the cutting board. Make slices of your desired thickness lengthwise through the prepared piece. Stack your slices and cut into thin, equal strips.

Garlic

THE EASIEST WAY TO PEEL AND CHOP OR MINCE GARLIC is to place a garlic clove on the cutting board, then use the side of a chef's knife to smash it. Remove the skin, and repeat the process with each clove you need for your recipe. Cut off the root ends and discard. Then, spread the peeled garlic across a cutting board, and chop by using your gripping hand to move the blade up and down in a rocking motion and your helping hand to steady the top of the blade, moving across the garlic cloves repeatedly until they are chopped or minced to your desired size.

Herbs

CHOP. Use your fingers to strip the leaves from the main stem. Discard the stems. Gather the leaves into a bundle and, using the "claw" grip, push them under your knife, using a rocking motion to chop them. Then, gather up all the chopped herbs, turn the pile 90 degrees, and chop them again for a rough chop. Repeat this process for finer pieces.

CHIFFONADE (ribbons) for basil, other leafy herbs, or greens. Pick the cleaned leaves from the stem and stack the leaves. Then, roll the leaves together into a tight roll or "cigar." Using your chef's knife, cut across the rolled-up bundle to make slices about ¼ inch thick. Keep the tip of your knife on the cutting surface and move the base of the blade in a rocking motion as you cut; this will provide stability and help the cutting go faster.

VEGETABLE PREPARATION

Start by washing your vegetables. For greens, take special care to clean them thoroughly. Leaves can accumulate a lot of soil, so don't just rinse them in a colander. Instead, submerge them in a large bowl or sink of cold water and gently swish them around, then remove them from the water, drain, and repeat with fresh water until there is no more dirt on the bottom of the bowl or sink. In the case of lettuce, adding some ice to the water will crisp up the leaves as well. Once clean, use a salad spinner to completely dry the greens, or dry with clean towels.

Raw. For salads especially, how you cut a vegetable can make a very big difference in texture and taste.

- For dense, tough vegetables, such as carrots or radishes, grate or thinly slice them. They'll become delicate, and by increasing surface area, you'll also provide a bigger exposure to dressing and other seasoning (flavor!).

- Make sure your greens are dry for salads, using a salad spinner or towels. This helps them stay crisp and hold onto dressing.

- Massage your kale. This tenderizes it and reduces its bitterness, and is a game changer for people who don't think they like kale salad. First, strip the leaves from the tough center rib, chop into strips, then massage with your hands, either dry or with salt and olive oil, until darker green and softened.

Cooked. The size of cuts for cooked vegetables depends on how quickly or slowly you will be cooking your vegetables. For slow methods, such as roasting or braising, 2- to 3-inch chunks will allow the vegetables to maintain their shape during long cooking. For quick sautés or stir-fries, cut thinly enough so that they can cook in a few minutes. Either way, make sure you cut your vegetables the same size so that they will cook evenly.

Healthy Cooking Methods

This section is to help you understand why you might choose one cooking method over another, depending on the ingredient and type of dish.

Blanching involves very briefly boiling vegetables in a large pot of salted boiling water until barely cooked, just a few minutes, then briefly shocking in an ice bath until just cooled (or else they'll get soggy), before drying on a towel. Blanching maintains color, texture, taste, and nutrition and is a great way to transform vegetables from raw to just cooked. This can also be done as a first step to reduce cooking time when sautéing greens or harder vegetables, to be followed by sautéing or roasting; for meal prep; or before freezing.

Boiling is one of the most basic of cooking techniques, whether it's to cook grains, pasta, or vegetables. For vegetables, I recommend this method for making soups or purees only.

Braising refers to cooking with a small amount of liquid over low heat for a long time—cooking slow and low. A heavy-bottomed pot, such as a Dutch oven, is best.

Frying can include panfrying, shallow frying, and deep-frying, the difference being increasing amounts of of oil. Of these methods, the only one I would consider healthy is panfrying in minimal oil, which is still an excellent method to develop crispiness and crunchiness for such things as firm tofu, tempeh, and battered vegetables.

Grilling, broiling, baking, and roasting are high-heat methods that bring out vegetables' sweetness. Grilling and broiling cook vegetables quickly. Baking and roasting are hands-off methods of cooking that allow you to prepare the rest of your meal while they sit in the oven. To get the best results when roasting vegetables, two key tips are (1) temperature—high heat (400° to 425°F, depending on your oven) is essential; and (2) not overcrowding. Allowing some space for air and heat to circulate around vegetables will prevent steaming, which does not bring out the same texture or flavor that roasting can.

Pureeing can be an excellent way to also use up vegetables near the end of their life span, since texture won't matter. To add flavor when using this method, start by sautéing some aromatics, such as onions, shallots, or garlic, until fragrant before adding the vegetables and water. This will ensure a flavorful puree or soup, as opposed to what would otherwise be most suitable as baby food.

Sautéing or stir-frying both use a minimal amount of cooking fat, high heat, and frequent movement to quickly cook vegetables until just tender. This quick method brings out a lot of flavor in vegetables while preserving nutrients.

Searing involves high heat to achieve browning and is used mainly for meat and fish but is also useful for mushrooms.

Simmering, the low-key version of boiling, is a gentle roll, with tiny bubbles barely breaking the surface of water, and a great method for long, slow cooking. This is good for beans, grains, and starchy vegetables.

Steaming is perhaps the simplest and quickest method of cooking vegetables, is environmentally friendly (for both water and energy use), and preserves the most nutrients. The easiest way to steam vegetables is to use a collapsible steamer basket inserted in any pot or pan with a lid, with about an inch of water on the bottom, then steaming for just a few minutes, until your desired tenderness. To enhance the flavor of steamed vegetables after cooking, drizzle them with flavorful olive oil or nut oil, and sprinkle with salt, spices and fresh herbs, and a little acid (lemon, lime, or vinegar), as desired.

TECHNIQUES FOR SPECIFIC INGREDIENTS
Spicing: Learn how to bring out the flavor from spices.

- Use ground spices early in the cooking process, not just sprinkling in at the end when their flavor won't be well integrated into the dish.

- Toast spices in a dry pan over low to medium heat, shaking periodically. To avoid burning them, take off heat as soon as you can smell the aroma because the residual heat will linger. For best flavor, toast immediately before using. Any remainder can be stored in a tightly covered container after cooling.

- Make a spiced oil (a process called blooming or tempering): Use ½ teaspoon of spice to 1 tablespoon or more of neutral oil for 30 seconds over low heat, and the oil will carry the flavors of the spices. The spiced oils in the Chilled Minted Pea Soup with Indian Spices (page 136), Magical Mango-Tamarind

Rasam (page 138), and Dal (page 287) are good examples. Store leftover spiced oil in a container in the refrigerator for up to a week.

- Make spice-infused vinegar: Using a 1:4 ratio of spices to liquid, warm the vinegar, then place whole spices in the warm liquid and transfer to a sterile glass jar or bottle. Let sit away from direct sunlight at room temperature for at least two weeks to slowly infuse their flavor. When ready, strain and store in a sterile glass container in a cool, dark place. Infused vinegar will keep up to 5 months at room temperature.

- Infuse whole spices in vodka or grain alcohol to make spice extracts, such as vanilla extract. Add 4 vanilla beans or cinnamon sticks, ¼ to ½ cup of other whole spices, or the rinds of two lemons to 8 ounces of vodka and place in a tightly sealed glass jar for at least a month. Taste and infuse for longer, depending on how intense you want the flavor to be. Store indefinitely in a cool, dark place.

- Use ground spices to flavor salt or sugar— combine in a mortar and pestle, spice grinder, or with your fingers, then store in an airtight container.

- Make spice blends (such as the Jerk Marinade, page 323) to season proteins. Or dip your bread into olive oil and either the Za'atar (page 253) or Dukkah (page 252).

Herbs: I enjoy them most fresh, but dried herbs also have earned their spot in the pantry and can add a taste of summer in the middle of winter. You can dry your own herbs using several methods, which include hanging them upside down by their stems; laying them on towels and putting them in a warm place out of direct sun; on a baking sheet or in a low oven; or microwaving briefly (in thirty-second intervals, for up to two minutes) between two layers of towels. Heartier herbs, such as rosemary, thyme, savory, marjoram, and oregano, retain the most flavor when dried; whereas more delicate herbs, such as cilantro and basil, are better preserved in pesto or herb oil.

BASICS OF COOKING WHOLE GRAINS

All whole grains can be cooked in a similar fashion to rice. I strongly recommend getting a rice cooker, which will make cooking whole grains a hands-off process. Fancier models come with multiple settings, but even an entry-level basic rice cooker, which costs $20 or less, can do the trick. Different whole grains require different amounts of water and time, so follow the directions on the package or by looking at the charts on the Whole Grains Council website. Before cooking whole grains using any of the following methods, add the appropriate amount of water or other seasoned liquid, if desired. Then, use one of these methods to cook:

- **Rice cooker method.** Add the grains and liquid and turn on the rice cooker. That's it!

- **Stovetop absorption method.** Bring the grains and liquid to a boil, then lower the heat to low and simmer, covered, until all the liquid is absorbed.

- **Cook it like pasta.** If you're not sure how much water to use, you can cook any whole grain in a large volume of water, as you would pasta, until it reaches your desired tenderness, and drain.

- **Bake it in the oven.** In this method, it is best to use an oven-safe pot with a tight-fitting lid, such as a Dutch oven. First, bring the water to a boil with a small amount of butter (about 1½ teaspoons per cup of uncooked grains) and salt, then add the rice or other whole grain. Cover the pot and transfer to a 350°F oven. Bake until steamed, which will be less than 30 minutes for refined grains and about an hour for whole grains.

- You can cook grains ahead of time and freeze them for 3 months.

- Consider soaking grains in warm water for several hours, or overnight, before cooking. Soaking grains before cooking can help neutralize phytic acid, a compound that is thought to decrease absorption of certain minerals, including zinc, phosphorus, calcium, and iron. Presoaking grains also helps break down hard-to-digest proteins, such as gluten, and will also allow grains to cook more quickly and fluffier.

- Consider toasting dry grains in a dry skillet before cooking, for additional flavor.

- After cooking grains, fluff with a fork.

- Think about flavoring your cooking liquid. Add or replace part of the water with broth, spices, or even apple cider.

An excellent resource describing whole grains, their nutrition, and how to prepare them is www.wholegrainscouncil.org/.

HOW TO COOK DRIED BEANS

No matter if you get your beans at your local grocery, health food, or ethnic store (a good source of less common beans) or online (ranchogordo.com is a great source of heirloom beans), cooking them is fairly simple. Note that dried beans sold in bulk bins are likely fresher than those in packages, which means they will cook more quickly.

❶ Decide on how many beans you want to cook. Most dried beans will triple in volume when cooked.

❷ Pour the beans onto a light-colored tray or baking sheet and pick through for rocks or other debris.

❸ Rinse and soak in water to cover for six hours or overnight (lentils and split peas do not need soaking).

❹ Drain and rinse, then put in a large pot, fill with water to cover by at least a few inches, boil for 5 minutes, skim away the foam, then simmer, partially covered, until tender, 1 to 3 hours, depending on type of bean. If desired, add aromatics, such as onion or garlic, and a bay leaf. Some people recommend adding salt at the end, to prevent them from being tough.

❺ If you use a pressure cooker, the cooking time will be shortened by up to 80 percent. If you use an electric pressure cooker, such as an Instant Pot, you can cook beans without soaking in an hour or less.

❻ Store in the fridge for up to 5 days or freeze for up to 3 months.

BEAN-COOKING TECHNIQUES TO REDUCE GAS

Beans contain a type of carbohydrate called oligosaccharides, for which humans lack the necessary digestive enzyme. As a result, digestion of beans occurs in the large intestine by bacteria, which results in the production of gas. Fortunately, since beans have been enjoyed for millennia, cooks have developed culinary techniques to reduce this issue.

- Boil beans in water with baking soda (about ¼ teaspoon per quart), then soak overnight and rinse thoroughly before cooking.

- Soak beans for 8 to 12 hours, changing the water (to get rid of the oligosaccharides) every 3 hours before cooking.

- When cooking beans, skim off the foam that forms, which comes from the oligosaccharides.

- For canned beans, drain and rinse the beans to reduce the amount of starch.

SPICES, HERBS, AND VEGETABLES THAT HELP WITH BEAN DIGESTION

- **Spices:** aniseeds, coriander, cumin, ajwain, asafetida (hing), ginger, and fennel.

- **Herb:** epazote (about 1 tablespoon per cup of dried beans); used in Latin American cuisine.

- **Vegetable:** kombu (kelp), about a 4-inch strip per pot of beans; used in Japanese cooking.

Making Healthy Cooking Delicious

Now that you have stocked your pantry and equipped your kitchen for healthy cooking, let's get cooking! Before you cook, set yourself up for success: Read the recipe all the way through before starting, and prep and organize your ingredients and equipment. Having everything you need for a recipe ready to go before you start cooking will save you time—and stress.

What makes food taste good? As of the early twentieth century, Western scientists thought there were only four basic tastes: salt, sour, bitter, and sweet, but now it's widely accepted that there is a fifth taste, umami (savory). Beyond these, Asian cultures have long recognized a few additional tastes. Ancient Chinese considered spiciness to be a basic taste, and in the ancient Indian healing system of Ayurveda, pungent and astringent are considered basic tastes in addition to the four basic tastes.

But taste is just what the tongue has receptors for. Flavor depends not only on taste but a combination of our other senses: aroma, texture, and temperature. Add crunch (and nutrition) with seeds and nuts. Enjoyment of food is also increased by visual appeal, so don't forget about presentation. Eating a wide variety of colorful vegetables is a good step in this direction because that means you will be "eating the rainbow." Even, or perhaps especially, if you are cooking for one, plate your food nicely, put away any electronic devices, play some nice background music, and soften the lighting—your food will taste even better.

Here are my tried and true tips to enhance all aspects of flavor:

Learn how to use spices. See page 9.

Learn how to use salt. Salt at the right times, and you'll need less. Start with a pinch at the beginning of cooking, and again at different parts of the recipe (e.g., to the aromatics at the beginning of a stir-fry, then again after the addition of the vegetables), and adjust at the end. For dishes that will be cooked for a long time, such as grains, beans, soups, and stews, salt very lightly at first. If you have oversalted a soup or stew, the easiest thing to do is to dilute with water. Potatoes or rice can also absorb some of the salt. If you need to cut down on sodium, use acidic flavorings, such as lemon juice and vinegar, for a salty taste without the sodium.

Do not fear fat. Fat is needed to absorb certain nutrients (A, D, E, and K) and helps with satiety (feeling full). It is necessary for browning and also carries flavors of aromatics and spices in a way that water cannot.

Use your senses, and also common sense! Cooking times will vary, depending on the freshness of ingredients, ambient temperature, humidity and altitude, the size and material of your pan, and, of course, your stove. So, use your eyes and ears, sense of smell, and taste to know when something is done. Is it browning? Is it making loud sizzling or boiling sounds? What does it feel like? The answers to these basic questions will help you develop your cooking intuition.

Taste, adjust, and taste and adjust again! As food cooks, its flavors will change, so you won't get the results you want unless you taste periodically and, most important, at the end. And the more you taste, the better your palate will become, and you will be a better cook. Balance the five tastes, and learn how to adjust. For example, is it too bitter? It might need another pinch of salt. Is it too sour? You might need some fat, sugar, or salt. Too sweet? Add acid or oil. Is something missing? It's probably umami. Add a source of umami, such as soy sauce, miso, tomato paste, mushroom stock, nutritional yeast, seaweed, or aged cheese.

MONDAY	**Pasta/Noodle/Rice Dishes** Mama's Chhá Bí-hún —Taiwanese Stir-Fried Rice Noodles (page 165)	**Pasta/Noodle/Rice Dishes** Mommy's Toishan-to-Trinidad Chow Mein (page 304)	**Pasta/Noodle/Rice Dishes** Eat Your Greens! Fried Rice (page 140)	**Pasta/Noodle/Rice Dishes** Pantry Pasta with Cherry Tomatoes, White Beans, and Sardines (page 223)
TUESDAY	**Tacos, Wraps, and Rolls** Roasted Salmon Tacos (page 88)	**Tacos, Wraps, and Rolls** Potato and Mushroom Tacos (page 87)	**Tacos, Wraps, and Rolls** Arepas "el Diablo" (page 93)	**Tacos, Wraps, and Rolls** Eat the Rainbow Fresh Spring Rolls (page 128)
WEDNESDAY	**Rice and Beans** Coconut Tofu with Spiced Coconut Rice (page 80)	**Rice and Beans** Mujadara (page 234)	**Rice and Beans** Pelau with Roasted Pumpkin (page 296)	**Rice and Beans** Rice Cooker Jamaican Rice and Peas (page 293)
THURSDAY	**Soups/Stews** Mexican-Spiced Roasted Butternut Squash Soup (page 70)	**Soups/Stews** Lentil Soup for a Small Planet (page 82)	**Soups/Stews** Saffron-Scented Mediterranean Fish and Fennel Stew (page 225)	**Soups/Stews** Chana and Aloo (page 310)
FRIDAY	**Breakfast for Dinner** Avocado Toast Variations (page 56)	**Breakfast for Dinner** Chilaquiles Verdes with Baked Tortilla Chips (page 58)	**Breakfast for Dinner** Shakshuka (page 197)	**Breakfast for Dinner** Buljol (page 263) with Coconut Bake (page 266)
SATURDAY	**Entrée Salads** Lemony Farro Salad with Avocado and Pistachios (page 65)	**Entrée Salads** Thanksgiving Kale Salad with Roasted Root Vegetables (page 69)	**Entrée Salads** Backpacker's Gado Gado (page 133)	**Entrée Salads** Salade Niçoise (page 231)
SUNDAY	**Stir-Fry or Sauté** Indian Spiced Kale with Coconut and Turmeric (page 146)	**Stir-Fry or Sauté** Kung Pao Tofu (page 158)	**Stir-Fry or Sauté** Ratatouille (page 229)	**Stir-Fry or Sauté** Spanish Spinach and Chickpeas (page 228)

SPICEBOX KITCHEN

MENU PLANNING AND MEAL PREP

If, like me, you have packed days, trying to balance work and home, cooking on a daily basis may seem overwhelming. Here's a guide to making this not only a possible task but an enjoyable one.

Plan Your Meals

Plan well, and you shouldn't have to shop more than once a week (for the most part), and won't have to decide what to eat for dinner when you're tired.

Once a week (for me it's on Saturday or Sunday morning), plan at least four or five dinner menus for the coming week, and make a grocery list from it. Try to plan a set of meals that have some ingredients in common, especially produce, to shorten your grocery list and reduce food waste. (I leave a couple days free for leftovers or eating out.)

One easy way to do this is to have a theme for each night, or think of five to seven core recipes or recipe types that you know how to make. Examples: entrée salads, stir-fry/sauté, pasta, grain salads/bowls, rice and beans/rice dishes, soups/stews, tacos/wraps. By swapping different proteins, vegetables, and spices/herbs, you can make many different variations on a theme: 7 recipe types x 4 variations = a month of different meals! On the opposite page is a sample meal plan using recipes from this book. (You'll want to supplement additional greens or add a protein to some of these.)

Expand Your Repertoire

Think of how you might change vegetables, proteins, or spices in any of the recipes to change its flavor profile. Examples of flavor profiles:

Mexican: cayenne, cumin, lime, oregano

Chinese: garlic, ginger, rice vinegar, sesame oil, soy sauce

Indian: coconut, cumin, curry, turmeric

Italian: basil, garlic, oregano

Trinidadian: coconut, curry, culantro, Scotch bonnet chili, thyme

Reconsider Leftovers

Leftovers can be flavorful prepared ingredients for a new dish if you don't like eating the same food more than once in a week. Also, leftovers = lunch. You can also use small amounts of any leftovers and add them to salad greens for a flavorful salad (and a way to make sure you're eating enough greens).

Look Ahead

Aside from getting the ingredients prepped and ready for the meal you are cooking, for me this also includes looking ahead to the next day's menu and taking any steps that need to be done in advance. This might include soaking beans and grains, marinating proteins, or defrosting.

Plan Your Shopping

You'll want to stock your pantry, and keep it stocked. **Make a master grocery list** (pages 33–34) of the essentials for your pantry and refrigerator, so you can very quickly take inventory before grocery shopping, and schedule grocery shopping into your calendar once per week. If grocery delivery makes sense for you, do that instead.

Meal Prep/Batch Cooking

In addition to planning your menu, prep and batch cooking mean very little active cooking time during busy workdays. These components can be made in advance, portioned into serving sizes, and stored in the refrigerator or freezer until ready to use in different recipes:

- Grains

- Beans, if cooking dried

- Vegetables

  - If using within 3 to 5 days, you can prewash, dry, and cut vegetables so they are ready to cook.

  - Shorten cooking time by precooking: blanch, parboil, roast. Blanched vegetables can be frozen and stored for 8 to 12 months.

- Stock and soup

- Sauces: vinaigrette, pesto, romesco, stir-fry sauce, marinade

TIPS FOR STORAGE

- Label with name of food and date.

- Use the "first in, first out" rule for rotating your food, so the oldest is in the front and will be used first.

- When freezing food, let foods cool completely before freezing to prevent the formation of ice crystals, the kiss of death for taste and flavor. Freeze food in portion sizes so that you only defrost what you need.

REDUCING FOOD WASTE

Besides eating less meat, another action we can take to protect the environment and also protect the world food supply is simple: Reduce food waste. Doing so will save money, and also conserve energy, water and other resources used to grow, manufacture, transport, and sell food. Many of the tips covered in previous sections (storage, meal planning and prep, and using the "first in, first out" rule) are simple things you can do to reduce food waste. You can also get creative with the food you have already purchased:

EXCESS FRESH PRODUCE

- Blanch and freeze.

- Slice and bake into chips.

- Preserve or ferment; make pickles (such as Pickled Red Onion, page 112), sauerkraut, Taiwanese Pickled Cabbage (page 174), kimchi (such as Quick Kimchi, page 177), Tepache (page 100), or kombucha. You can even save and combine leftover pickling brine from various jars and reboil to pour over cut-up veggies for a quick pickle.

- Dry herbs, make them into pesto, or puree them in oil and keep in the freezer.

- Be flexible, and learn to make swaps with a similar vegetable you have rather than buying the exact ingredient called for. For example, you can swap any of these foods for another in the same category: greens, root vegetables, mushrooms, beans.

WILTED OR OVERRIPE PRODUCE

- Wilted salad greens can be quickly sautéed with garlic and salt.

- Bruised overripe tomatoes can be used to make tomato soup, sauce, or gazpacho.

- Berries past their prime are perfect for jams, pie filling, compote, or purees, which can be mixed with sparkling water for homemade soda, or to add to smoothies or baked goods.

- Ripe bananas make great banana bread, and you can also freeze them in chunks to use for smoothies or banana "nice" cream.

SCRAPS

- Save vegetable tops and scraps and meat bones to make stock; keep a container in the freezer and add scraps; when you have enough, make stock.

- Root vegetable greens can be made into pesto, such as carrot tops, or sautéed as you would other greens, such as radish and beet greens.

- Parmesan rinds are great for flavoring soups; store in the freezer.

- Leeks and scallions can be regrown by placing their roots in water or dirt.

- Stale bread can be made into croutons or bread crumbs, or used to make panzanella, bread pudding, or vegetable strata.

- Stale tortilla chips are perfect for chilaquiles.

GET A FRESH PERSPECTIVE ON LEFTOVERS

- Leftovers = seasoned meal prep. Add leftovers into casseroles, stir-fries, frittatas, and soups.

- Rice or other cooked grains can be used to make fried rice or rice pudding, or as a base for veggie burgers.

- Risotto can be used to make arancini.

- Tortillas can be fried or baked into homemade tortilla chips.

UNDERSTAND DATES ON PACKAGED GOODS

- "Use by" indicates a date by which the food is safe to be eaten.

- "Best before" means the food's quality is best prior to that date, but it is still safe for consumption after it.

- "Sell by" date is helpful for stock rotation by manufacturers and retailers but is not an indicator of expiration.

OTHER TIPS

- Purchase fresh but cosmetically nonstandard produce that doesn't fit strict retail standards for size and shape. This is easy to do if you purchase from a farmers' market or farm stand, or subscribe to a CSA, especially one that specifically selects for this less cosmetically desirable produce.

- Compost what you can't save.

- Donate shelf-stable goods to food banks.

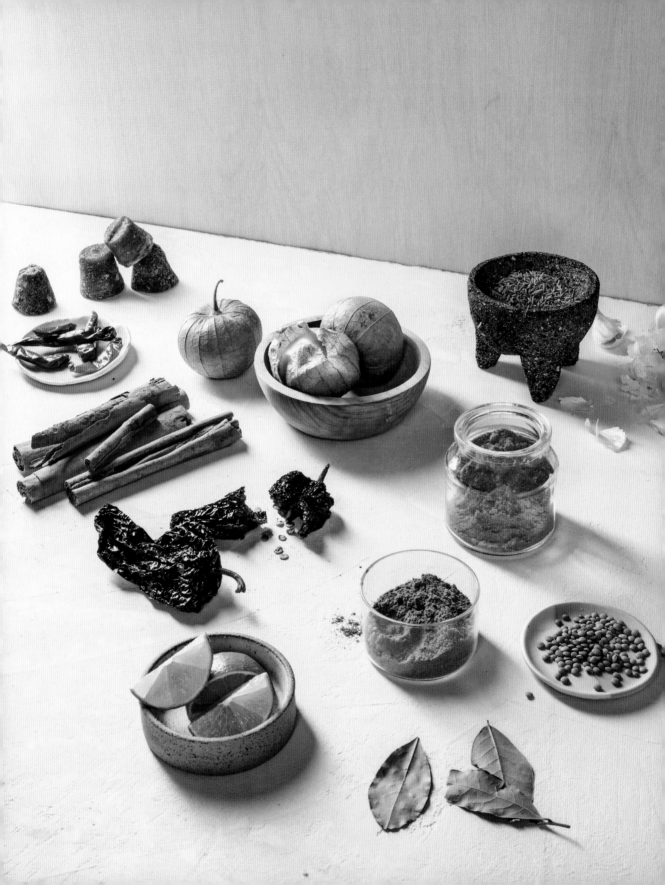

PART TWO

RECIPES

CALIFORNIA

CALIFORNIA PANTRY

spices

cayenne

cinnamon

cloves

cumin

garlic

ginger

oregano

vanilla

herbs

basil

bay leaf

cilantro

mint

fat

olive oil

acids

apple cider vinegar

lemon

lime

CALIFORNIA

W̷HEN I WAS SEVENTEEN, I visited San Francisco for the first time. This hilly city in the fog caught my attention and captured my heart, and I decided then that one day, I would make San Francisco my home. Nearly ten years later, I made good on my promise and have since explored all the diverse quirkiness that initially beckoned me, and beyond.

My first visit took me throughout the still ungentrified Mission District, where I had my first San Francisco–style burrito at Pancho Villa. I had Brittany-style crepes at Ti Couz, where I enjoyed the chewy nuttiness of buckwheat flour for the first time. I was awestruck by the seemingly endless aisles at Rainbow Grocery, which had ingredients I had never seen nor imagined. I left sipping a bottle of freshly pressed ginger juice, whose intense spiciness mirrored my wide-eyed enchantment with the city. San Francisco is a well-known food lover's paradise, with bountiful farmers' markets, artisanal producers of anything you might want to eat, and a diverse population that literally brings the world to your doorstep.

When I moved to San Francisco after medical school, I suddenly had more choices than days of the week—ranging from Salvadoran *pupuserias*, Vietnamese pho restaurants, North and South Indian restaurants, dim sum, and endless others. We moved in next door to an elderly Mexican American couple, who shared child-rearing tips, lemons, homemade chilaquiles, tamales, and recipes. There was also California cuisine, from the simple perfection at the temple of California cuisine, Chez Panisse, to the blissful vegetarian from the Zen restaurant Greens. The lettuce was so tender and fresh, I wondered how it could be the same thing I had eaten in the previous two decades of my life. That's how I felt as I cruised the vendors at the farmers' markets, curiosity and taste buds piqued by the technicolor array of produce, all local, which was either new to me (tatsoi, Vietnamese fish herb) or nothing like the mass-produced equivalents I had previously only known (lettuce, figs, Meyer lemons).

The following recipes are the result of the love affair with food I've cultivated in the last two decades of making my home in Northern California, and are my version of California cuisine—simple and fresh, celebrating the bounty of our farms and the diverse flavors of our multicultural community, which make it a joy to cook deliciously healthy food.

2 cups Scottish porridge oats or quick rolled oats

8 cups water

1½ to 2 teaspoons ground ginger, plus more to taste

Pinch of salt

2 oranges

Garnishes: chopped walnuts, splash of milk (any type)

THERE'S NOTHING MORE COMFORTING than a bowl of oatmeal. Scottish porridge oats cook up quickly into a creamy bowl of hot cereal. If you can't get them, McCann's Quick Oats or Bob's Red Mill Rolled Oats make good substitutes. The key here is to use a lot more water than you expect to, and to stir and stir, as you would with polenta, to make the oats extra smooth and creamy. The ginger and orange zest dress it up with little effort. Consider using different colors of oranges, including rosy Cara Cara and crimson blood oranges, to make this simple breakfast both sophisticated and beautiful.

SOPHISTICATED GINGER-ORANGE OATMEAL

Makes 6 to 8 cups oatmeal

Place oats and water in a saucepan along with ginger and salt, stir well, and bring to a boil.

Lower heat to a simmer and cook, uncovered, stirring every few minutes, until thickened and creamy, 5 to 10 minutes. Add more water, to desired consistency, if needed.

Meanwhile, zest oranges and set zest aside. Then, use a knife to cut off rest of peel from oranges, removing all pith (white membrane). Slice peeled oranges crosswise into disks, then cut those in half.

When porridge is ready, remove from heat, add additional ginger to taste, and stir in orange zest.

Serve hot in individual bowls with garnishes of orange disks, walnuts, and an optional extra pinch of ground ginger and a splash of milk.

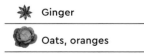

Ginger

Oats, oranges

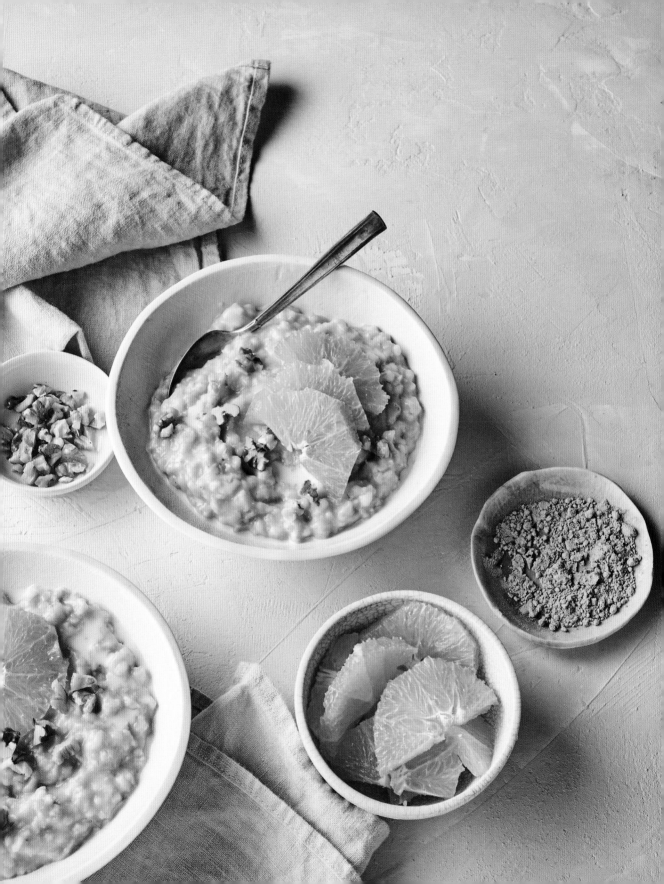

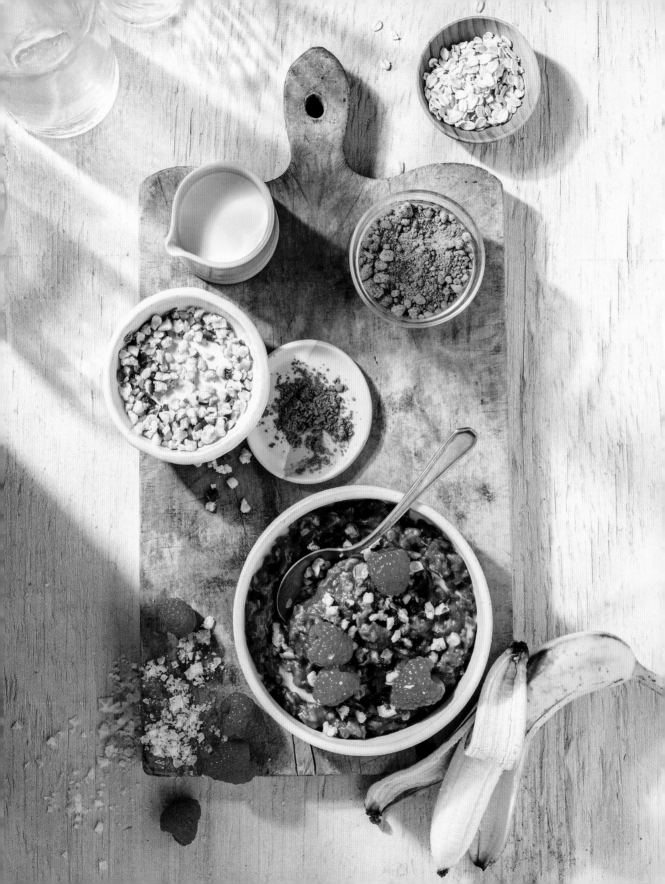

1 cup rolled or quick oats,
not steel-cut

2 very ripe bananas, mashed

2½ to 3 cups water

2 to 3 tablespoons
unsweetened cocoa powder

GARNISHES

Drizzle of nondairy milk

1 to 2 tablespoons chopped,
toasted hazelnuts

Pinches of jaggery

Pinches of fleur de sel

Fresh berries (optional)

THIS SOPHISTICATED yet simple recipe can serve as a decadent breakfast, snack, or even dessert. Jaggery, a brown sugar found in Indian markets, is made from boiling sugarcane juice. Its flavor has hints of molasses and caramel. Mexican *piloncillo*, Southeast Asian *gula melaka*, or regular dark brown sugar may be substituted. And since you're just using a pinch here, doesn't push this into unhealthy!

VEGAN CHOCOLATE BANANA OATMEAL WITH HAZELNUTS, JAGGERY, AND FLEUR DE SEL

<u>Serves 2</u>

Combine oats, bananas, water, and cocoa powder in a saucepan and stir.

Bring to a low boil over medium heat, stirring often. Cook for about 5 minutes, to your desired consistency, mashing bananas as you stir. Add more water, if desired.

Serve in individual bowls. Garnish each portion with a drizzle of nondairy milk, a sprinkling of nuts, pinches of jaggery and fleur de sel, plus berries, if desired.

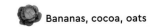 Bananas, cocoa, oats

3 cups rolled oats, certified gluten-free if needed

1 cup raw hulled sunflower seeds

1 cup raw hulled pumpkin seeds (pepitas)

1 cup unsweetened flaked coconut (such as Bob's Red Mill brand)

¾ cup pure maple syrup

½ cup extra-virgin olive oil

1 teaspoon salt

1 tablespoon ground cardamom

1 tablespoon ground ginger

1 cup roasted black sesame seeds (available from Asian groceries or online)

THIS GRANOLA was adapted from the Genius Granola on the recipe website Food52. I've made it gluten- and nut-free, replacing the nuts with seeds. Cardamom, ginger, and toasted black sesame seeds add warm flavors to this granola, which makes a fantastic breakfast or snack.

SPICED GRANOLA

Makes 7 cups granola

Preheat oven to 300°F.

Line two rimmed baking sheets with foil, parchment paper, or a silicone mat.

Stir together oats, sunflower seeds, pumpkin seeds, coconut, maple syrup, olive oil, salt, cardamom, and ginger in a bowl until well combined. Then, transfer to prepared baking sheets and spread evenly in a thin layer.

Bake for 20 to 30 minutes, stirring every 10 minutes for even browning and rotating pans at halfway point. Remove from oven when oats are golden brown.

While granola is still hot, stir in black sesame seeds. Adjust salt to taste.

Allow to cool completely before storing in a tightly sealed jar or container for up to 1 month.

Cardamom, ginger

Oats, pumpkin seeds, sesame seeds

1 cup arugula, baby kale, or spinach

1 cup frozen cubed mango

½ very ripe banana, frozen preferred

1 cup plain kefir

¼ teaspoon ground cardamom

¼ to ½ teaspoon ground ginger

Honey or agave nectar (optional)

BLENDING LEAFY GREENS into a smoothie is a great way to incorporate a serving of these nutritional powerhouses into your diet. In contrast to more commonly used neutral greens, such as kale and spinach, arugula lends an unexpected peppery bite to this bold breakfast smoothie, which gets additional character from cardamom and ginger. Think of this as a green smoothie crossed with a mango lassi. *Note:* A high-speed blender is best for making green smoothies.

SPICED GREEN SMOOTHIE WITH ARUGULA AND MANGO

Makes 2 cups (1 large or 2 small smoothies)

In a blender, blend together all ingredients, except sweetener, until smooth. Add sweetener, if desired.

Serve immediately or keep refrigerated until serving.

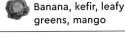 Cardamom, ginger

Banana, kefir, leafy greens, mango

½ cup coconut milk + ½ cup water, or 1 cup light coconut milk

1¼ cups cubed fresh pineapple

1 cup baby kale

2 ice cubes

½ frozen banana, sliced (optional, if your pineapple isn't very sweet)

WITH COCONUT MILK and pineapple, this nonalcoholic tropical treat can be enjoyed at breakfast or as a dessert (a splash of rum wouldn't be inappropriate at cocktail hour).

The kale adds a vibrant color while also contributing a serving of greens.

PIÑA KALEADA

Serves 2

Place all ingredients in a high-speed blender and blend until smooth.

 Kale, pineapple

TRENDY OR NOT, I think avocado toast is a good template for a nourishing light breakfast, lunch, or snack, if you think of it as a platform for some tasty, nourishing toppings.

First, start with the bread. If you're lucky enough to live in San Francisco, get a good whole-grain loaf, such as Tartine bread. Other good options include the 21-seed Dave's Killer Bread, sold sliced on the shelves of most supermarkets, or other whole-grain breads. They will not only provide the fiber and other nutrients of whole grains but be sturdy enough to hold your toppings.

Next, the avocado. It doesn't matter if you have the bumpy, black-skinned Mexican variety or the smoother, green-skinned variety—make sure your avocado is not overripe and mushy but just right: slightly firm and sliceable. You can either arrange it in slices, or if it's a bit softer, dice it, place it on your toast, and then use a fork to smash it.

Toppings are your chance to get creative. Add spices. Add leftovers. Add things you would put into a salad. You need just a few tablespoons per piece of toast, so this is a good way to use up those odds and ends/ leftovers that have a lot of flavor to contribute but are not enough to make a meal.

AVOCADO TOAST VARIATIONS

HERE ARE SOME SUGGESTIONS:

THE CLASSIC: Whole-grain toast, avocado, red pepper flakes, squeeze of lemon juice, pinch of salt, and drizzle of olive oil.

SALAD DAYS: Whole-grain toast, avocado, arugula, thin slices of radish, pinch of salt, and drizzle of olive oil.

ITALIAN: Whole-grain toast, avocado, sliced cherry tomatoes, fresh basil, red pepper flakes, squeeze of lemon juice or several drops of balsamic vinegar, pinch of salt, and drizzle of olive oil.

SPANISH: Whole-grain toast, avocado, Smoky Spanish Chickpeas (page 106), squeeze of lemon, pinch of salt, and drizzle of olive oil.

 Chile peppers, za'atar, harissa

Avocado

MOROCCAN I: Whole-grain toast, avocado, thinly sliced bell pepper, za'atar, squeeze of lemon juice, pinch of salt, and drizzle of olive oil.

MOROCCAN II: Whole-grain toast, avocado, thinly sliced preserved lemon rind, harissa, squeeze of lemon juice, cilantro, pinch of salt, and drizzle of olive oil.

EGYPTIAN: Whole-grain toast, avocado, dukkah, squeeze of lemon juice, pinch of salt, and drizzle of olive oil.

SMOKY: Whole-grain toast, avocado, pimentón, black salt, squeeze of lemon juice, and drizzle of olive oil.

MEXICAN: Whole-grain toast, avocado, thinly sliced jicama, cayenne, squeeze of lime juice, pinch of salt, and drizzle of olive oil.

KOREAN: Whole-grain toast, avocado, gochugaru, toasted sesame seeds, several drops of rice vinegar, pinch of salt, and drizzle of toasted sesame oil.

JAPANESE: Whole-grain toast, avocado, furikake, togarashi (Japanese chili powder), few drops of rice vinegar, pinch of salt, and drizzle of toasted sesame oil.

TAIWANESE: Whole-grain toast, avocado, thinly sliced cucumber, several drops of seasoned rice vinegar, pinch of salt, drizzle of toasted sesame oil, scattering of thinly sliced scallions, and crispy fried shallots.

1 tablespoon canola oil

1 quart salsa verde, cooked version (recipe follows)

1 (14-ounce) bag corn tortilla chips, preferably thick and unsalted (or bake your own; recipe follows)

½ cup shredded Monterey Jack cheese

Optional toppings: shredded leftover cooked chicken or turkey breast, or fried eggs

GARNISHES

2 tablespoons crumbled queso fresco

3 tablespoons finely chopped white onion

1 tablespoon finely chopped fresh cilantro

Crema or Cashew Lime Crema (page 107)

Canola or other neutral oil

 Chile pepper, garlic

Cilantro, corn, tomatillos

MEXICAN BREAKFAST FAVORITE chilaquiles are made of corn tortilla chips cooked in red or green salsa and topped with cheese, onions, and cilantro. The chips absorb the flavor of the salsa, and in some versions they're cooked long enough that they become completely soft. I prefer an in-between version that is both crisp and softened. Typically, this dish is served like a hash, topped with sunny-side up or fried eggs, melted cheese, and some fresh herbs and onions. Our neighbor, Teresa (Risa to my kids, who considered her their honorary *abuela*) used to surprise us periodically with her excellent home cooking—pies baked with apples from her tree, rice pudding, and—best yet—a platter of her chilaquiles with red salsa. When Teresa stopped cooking due to illness, the tables turned and I began to cook for them when possible; it was a big challenge for her husband, Rick, to start cooking in his mideighties. Since Teresa is no longer with us, I try to cook for him more often. Rick always appreciates what I share but also rates my food informally. He calls immediately after we bring over my food if he loves it; and if he really loves it, follows up by leaving a handwritten note and bag of lemons or apples from their trees on my doorstep. But he might not call at all if it was a dud (apparently he's not a fan of mochi). When I made my first batch of chilaquiles for him, I decided it would be a surprise. Peter brought them over but didn't tell Rick what it was. Within seconds of the delivery, the phone rang. "These taste like Mexican chilaquiles," he said. Rick, who grew up in a Mexican family but didn't cook, even asked about the type of chiles I used and made a paternal suggestion that I could buy premade tortilla chips to save myself a step. He told me he loved them, but more than what he said, I interpreted his excited questioning about them as the equivalent of a five-star review.

CHILAQUILES VERDES WITH BAKED TORTILLA CHIPS

Serves 4

Place a wide pot or sauté pan over medium-high heat and add oil. When oil is shimmery, pour in salsa verde; it will bubble a bit. Lower heat to medium and simmer, stirring occasionally, until sauce is slightly thickened, 10 to 15 minutes.

continued ⟼

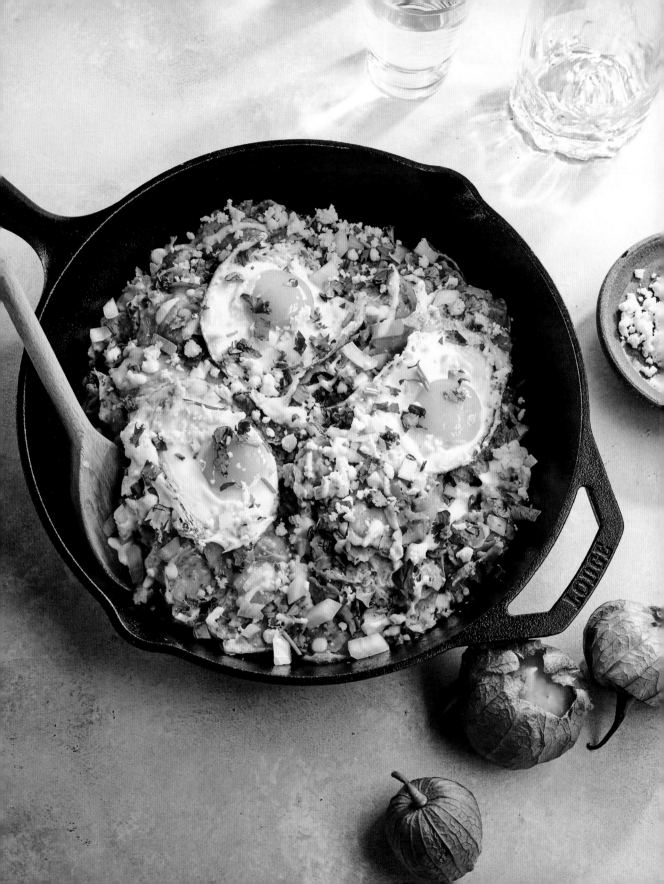

Immediately add chips to salsa, tossing gently until they have absorbed enough sauce to become soft. Take care not to break chips. Sprinkle Monterey Jack cheese on top and let it melt.

Divide chilaquiles among four plates.

Top with shredded chicken or turkey, or fried eggs, if desired.

Sprinkle with queso fresco, chopped onion, and cilantro. Garnish with crema and serve immediately. Share with your neighbors!

Salsa Verde

Makes 1 quart salsa verde

1 jalapeño pepper, stemmed, or more to taste

10 tomatillos, husked

2 to 3 garlic cloves

1 small onion, sliced

½ cup fresh cilantro

Salt

Place all ingredients, except cilantro and salt, in a large saucepan, cover with water, and bring to a boil.

Boil for 5 to 10 minutes, or until tomatillos yield to a fork.

Drain off liquid, transfer cooked vegetables to a blender, and blend for 30 seconds to a minute, or until coarsely blended.

Add cilantro and salt to taste, and blend again for a few seconds.

May be stored in a covered container for a week in refrigerator.

Baked Corn Tortilla Chips

Makes 160 chips (equivalent to a 14-ounce bag of store-bought chips)

Preheat oven to 350°F. Brush two or three baking sheets with a thin coating of oil and set aside.

Place a tortilla on a cutting board, then brush its top with a thin layer of oil, making sure to cover all the way to edges. Place another tortilla on top of that, and brush its top with oil. Continue with remaining tortillas.

Cut stack of oiled tortillas into eight wedges.

Place wedges in a single layer on prepared baking sheets, leaving a little room around each so that they can crisp up. Sprinkle with salt.

Bake for 8 to 12 minutes, rotating pans after 5 minutes. Chips are done when their edges are crisp and dry. Remove from oven. Chips will continue to crisp as they cool. Best enjoyed on first day, but may be kept in a sealed container for up to 3 days before they lose their crunch.

Canola oil

20 small corn tortillas

Salt

1 medium-size cucumber

1 tablespoon fresh mint leaves

1 ripe avocado

6 ounces arugula

1½ cups ripe blackberries

Fine kosher salt and freshly ground black pepper

Extra-virgin olive oil (Persian lime—or Meyer lemon–infused olive oil really make the dressing pop, but if you can't find these, just use the grassiest-tasting extra-virgin olive oil you can get)

WHILE SAN FRANCISCO is definitely urban, even gritty, it also has pockets of nature everywhere you go. My neighborhood is bordered on one end by a park filled with geese, herons, ducks, egrets, and other wildfowl. In the other direction, there are two coyotes who make the big, dusty hill their home. And even on the streets, I sometimes see raccoons, possums, and skunks confidently walking up the sidewalk of the steep hill we live on, like they own it. Best yet, in July and August, wild blackberries spring up wherever there is a patch of dirt, there for the foraging—and they inspired this salad. Peppery arugula contrasts nicely with these sweet and tart berries while cucumbers bring in some juiciness, and creamy avocado ties it all together for a light and refreshing dish.

SAN FRANCISCO SUMMER ARUGULA SALAD WITH BLACKBERRIES, AVOCADO, AND CUCUMBER

Serves 4

Peel and slice cucumber into thin disks (or half-moons, if very large).

Chiffonade mint leaves. To do this, stack leaves into one pile, then roll tightly from stem to tip. Cut across this roll of leaves into thin strips, then fluff into ribbons.

Peel, pit, and cut avocado into thin, pretty slices.

To assemble salad:

- Get a pretty platter and scatter arugula over it.
- Sprinkle mint over arugula.
- Place cucumbers evenly over greens.
- Arrange avocado slices on top.
- Top with blackberries.
- Garnish with a pinch of salt and pepper and a light drizzle of olive oil.

 Black pepper

Arugula, avocado, mint

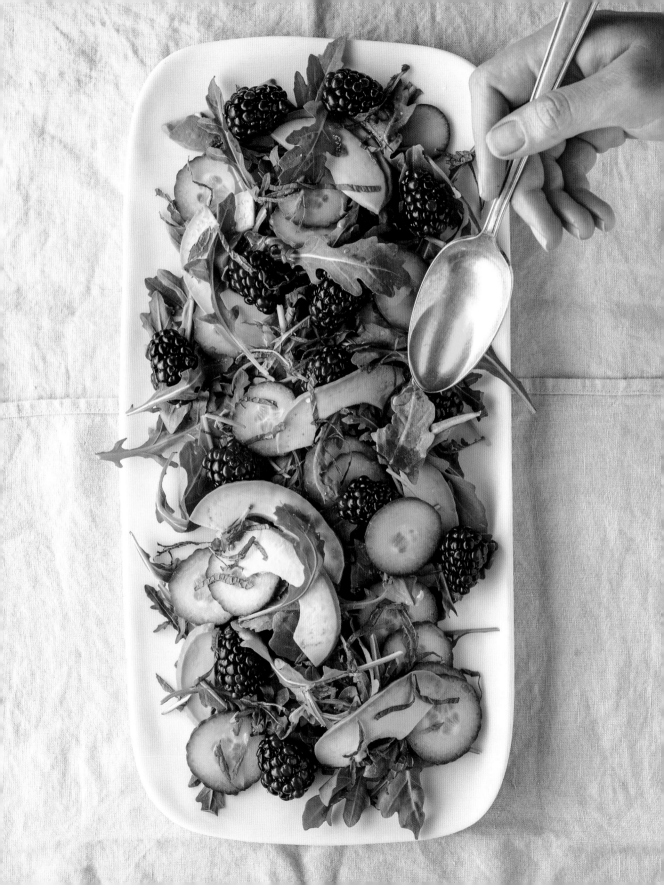

1 cup arugula

1 pound yellow peaches, pitted and sliced into wedges

8 ounces burrata or fresh mozzarella, sliced or torn into half-moons

1 teaspoon olive oil

Pinch of salt

A few grinds of black pepper

A few pinches of harissa

2 tablespoons torn fresh basil, mint, or tarragon leaves

CLASSIC ITALIAN CAPRESE SALAD is made with summer garden tomatoes, fresh mozzarella, and basil; this version swaps in stone fruit for tomatoes (which are technically fruit). Since burrata is basically fresh mozzarella filled with cream, the idea seemed natural—peaches and cream. Different herbs work well here—basil, mint, or tarragon are a few I've tried. To round out the salad and make it more substantial, I serve it on a bed of peppery arugula, which plays nicely off the sweetness of the peaches. A sprinkling of harissa at the end adds an unexpected smoky and slightly spicy note. Make sure to use ripe, ideally farmers' market or farm stand peaches for the best results—their juices add to the dressing.

SUMMER PEACH BURRATA CAPRESE WITH HARISSA

Serves 6

Scatter arugula on a platter.

Arrange peach slices and burrata on bed of arugula.

Drizzle with olive oil, a pinch of salt, some pepper, and a few pinches of harissa. Garnish with your choice of herbs.

 Harissa (chile peppers, coriander, cumin, garlic)

Arugula, herbs, peaches

1 cup uncooked farro perlato

1 cup thinly sliced lacinato kale

1 cup arugula

1 cup fresh basil, chopped

1 tablespoon finely sliced chives

1 avocado, peeled, pitted, and sliced

¼ cup crumbled feta (leave this out to make vegan)

½ cup pistachio nuts, coarsely chopped

VINAIGRETTE

Grated zest of 1 lemon

2 tablespoons freshly squeezed lemon juice

6 tablespoons olive oil

½ teaspoon ground cumin

¼ teaspoon sea salt

Freshly ground black pepper

PERFECT AS A STARTER or as a light lunch, this summery grain salad has many different textures, from chewy farro to creamy avocado to crunchy pistachio. The two types of lemon—freshly squeezed juice and zest—brighten and lighten up this salad.

LEMONY FARRO SALAD WITH AVOCADO AND PISTACHIOS

<u>Serves 6</u>

In a large saucepan, bring 3 quarts of salted water to a boil. Add farro perlato. Lower heat and simmer, covered, until tender, about 20 minutes. (You can use regular farro, but cooking time will double.) Drain as you would pasta, then spread on a baking sheet to cool.

While farro is cooking, massage kale with your fingers until wilted.

To make vinaigrette, whisk together lemon zest and juice, oil, cumin, salt, and pepper in a small bowl.

After farro has cooled, toss it in a bowl with kale and arugula, then use your fingers to evenly distribute greens through farro.

Pour vinaigrette over farro and greens, add basil and chives, and toss gently to coat.

To serve, spoon greens mixture onto a platter. Lay slices of avocado over salad, sprinkle feta and pistachios over top, and serve. If not serving immediately, refrigerate salad, but let it come to room temperature before serving.

✳ Cumin

 Avocado, basil, farro, leafy greens, pistachios

1 pound sweet potato, peeled

1 tablespoon olive oil

Kosher salt

1 ear corn

½ to 1 teaspoon grated fresh ginger

1 tablespoon rice vinegar

½ teaspoon ground white pepper

Green onions, thinly sliced into rings

I FIRST MADE THIS RECIPE for a weekend at a friend's ranch in Petaluma, a farming community about an hour north of San Francisco with a large population of cows and chickens, surprisingly close to Highway 101. This was in the days when our children were small, and it was a chance for them to experience relative freedom on grassy hills under sunny skies, outside the city. This is a sweeter variation on potato salad that makes a great accompaniment to a summer barbecue. The ginger, green onion, and rice vinegar lighten it up and add a subtle Asian flavor. To make this even more interesting, consider cooking the corn and sweet potato on the grill to catch some of the smokiness from the fire.

ROASTED SWEET POTATO AND CORN SALAD

Serves 4

Preheat oven to 400°F.

Dice sweet potato into ½-inch cubes, toss in a bowl with olive oil and a pinch of salt, then arrange in a single layer on a baking sheet. Bake until tender, about 20 minutes, turning at 10-minute point. Meanwhile, cut the kernels off the cob of corn and place in a medium bowl.

Transfer the roasted sweet potato cubes to the bowl and add grated ginger, rice vinegar, white pepper, and salt to taste. Allow to cool to room temperature, then garnish with green onions.

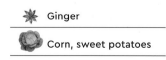

Ginger

Corn, sweet potatoes

2 Fuyu persimmons, cut into thin slices

1 medium-size jicama, peeled and cut into thin slices

2 celery stalks, cut into thin diagonal slices

A few tablespoons of pomegranate arils

Pinch of sea salt

Freshly ground black pepper

Drizzle of extra-virgin olive oil

WHILE THE HOLIDAYS can be a time of decadence and feasting, I like to include lighter dishes to balance it all out (as well as add hydration, fiber, and vitamins and minerals). This composed salad provides some table eye candy with its colorful seasonal fruits, including pomegranate arils, which are like little rubies or Christmas lights. Fuyu are the crunchy, flat-bottomed variety of persimmons; they have a sweet taste and slightly jellylike interior. (If you can't get them where you live, feel free to substitute another seasonal fruit, such as apples or pears.) This is not really a recipe but a guideline. Use more or less of each fruit as you desire, or make a colorful substitution. Apples and Asian pears are also nice substitutions for the jicama, which is a crunchy, slightly sweet, and nutty-tasting root vegetable.

JEWEL BOX HOLIDAY SALAD

Serves 4

Arrange fruits artfully on a platter, then sprinkle with seasonings and drizzle with olive oil.

Black pepper

Celery, jicama, persimmons, pomegranate

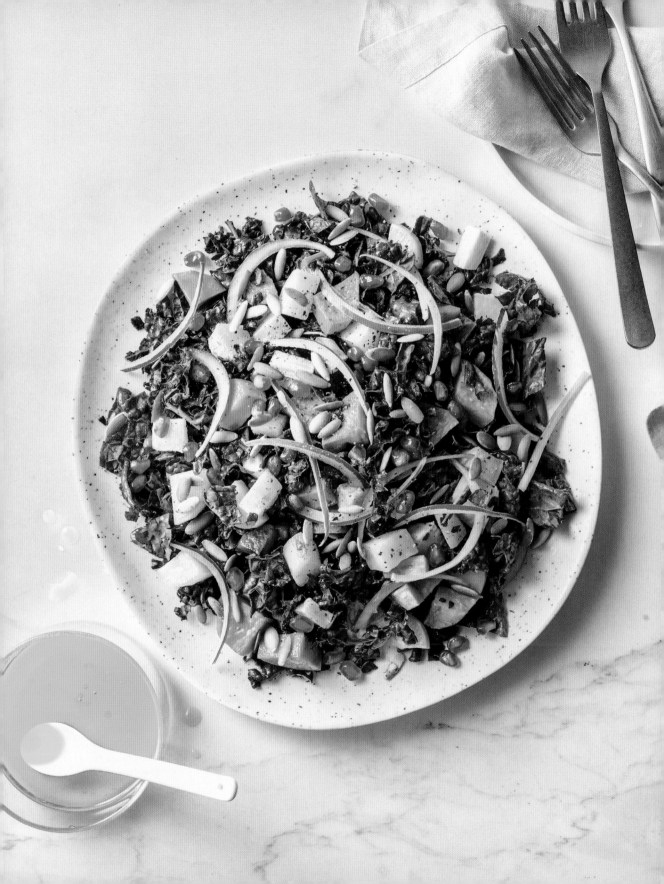

YES, EVEN ON THANKSGIVING, I serve my family and friends kale salad. This is a vibrant and robust taste of fall, full of hearty, seasonal root vegetables, a hint of maple syrup, and the crunch of pumpkin seeds. You'll "Eat the Rainbow" when you eat this salad, which is hearty enough to make a meal for your vegetarian guests, served with a side of quinoa or farro.

THANKSGIVING KALE SALAD WITH ROASTED ROOT VEGETABLES

Serves 12

Heat oven to 400°F. Line two baking sheets with parchment paper. Peel root vegetables, as desired (no need to peel delicata), and then cut into ¼- to ½-inch-thick slices. Toss with olive oil and salt in a bowl, then arrange in a single layer, with some space between vegetables, on prepared baking sheets. Cook until tender, about 20 minutes, flipping over at 10-minute point. When vegetables are light brown around edges and you're able to pierce them with a fork, remove from oven and allow to cool.

Thinly slice or tear kale into bite-size pieces and place in a salad bowl. Massage kale with your hands for about a minute, or until it has softened and is glossy and darker green.

Prepare dressing: Combine all dressing ingredients in a small bowl and whisk, or pour into a jar, tightly close lid, and shake until combined. Pour dressing onto prepared kale and toss to cover.

Toast pumpkin seeds for garnish: Place in a single layer in a small, dry skillet and heat over medium-low heat, shaking often, until pumpkin seeds puff up a bit and change from green to tan. This will take 30 to 60 seconds. Remove from heat and allow to cool.

When vegetables have cooled, arrange them atop dressed kale salad. Scatter with toasted pumpkin seeds, pomegranate arils, and red onion.

1½ pounds assorted root vegetables, such as sweet potato, delicata squash, and parsnip (about 2 small sweet potatoes, 1 delicata, 1 parsnip)

2 tablespoons olive oil

Pinch of salt

1 bunch curly green kale, center rib removed

DRESSING

1 tablespoon pure maple syrup

2 tablespoons apple cider vinegar

2 tablespoons extra-virgin olive oil

Pinch of salt

Freshly ground black pepper

GARNISHES

¼ cup raw hulled pumpkin seeds (pepitas)

¼ cup pomegranate arils

2 tablespoons thinly sliced red onion

Black pepper

Kale, pumpkin seeds, pomegranate, winter squash

1 (2½-pound) butternut squash, peeled, seeded, and cut into 1-inch cubes (if buying already prepped, about 4 cups)

1 large carrot, peeled and cut into 1-inch chunks

¼ cup olive oil

1 large yellow onion, thinly sliced

4 garlic cloves, thinly sliced

4 cups low-sodium vegetable stock

1 bay leaf

½ teaspoon fine kosher salt

Freshly ground black pepper

⅛ to ¼ teaspoon ground cinnamon

⅛ to ¼ teaspoon cayenne pepper

GARNISHES

1 recipe Cashew Lime Crema (page 107)

1 recipe Orange Spiced Pepitas (page 111)

BUTTERNUT SQUASH SOUP is a fall classic and a good way to introduce pureed soups into your repertoire. I created this version with Mexican spices and garnishes in honor of Day of the Dead, when calabaza, a kind of pumpkin, is a featured ingredient. Roasting the vegetables brings out all the warm and deep flavors and creaminess (without cream). Once you're comfortable making this soup, consider substituting other root vegetables, such as sweet potato or parsnip, using the same technique, and feel free to swap out other spices.

MEXICAN-SPICED ROASTED BUTTERNUT SQUASH SOUP

Serves 4 to 6

Preheat oven to 425°F. Toss squash and carrot with 2 tablespoons of olive oil and arrange in a single layer on two baking sheets, being sure not to overcrowd pans. Roast until squash and carrot are very well browned on a couple of sides, about 30 minutes, turning vegetables after 10 to 15 minutes.

While vegetables are roasting, make Cashew Lime Crema and Orange Spiced Pepitas. Set aside.

Once vegetables are roasted, heat remaining 2 tablespoons olive oil in a large saucepan or Dutch oven over medium heat. Add onion and garlic and sauté until soft and lightly golden, about 10 minutes.

Add roasted vegetables to saucepan along with stock and bay leaf. Bring to a low boil, then lower heat and simmer, covered, until vegetables are very soft, about 20 minutes. Discard bay leaf.

Using a blender or immersion blender, blend soup until completely smooth. Return soup to saucepan and thin with water, if needed, until it reaches your desired consistency. Season with salt, black pepper, cinnamon, and cayenne to taste.

Ladle soup into bowls, then garnish with a dollop of Cashew Lime Crema and top with Orange Spiced Pepitas. Serve right away, swirling in crema with your spoon.

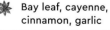

Bay leaf, cayenne, cinnamon, garlic

Carrots, pumpkin seeds, winter squash

I FIRST HAD CEVICHE in college on my first trip to Mexico, which was just a day trip with a college roommate who lived in San Diego, just over the border. I remember having a debate about whether lime juice actually cooks the seafood (technically not), then worrying whether I had made a good choice from a food hygiene perspective. I was fine, of course, and have since grown to love this simple way of showcasing the flavor of fresh seafood. This recipe is a fancier version of my first ceviche, with a balance of flavors and textures. In Mexico, ceviche is often served with saltine-type crackers, or you could enjoy this with tortilla chips.

MEXICAN SHRIMP CEVICHE

Serves 6 to 8 as an appetizer

Place shrimp in a bowl and sprinkle with a pinch of salt. Stir in lime juice and marinate for 15 minutes. Shrimp will become opaque once it has "cooked."

Add all remaining ingredients, except avocado, cilantro, and tortilla chips, and including salt and cayenne to taste.

Just before serving, gently fold in avocado and cilantro.

Serve with tortilla chips.

8 ounces fresh or frozen raw shrimp, defrosted if frozen, cut into ¼-inch dice

Salt

½ cup freshly squeezed lime juice

1 to 2 oranges or ½ ruby grapefruit, peel cut away, seeded, and diced

¾ cup peeled, seeded (unless using English or Persian), and diced cucumber (¼-inch dice) or equivalent amount of jicama

½ cup diced white onion (¼-inch dice)

1 to 2 serrano chiles, stemmed and seeded, minced finely

Cayenne pepper

Zest of 1 to 2 limes

1 firm-ripe avocado, peeled, pitted, and cut into ¼-inch dice

¼ cup fresh cilantro, finely chopped

Tortilla chips or saltine crackers, for serving

 Cayenne

Avocado, cilantro, cucumber, oranges, shrimp

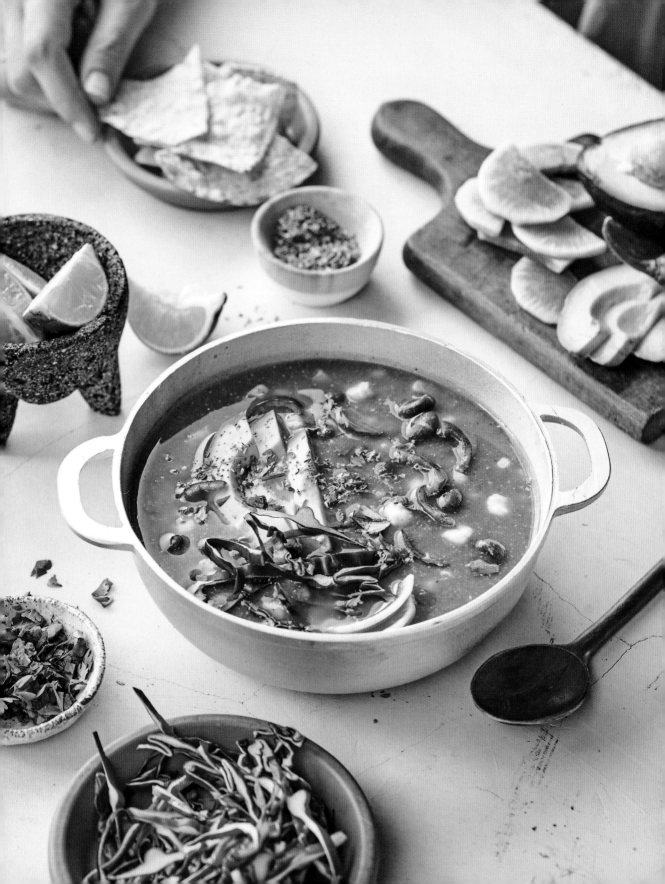

THERE ARE THREE main types of this nourishing, soothing, hominy-based soup, the most popular being red, as well as white, and the one I'm presenting here, green. Pozole is a dish of pre-Hispanic origins in Mexico, and a dish reserved for special celebrations and religious ceremonies. This meat-free version uses pepitas, tomatillos, and green chiles for its hue, and calls for roasting the chiles and aromatics for its flavor. The garnishes are definitely not optional; they add even more color, texture, and flavor. *Note*: Chayote is a light-green, pear-shaped, crunchy, sweet-tasting squash that can be eaten raw or cooked. If unavailable, feel free to replace with zucchini or summer squash.

POZOLE VERDE

Serves 8

Preheat oven to 400°F.

Cut onion and chiles in half. Place on baking sheet with unpeeled tomatillos and garlic. Roast until soft and beginning to brown, about 30 minutes. Remove from oven and let cool for 10 minutes.

Stem and seed chiles. Remove tomatillo husks and peel garlic and onion. Place roasted vegetables, pumpkin seeds, cilantro, and greens in a blender or food processor and pulse for a minute or so, until you have a coarse paste with the texture of relish.

Place blended pozole paste in a medium-size pot. Add stock and water, as needed, until you get a stewlike consistency. Season with salt to taste, cumin, and oregano. Bring to a boil over medium heat, then lower heat to low and simmer for 10 minutes.

Add hominy and beans and simmer for another 5 minutes. Add corn and chayote and simmer for 1 to 2 more minutes, or until mixture is heated through, but chayote remains crunchy.

To serve, ladle pozole into bowls and top with a drizzle of olive oil. Serve with plates of garnishes.

1 white onion

2 poblano chiles

3 serrano chiles

4 medium-size tomatillos (about 8 ounces)

6 garlic cloves

½ cup raw hulled pumpkin seeds (pepitas)

½ cup fresh cilantro, roughly chopped

1 cup leafy greens, such as spinach or kale

8 cups vegetable stock

Salt

¼ teaspoon ground cumin

¼ teaspoon dried Mexican oregano

1 (29-ounce) can white hominy, drained and rinsed

1 (15-ounce) can pinto beans, drained and rinsed

Kernels from 3 large ears of corn (about 2 cups)

1 chayote, pitted and diced into bite-size pieces

Olive oil, for drizzling

GARNISHES

2 avocados, peeled, pitted, and sliced

1 cup finely shredded red cabbage

½ cup sliced serrano chiles

¼ cup dried Mexican oregano

3 limes, cut into quarters

1 watermelon radish, thinly sliced into bite-size wedges

Tortilla chips

Roughly chopped fresh cilantro

✳	Chile peppers, cumin
🥬	Beans, chayote, cilantro, corn, leafy greens, oregano, pumpkin seeds, tomatillos

6 tablespoons pine nuts

5 tablespoons olive oil

1 medium-size onion, thinly sliced

Salt

2 garlic cloves, coarsely chopped

2 pounds Brussels sprouts, stems trimmed, sliced in half lengthwise

Freshly ground black pepper

¼ cup water, plus more if needed

¼ cup pure maple syrup, preferably Grade A (medium amber) or Grade B

IF YOU'RE UNCERTAIN about Brussels sprouts, these maple syrup–glazed sprouts will make you fall in love. This is one of the first recipes I developed for my cooking classes, and by the end of the first class, I had avowed Brussels sprouts haters eating them with their hands and licking the plate. The trick with Brussels sprouts is to avoid overcooking them, or else they will be mushy and won't smell appetizing. The added sweetness of caramelized onions and maple syrup mellow out any potential bitterness, and the pine nuts add crunch and richness.

Note: Depending on the size of your pan, you may need to cook this in two batches.

GATEWAY BRUSSELS SPROUTS

Serves 12 as a side dish

Heat a small, dry skillet over medium-low heat, then add pine nuts. Allow to toast until golden, about 5 minutes, stirring or sautéing every minute or so to prevent burning. Remove from heat when toasted.

Heat 2 tablespoons of olive oil in a medium skillet with a lid over medium-low heat, then add onion and a pinch or two of salt. Cover and allow to cook slowly until caramelized, about 30 minutes, stirring every 5 minutes, each time adding a bit of water if onion begins to dry out. Remove from heat when onion is browned and soft.

In a large skillet with a lid, heat remaining 3 tablespoons of olive oil over medium heat. Add garlic and sauté until golden, then transfer to a plate and set aside. Next, add Brussels sprouts, cut side down, to same pan in a single layer, and cook, uncovered, over medium-high heat. Some leaves may fall off—add these too. Sprinkle evenly with a few pinches of salt and pepper. After a minute, check to see whether cut sides have browned. When lightly golden, turn over Brussels sprouts with a spatula.

Add ¼ cup of water, cover pan, lower heat to medium-low, and cook for about 3 minutes, or until most of liquid has evaporated and Brussels

✳ Black pepper

🌸 Brussels sprouts

continued ⟶

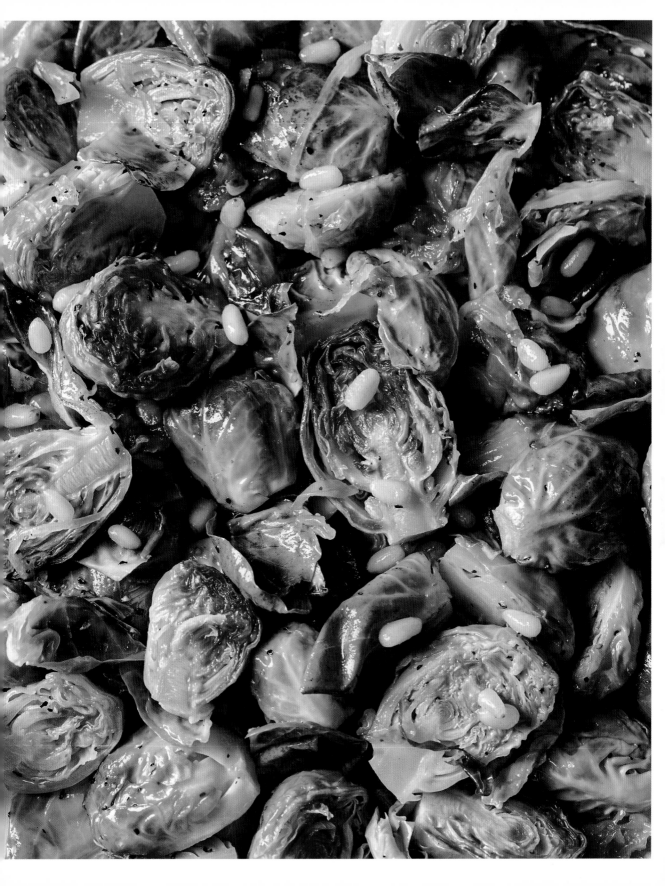

sprouts are fork-tender. If they are not tender, add another tablespoon of water and cook for another minute. (Brussels sprouts should be al dente and bright green, not soft and mushy.)

Now, add maple syrup, stir, increase heat to medium, and cook, uncovered, until syrup begins to bubble, a minute or less.

Turn off heat, add sautéed garlic, caramelized onion, and pine nuts, and toss together.

½ head red cabbage, shredded

1 red apple, skin on, cored and cut into ½-inch chunks

½ small red onion, thinly sliced

1 teaspoon salt, or to taste

Freshly ground black pepper

2 tablespoons butter or vegan butter

¼ cup fried shallots

CABBAGE may not seem like a glamorous vegetable, but maybe red cabbage, which turns purple when cooked, might win you over. This is a fabulous and simple winter side dish that Emma, my older daughter, loves more than you might imagine a teenager would. In fact, one of her favorite lunchbox sandwiches is red cabbage on a buttered ciabatta roll. The butter in this dish really enhances and mellows out the flavor of the cabbage, and also plays a nutritional role—fat is necessary to absorb the vitamin K, which is abundant in this vegetable.

EMMA'S ROASTED RED CABBAGE WITH SHALLOTS AND APPLES

Serves 4 to 6 as a side dish

Preheat oven to 350°F.

Place cabbage, in an even layer, on the bottom of a 9 x 13-inch baking pan, then scatter apples and onion evenly on top. Season with salt and pepper to taste and then dot with tiny pieces of butter.

Seal baking pan tightly with a piece of foil and bake for 20 minutes.

After 20 minutes, remove pan from oven and carefully remove foil, making sure not to burn yourself with steam. Gently stir cabbage mixture, which should now have softened, taste, and adjust seasoning. Replace foil and place back in oven to bake for another 10 to 15 minutes, or until completely softened.

Transfer to a platter, and just before serving, scatter fried shallots on top.

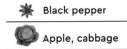

Black pepper

Apple, cabbage

1 tablespoon olive oil

½ white onion, sliced

Salt

2 Hatch or Italian green chiles or 1 Anaheim chile, stemmed and seeded and quartered lengthwise (about 1½ cups)

Kernels from 1 ear of corn

3 tomatillos, husked and cut into 8 wedges

¼ to ½ teaspoon cayenne pepper, to taste

Juice of 1 lime

THIS RECIPE started out as a version of *esquites*, corn kernels slathered in cheese, chili powder, and lime. I supplemented it with other Mexican produce I happened to have in the kitchen, including some lovely green chiles, and a tomatillo with a bite taken out of it. Let me explain. My daughter had read a passage in a book about a girl picking a sun-warmed tomatillo off the vine in her mother's garden, and taking a juicy bite out of it, right then and there. Captivated by this sensuous image, my daughter took a bite out of a tomatillo. Since it had probably been picked weeks before from a vine in Mexico, it tasted disappointingly sour in our fog-cooled San Francisco kitchen. It's all about the context. But the tomatillo didn't get thrown into the compost bin. Instead, I took inspiration from the challenge and created this lovely end-of-summer side dish.

MEXICAN CORN WITH TOMATILLOS AND GREEN CHILES

Serves 4 as a side dish

Heat a medium-size sauté pan, then add oil and heat over medium-high heat until shimmery. Add onion along with a pinch of salt and sauté until translucent.

Increase heat to high, then add sliced chiles and sear until browned and blistered in some spots.

Add corn and tomatillos and cook for 30 seconds.

Add salt and cayenne to taste. Squeeze lime juice on top just before serving.

Serve as a side dish or as a topping for Roasted Salmon Tacos (page 88).

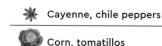

Cayenne, chile peppers

Corn, tomatillos

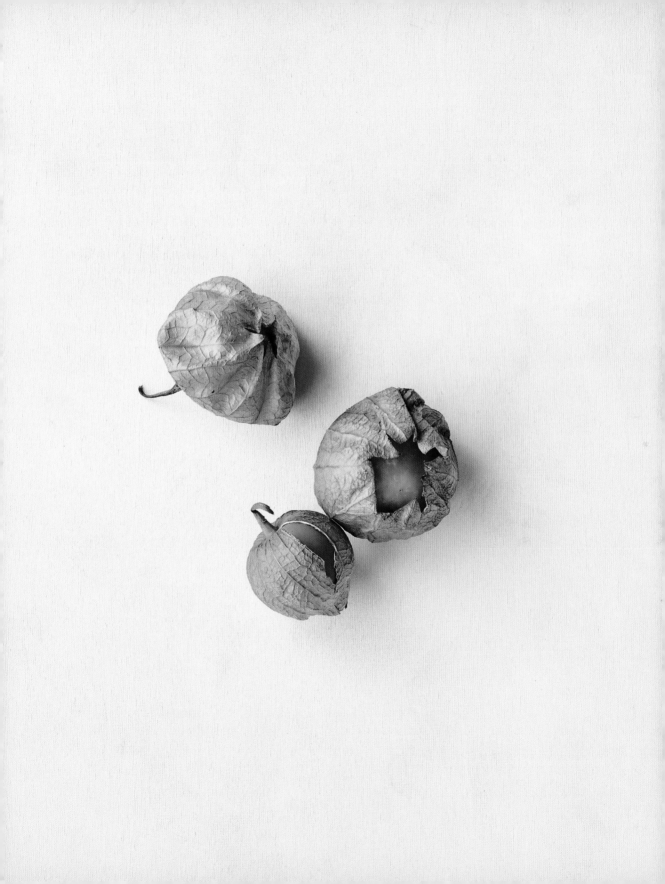

COCONUT TOFU

14 ounces firm tofu

1½ tablespoons low-sodium soy sauce

2 tablespoons pure maple syrup

1 tablespoon sesame oil

1 teaspoon garlic powder

½ teaspoon freshly ground black pepper

¼ cup unsweetened shredded coconut

SPICED COCONUT RICE

2 cups uncooked brown jasmine or basmati rice

1½ cups coconut milk

1½ cups water

1 teaspoon fine kosher salt

2 bay leaves

3 cardamom pods, lightly crushed

1 cinnamon stick

Bay leaf, cardamom, cinnamon

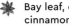 Whole grains, tofu

THIS MEAL was inspired by an eight-year-old vegan. In second grade, my daughter had a friend, Caycie, who has been a vegan as long as she remembers. There's only one problem: Caycie didn't like most vegetables! I thought, *What does she eat?* The answer came many months later when my daughter came home asking for Caycie's lunch: coconut tofu with coconut rice. We pieced the ingredients together through Google images (kids these days!), and I created this recipe. I've paired it with brown jasmine rice steamed with coconut milk and aromatic spices. This is a delicious and satisfying meal when served with sliced cucumbers or a side salad. One day, I'll get Caycie to eat the salad too.

COCONUT TOFU WITH SPICED COCONUT RICE

Serves 4

Thirty minutes before starting, press tofu: Drain tofu, wrap in two layers of paper towels, and press between two heavy cutting boards. Pat dry with paper towels.

While tofu is pressing, prepare spiced coconut rice: Combine rice with coconut milk, water, salt, bay leaves, cardamom pods, and cinnamon stick in a rice cooker and cook according to manufacturer's instructions. Alternatively, you can make this on stovetop by bringing all coconut rice ingredients to a boil in a large pot and then simmering, covered, until all liquid is absorbed. Remove bay leaves, cardamom pods, and cinnamon stick before serving.

Prepare coconut tofu: Whisk together soy sauce, maple syrup, sesame oil, garlic powder, and pepper in a bowl.

Cut pressed tofu into 1-inch cubes.

Place tofu cubes in a container with a lid, then pour in prepared marinade. Seal and shake to coat; marinate for at least 15 minutes. While tofu marinates, preheat oven to 350°F and line a baking sheet with foil.

Spread shredded coconut on a plate and dredge marinated tofu cubes until evenly coated. (*Note*: Coconut will not stick very much; you'll scatter remainder over top before baking.) Place tofu cubes on prepared baking sheet. Sprinkle remaining coconut on top. Reserve leftover marinade to use as a dipping sauce or for a dressing for salad greens, shredded kale, or sliced cucumbers to serve as a side.

Bake tofu for 20 to 25 minutes, or until golden brown. Serve with spiced coconut rice.

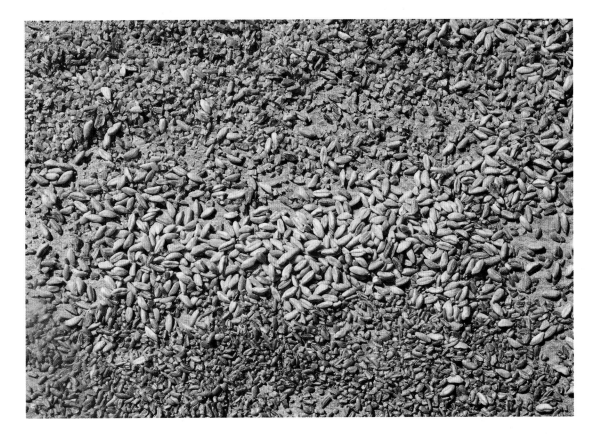

¼ cup olive oil

2 large onions, chopped

1 carrot, chopped

1½ teaspoons fresh thyme, finely minced, or ½ teaspoon dried

1½ teaspoons fresh marjoram, finely minced, or ½ teaspoon dried

3 cups no-salt added vegetable stock

1 cup dried lentils, rinsed (to shorten cooking time, precook lentils for about 20 minutes by boiling in water, then drain)

Salt and freshly ground black pepper

¼ cup chopped fresh flat-leaf parsley

1 (16-ounce) can no-salt added diced or crushed tomatoes

¼ cup dry sherry

Garnishes: ⅔ cup grated Swiss cheese, chopped flat-leaf parsley

Black pepper

Herbs, lentils, tomatoes

CAN A BOWL of soup save the world? The sustainability of our food supply has become an urgent question. It's clear that the easiest way to ensure that we all have food to eat in the future is to eat a plant-based diet. This echoes the work of Frances Moore Lappé, activist and author of 1971's *Diet for a Small Planet*. This recipe is adapted from one in that book, Lentils, Monastery Style, but its rich flavorings are anything but ascetic. Herbs, sherry, and a rich garnish of Swiss cheese make this not only a balanced vegetarian meal but are the perfect accents to the earthy flavor of the lentil base. This recipe is a good example of how eating conscientiously doesn't mean eating blandly; you can make endless variations by substituting different herbs and spices (and it can be doubled and frozen for later). My suggestions follow.

LENTIL SOUP FOR A SMALL PLANET

Serves 4 to 6

Heat oil in a large pot and sauté onions and carrot for 3 to 5 minutes, or until onions are soft and translucent.

Add thyme and marjoram and sauté for 1 minute.

Add stock, lentils, salt and pepper to taste, parsley, and tomatoes and cook, covered, until lentils are tender, about 45 minutes.

Add sherry, and adjust salt to taste.

Ladle into bowls and garnish with grated Swiss cheese and extra parsley.

SUGGESTED ACCOMPANIMENTS
Cornbread or a crusty loaf of bread.

GLOBAL VARIATIONS
Indian: Substitute cumin seeds and ground turmeric for thyme and marjoram, and cilantro for parsley; omit Swiss cheese and substitute a dollop of yogurt.

Mexican: Substitute oregano and chili powder for thyme and marjoram, and cilantro for parsley; substitute queso fresco for Swiss cheese.

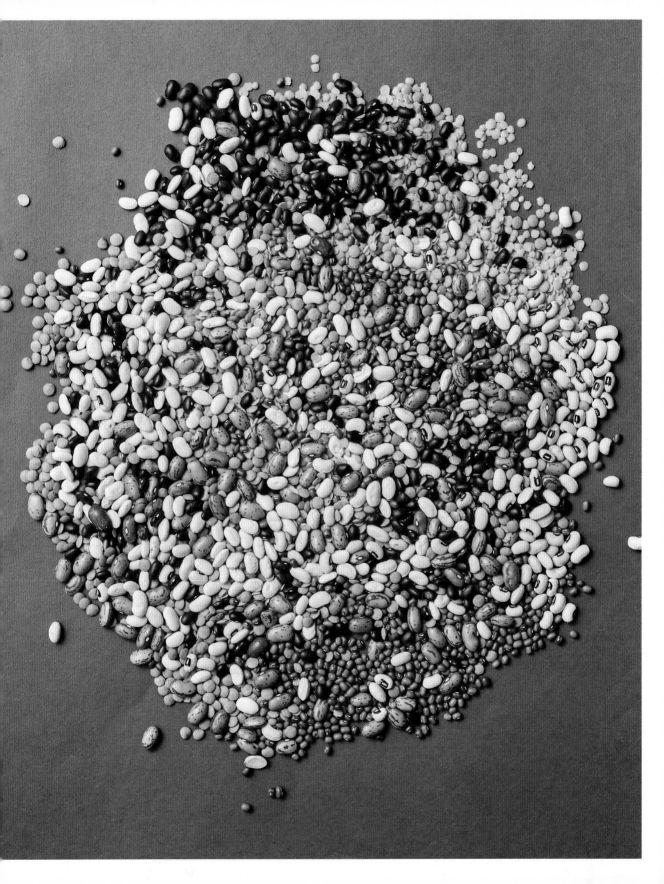

8 ounces dried Vaquero or pinto beans, soaked in water overnight

1 tablespoon canola oil

1 to 2 chipotles in adobo, finely diced

½ onion, finely diced

½ bell pepper, seeded and finely diced

1 carrot, finely diced

1 teaspoon ground cumin

½ teaspoon cayenne pepper

1 (14.5-ounce) can diced fire-roasted tomatoes, no or low-sodium preferred

5 cups water

1 teaspoon dried oregano

Salt

1 ounce dark chocolate

Optional garnishes: chopped fresh cilantro, shredded cheese

Cornbread, for serving

THIS IS a flavorful and satisfying smoky, meatless chili, with a surprise ingredient (chocolate!). I'm featuring Vaquero beans, also known as Orca beans, which are a playful black and white, resembling a cow. They're fun to cook with because even after cooking and giving off an inky pot liquor, they maintain their dappled markings. If you have trouble obtaining these lovely beans, pinto beans make a fine, though less playful, substitute. (I recommend Rancho Gordo for a source of high-quality heirloom and hard-to-find dried beans, ranchogordo.com.)

SMOKIN' HOT VEGAN VAQUERO CHILI

Serves 4 to 6

After beans have been soaked, drain from soaking liquid and set aside.

Heat canola oil in a heavy pot over medium-high heat, add chipotles, onion, bell pepper, and carrot, and cook stirring, for about 5 minutes, or until vegetables have softened.

Add cumin and cayenne and fry for another minute.

Add beans, tomatoes, water, and oregano and bring to a boil. Then, lower heat and simmer for 1 to 2 hours, until beans are soft. (Cooking time will depend on the age of your beans.)

Add salt to taste. Just before serving, add chocolate and stir well (heat will melt chocolate).

Ladle into bowls and top with garnishes, if desired. Serve with cornbread.

Leftovers will keep in refrigerator for up to 5 days, or frozen for up to 3 months.

Cayenne, chile peppers, cumin

Beans, chocolate, oregano, tomatoes

1 baguette

Cream cheese

Leftover Chinese Eggplant with Black Vinegar and Thai Basil (page 148)

English or Persian cucumber, thinly sliced

Arugula

Salt and freshly ground black pepper

THIS SANDWICH came about due to one of my daughters' openness to trying new flavor combinations (also known as refusal to eat the same thing more than once a month!), plus my zeal for repurposing leftovers. And voilà—her favorite sandwich was born. Immigrants have always figured out how to use local ingredients to substitute for what they cannot get in their new home. I've named this the Chinese American eggplant sandwich because this is a combination of the flavors of Chinese cuisine with ingredients found only on our shores, just like the Chinese American dishes that were created out of necessity in San Francisco's Chinatown during the gold rush.

CALIFORNIA GOLD RUSH CHINESE AMERICAN EGGPLANT SANDWICH

Makes 1 sandwich (though you can scale up as your leftovers indicate!)

Cut baguette into desired length, then split and toast cut sides.

Spread a layer of cream cheese on both toasted sides of baguette. Place both halves, cream cheese side up, on a cutting board.

Place pieces of leftover eggplant, draining away most of sauce, onto bottom half. Top with cucumber slices and arugula. Add a pinch of salt and pepper to taste. Top with other baguette half. Press together tightly.

※ Black pepper

Arugula, eggplant

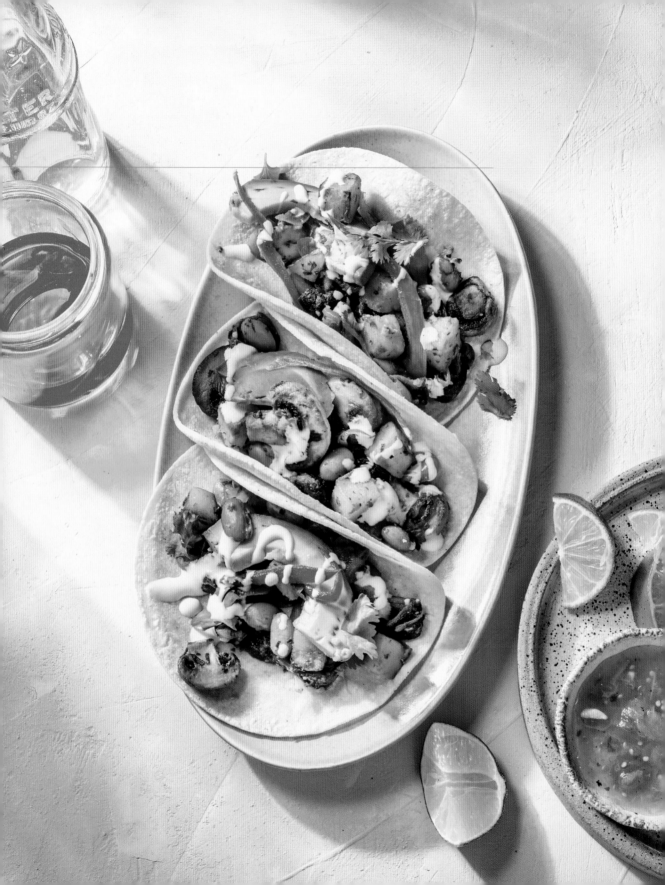

THE FIRST TIME I had a potato and mushroom taco, I was surprised by how meaty it tasted. In my version, I have added roasted poblanos and pinto beans to make this truly satisfying. Don't forget the *crema*, whether dairy or Cashew Lime Crema (page 107).

POTATO AND MUSHROOM TACOS

Serves 6 to 8

Roast poblanos directly over flame of a gas burner or under broiler until completely charred, turning with tongs, after about 10 minutes. Transfer to a bowl and cover with a plate or plastic wrap, or place in a paper bag and fold shut, and let steam until cool enough to handle, about 10 minutes. Scrape off charred skin with a paring knife; remove and discard stems and seeds. Slice into strips and set aside.

Meanwhile, put potatoes into a large, nonstick skillet and cover with cold water; add ½ teaspoon of salt. Bring to a simmer over medium-high heat and cook until just tender, 5 minutes, then drain. Set potatoes aside and wipe skillet dry.

Heat 2 tablespoons of canola oil in same skillet over medium-high heat. Add drained potatoes and cook until golden and crisp, about 4 minutes per side. Remove with a slotted spoon and drain on a paper towel–lined plate. While potatoes are still hot, sprinkle with half of cilantro and parsley and salt to taste. Set aside. Wipe out skillet.

Heat same skillet over high heat, add mushrooms and sear on both sides until golden, a few minutes per side. Transfer to a plate.

Add remaining tablespoon of oil to same skillet, allow it to heat over medium-high heat for a few seconds, then add onion and a pinch of salt and cook, stirring occasionally, until translucent, about 5 minutes. Stir in remaining cilantro and parsley and garlic and cook for another minute.

Add roasted poblanos and pinto beans along with lime juice and cayenne. Stir to combine and cook for 1 to 2 minutes. Stir in potatoes and mushrooms and season with salt and pepper to taste.

Serve in warmed tortillas with garnishes.

4 medium-size poblano chiles

3 medium-size Yukon Gold potatoes, cut into ½-inch pieces

Kosher salt

3 tablespoons canola oil

2 tablespoons finely chopped fresh cilantro

2 tablespoons finely chopped fresh parsley

12 ounces cremini and/or white mushrooms, thinly sliced

1 large white onion, thinly sliced

1 garlic clove, minced

1 (14.5-ounce) can pinto beans, drained and rinsed

Juice of 2 limes

½ teaspoon cayenne pepper

Freshly ground black pepper

Corn tortillas, warmed

GARNISHES

½ cup Mexican crema or Cashew Lime Crema (page 107)

Pickled Red Onion (page 112)

Peeled, pitted, and sliced avocado

Limes

Fresh cilantro

Salsa of your choosing (see page 110 to make your own)

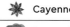

Cayenne, chile peppers

Beans, herbs, mushrooms, potatoes

Canola oil

2 pounds center-cut, fresh skinless salmon fillet

1 teaspoon chipotle powder

1 teaspoon ground cumin

Grated zest of 1 lime

1½ teaspoons kosher salt

Juice of 1 lime

Corn tortillas, warmed

SUGGESTED GARNISHES

Mexican Corn with Tomatillos and Green Chiles (page 78)

Grilled Pineapple Salsa (page 111)

Cashew Lime Crema (page 107)

Pickled Red Onion (page 112)

Shredded green cabbage

Peeled, pitted, and sliced avocado

Squeeze of lime juice

SALMON is definitely a North of the Border filling for tacos, but it works well. This recipe packs flavor from a simple spice rub and cooks quickly in the oven. As with most tacos, or at least in my opinion, the garnishes make this. Follow my suggested toppings below, but feel free to swap out for your favorites (or whatever you have). This makes an easy, sophisticated-tasting, but simple meal for Taco Tuesday.

ROASTED SALMON TACOS

Serves 8

Preheat oven to 425°F. Brush a foil-lined baking sheet with oil and place salmon on it.

Make spice rub: Mix together chipotle powder, cumin, lime zest, and salt in a small bowl.

Squeeze lime juice evenly over top of salmon, then rub with spice rub.

Roast for 12 to 15 minutes, depending on thickness of salmon, or until just cooked through. It will flake easily with a fork when done.

Slice into bite-size strips, then place on a serving platter.

Serve with suggested garnishes, and allow everyone to assemble their own tacos. *¡Buen provecho!*

✳ Chipotle, cumin

🥬 Salmon

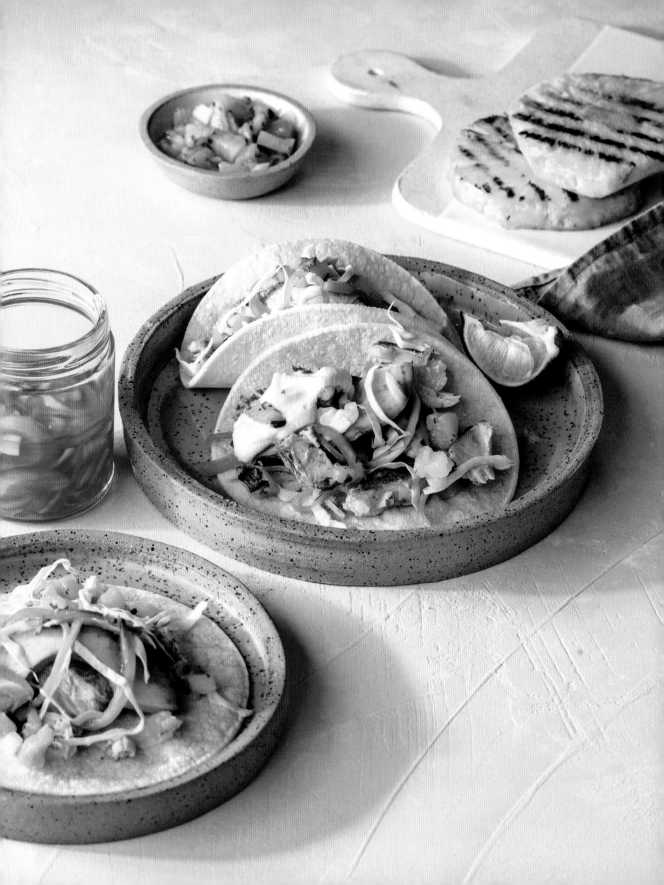

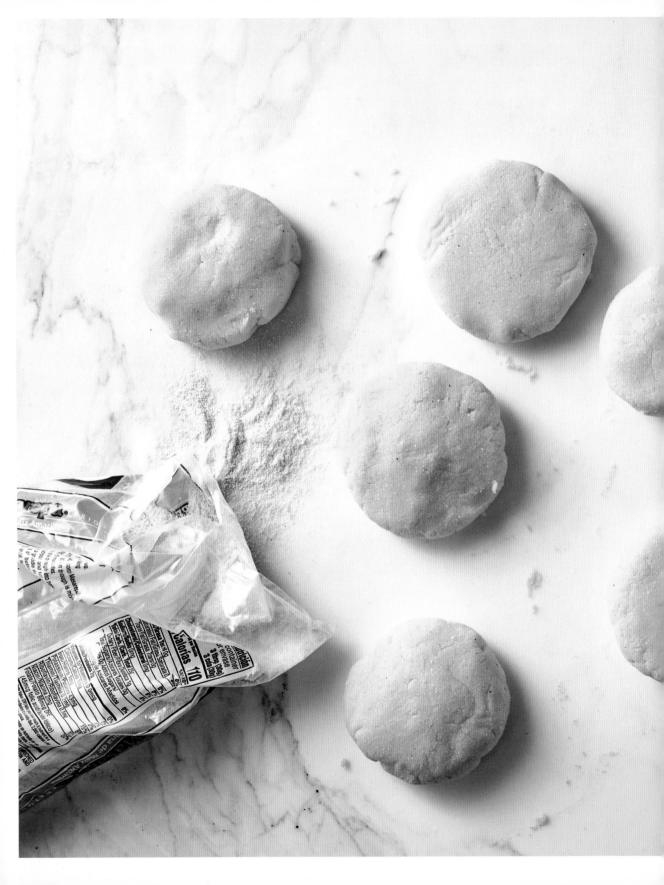

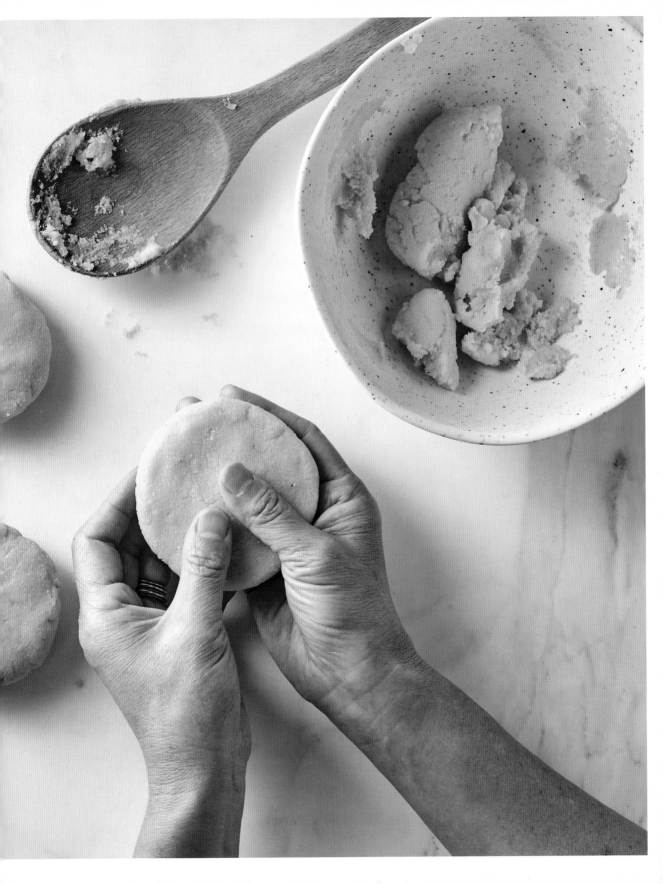

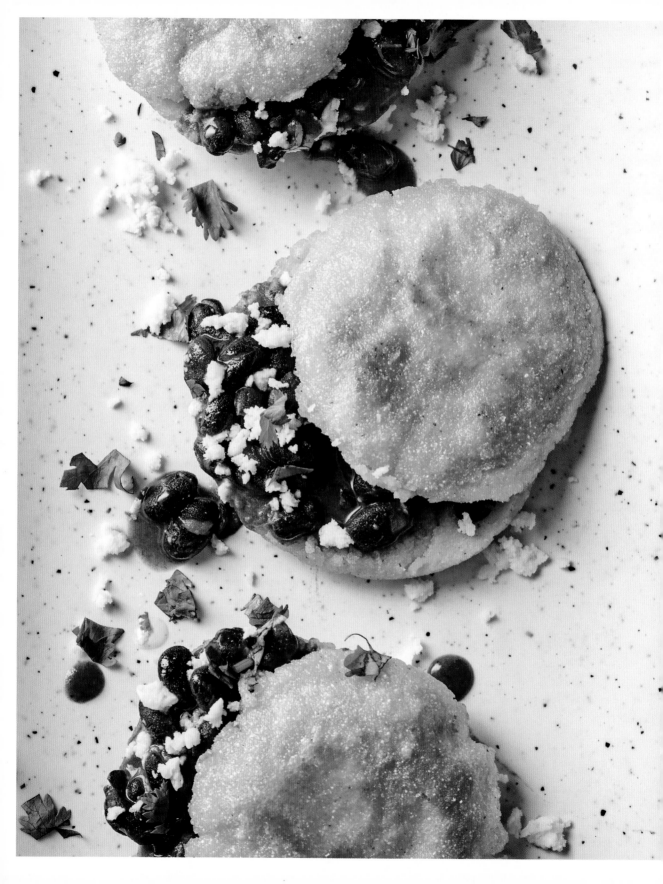

AREPAS are corn pockets, like pitas, that have origins in the indigenous tribes of South America. A popular street food or snack in Venezuela and Colombia, they can be eaten plain but are usually split and stuffed with savory fillings. This filling is a classic combination of black beans and queso fresco, but you can fill these with anything you like. Other suggested fillings include shredded cooked chicken or pork, corn salad with onion and fresh herbs, tomatoes, and avocado. Note that this calls for arepa flour, which is precooked yellow or white cornmeal. Sometimes sold as *masarepa* or *harina precocida*, it can be found in Latin American markets and some supermarkets, and is not the same as masa harina.

This recipe is gluten-free and, if the cheese is left out, vegan.

AREPAS "EL DIABLO"

Makes 8 arepas

Prepare filling: Heat oil in a small saucepan over medium-high heat and add onion and garlic. Cook until softened, 1 to 2 minutes. Add beans, water, salt, red pepper flakes, and oregano, cook for 3 to 5 minutes, then remove from heat and set aside, covered.

Prepare arepas: Combine arepa flour and salt in a medium-size bowl. Make a well in center and add warm water. Using a wooden spoon, gradually incorporate dry ingredients, stirring until no dry lumps remain. Let rest for 5 minutes to hydrate.

Knead dough a few times in bowl, then divide into eight equal pieces. Roll each piece into a ball on a work surface, then gently flatten to about ½ inch thick.

Heat 1 tablespoon of oil in a large, nonstick skillet with a lid over medium heat. Add four arepas, cover, and cook until bottoms are golden brown, 6 to 8 minutes. Uncover, flip, and cook (keep uncovered) until other sides are golden brown, 6 to 8 minutes. (When they're done, you'll get a hollow sound when you tap on the arepa.) Transfer arepas to a wire rack. Repeat with remaining 1 tablespoon oil and remaining dough.

When ready to serve, split arepas by slicing horizontally almost all the way through, as you would a pita, and stuff with prepared bean filling and queso fresco; serve with a squeeze of lime juice and some cilantro.

FILLING

2 tablespoons olive oil

3 tablespoons minced white onion

2 garlic cloves, minced

2 (15-ounce) cans no-salt-added black beans (drained but *not* rinsed)

½ cup water

½ teaspoon salt

¼ to ½ teaspoon crushed red pepper flakes

½ teaspoon oregano leaves

AREPAS

2 cups arepa flour

2 teaspoons kosher salt

2½ cups warm water

2 tablespoons vegetable oil

4 ounces queso fresco (available from Latin American markets) or mild feta, to serve

Garnishes: lime wedges and cilantro sprigs

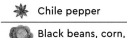

✳ Chile pepper

Black beans, corn, garlic, oregano

12 ounces washed and pitted super ripe Italian prunes or other plums, washed and pitted

2 cinnamon sticks

1 quarter-size slice fresh ginger, peeled

2 to 4 tablespoons demerara sugar, or to taste

2 tablespoons chia seeds, plus more if needed to thicken

THE HOME we've lived in for twenty years boasts four decades-old Italian prune trees. They're the most reliable markers of the season we know—without fail, they bear their sweet fruit for the first two weeks of July. After a week, the plums get too soft, even in the refrigerator. Years of experience with this phenomenon has led me to create a jam to preserve our plums long after summer has ended. Cinnamon and ginger balance the tartness of the plums, while demerara sugar can sweeten, if needed. Adding chia as a thickener instead of pectin is a way to reduce the amount of sugar needed and also add fiber, protein, and omega-3 fatty acids. This will keep for up to two weeks in the refrigerator, or for longer using standard canning methods.

SPICED PLUM-GINGER CHIA JAM

Makes 1½ to 2 cups jam

Place pitted plums, cinnamon sticks, and ginger in a heavy pot.

Slowly bring to a boil over medium-low heat (without additional water), then lower heat to a simmer. Add demerara sugar, stir, and adjust to taste.

Simmer for an hour, covered, stirring occasionally.

Meanwhile, if you will be canning jam, prepare jars for canning, using proper technique.

After an hour or so, you should have an incredibly fragrant and irresistible sauce. To thicken, first remove ginger and cinnamon sticks, then stir in chia seeds and let stand for 5 minutes. Check thickness. If you'd like a thicker consistency, stir in more chia seeds, 1 teaspoon at a time.

Pour hot jam into prepared jars and can for later use. Alternatively, if you are planning to eat this up quickly, place in clean jars, let cool, then refrigerate. Enjoy with toast, Greek yogurt, over vanilla ice cream, or if you're like my kids, by the spoonful!

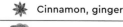

✳ Cinnamon, ginger

🌸 Chia, plums

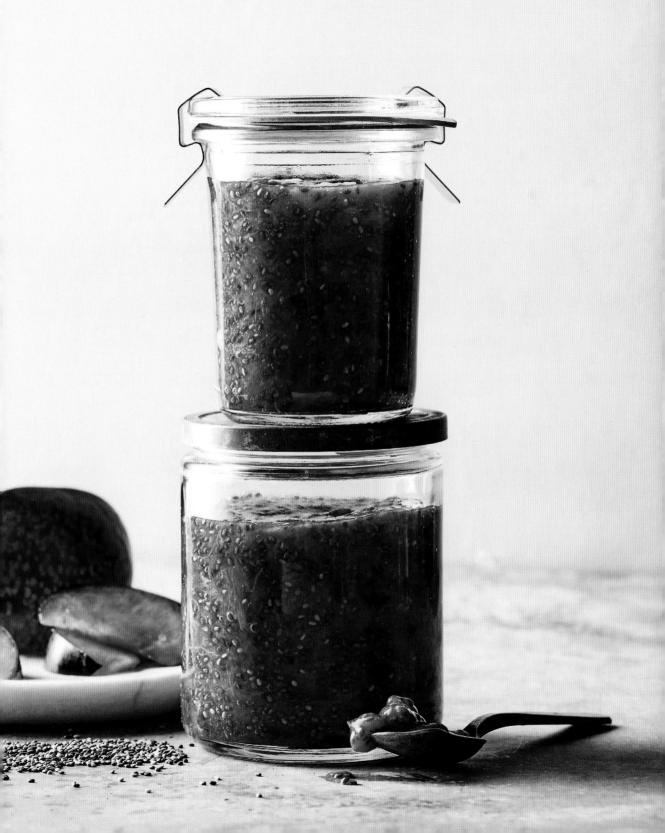

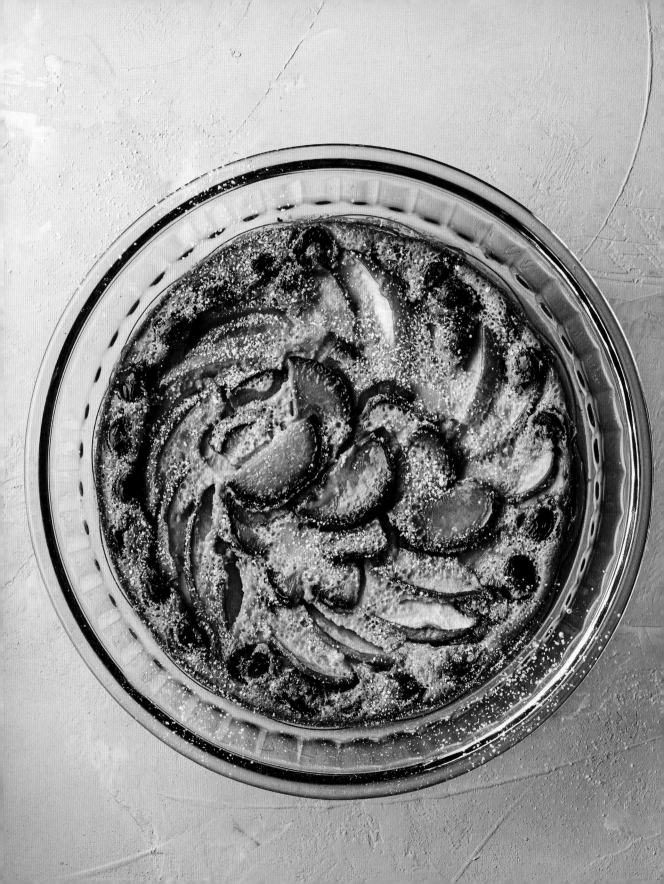

TO MAKE a seasonal variation on the classic clafoutis, a custardy French dessert that typically contains only cherries, I combined cherries with slices of other local stone fruit: plum and white nectarine, whose sweetness is balanced by the bite of ginger. This is a very simple dessert—all you need to do is pour and bake.

CHERRY, PLUM, AND NECTARINE CLAFOUTIS

Serves 6

Butter, for pan

8 ounces cherries, stemmed and pitted (if using frozen, defrost and towel dry before using)

1 firm-fleshed ripe plum

1 firm-fleshed ripe white nectarine

3 large eggs

½ cup granulated sugar

1 teaspoon ground ginger

Pinch of salt

2 teaspoons pure vanilla extract

½ cup all-purpose flour

1¼ cups whole milk

Confectioners' sugar, for garnish (optional)

Butter a 9-inch deep-dish pie plate and preheat oven to 350°F.

Slice and arrange fruit in an even layer in prepared pie plate.

Whisk or blend together eggs and granulated sugar in a medium bowl; add ginger, salt, and vanilla; then flour; and last, milk, mixing until you have a smooth and airy batter. Pour batter over fruit.

Bake for 35 to 40 minutes, or until puffy and lightly browned and a knife inserted into center comes out clean.

Remove from oven, let cool on a wire rack, and serve just slightly warm or refrigerate and serve cool (will be easier to slice as it cools further). Dust with confectioners' sugar before serving, if desired.

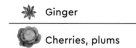

Ginger

Cherries, plums

1 (15-ounce) can pure
pumpkin puree

1⅔ cups coconut milk
(1 [13.5-ounce] can)

3 tablespoons cornstarch

2 tablespoons pure maple
syrup

¼ cup brown sugar (light or
dark, your preference)

½ teaspoon ground
cinnamon

½ teaspoon freshly grated
nutmeg

½ teaspoon ground ginger

1 teaspoon pure vanilla
extract

**COCONUT WHIPPED CREAM
(OPTIONAL, MAKES ½ CUP)**

1 (13.5-ounce) can full-
fat coconut milk, chilled
overnight in refrigerator

1 teaspoon pure vanilla
extract

OPTIONAL GARNISHES

Minced candied ginger

Orange Spiced Pepitas
(page 111)

POT DE CRÈME is a dense, rich pudding, usually made with heavy cream and eggs. This is a healthier, but still decadent, pumpkin version. Because it is vegan (egg- and dairy-free), it's suitable for many dietary restrictions. It tastes like pumpkin pie without the crust.

PUMPKIN POTS DE CRÈME

Serves 4

Whisk all pots de crème ingredients together in a medium-size bowl until smoothly combined.

Pour into a saucepan and simmer over medium-low heat until thick, 6 to 8 minutes, stirring frequently to avoid lumps.

Transfer into individual serving cups or jars (small mason jars are a nice touch) and chill in refrigerator until firm, about 1½ hours.

Prepare coconut whipped cream (if using): After chilling can of coconut milk in refrigerator overnight, open it and scoop out only solidified coconut cream on top. (Reserve remaining coconut milk for another use.) Place cream in a medium-size bowl, and use an electric hand mixer on high speed to whip until it forms soft peaks, 3 to 4 minutes. Stir in vanilla. Refrigerate whipped cream until ready to use. It will harden a bit, so gently stir it again before serving.

Immediately before serving, top pots de crème with a dollop of whipped cream and/or a few sprinkles of minced candied ginger or Orange Spiced Pepitas.

✳ Cinnamon, ginger,
nutmeg

🎃 Pumpkin, pumpkin
seeds

AT OUR QUARTERLY dinner event, Spicebox Supperclub, four couples take turns presenting dinners on a theme. Inspired by a Nigel Slater recipe served at our Eastern European supperclub, my recipe is flourless and gluten-free. The beets add both moistness and a subtle earthiness, while allspice will keep your guests guessing about the secret ingredient.

1 small beet (4 ounces)

8 tablespoons (1 stick) unsalted butter, plus more for pan

Unsweetened cocoa powder, for dusting

8 ounces bittersweet chocolate, chopped

5 large eggs

⅔ cup granulated sugar

¼ cup hot espresso or strong coffee

½ teaspoon ground allspice

Optional garnishes: crème fraîche and confectioners' sugar

SPICEBOX SUPPERCLUB FLOURLESS CHOCOLATE BEET CAKE

<u>Serves 8</u>

Cook beet (unpeeled) by placing in a saucepan with water to cover, adding a splash of vinegar (to maintain color), and boiling for about 45 minutes, or until tender. Immediately drain and plunge into cold water to cool. Once beet has cooled, use fingers to remove skin (it should slip off easily). Cut into chunks and puree in a food processor or blender until very smooth (add a little water, if needed).

Meanwhile, preheat oven to 325°F.

Prepare a 9-inch springform pan by buttering sides and bottom and dusting with cocoa powder.

Melt remaining butter in another pan, then add chopped chocolate and melt over low heat, stirring with a whisk periodically. Remove from heat and set aside.

Beat eggs and granulated sugar together in a bowl with an electric hand or stand mixer until frothy. Fold in beet puree, chocolate mixture, espresso, and allspice.

Pour batter into prepared pan and bake for 30 to 40 minutes, or until cake begins to pull away from sides of pan and springs back when touched lightly with your finger.

Let cool in pan on a wire rack for 10 minutes, then serve warm or at room temperature with a dollop of crème fraîche and a dusting of confectioners' sugar.

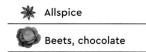

✳ Allspice

🪷 Beets, chocolate

1 ripe pineapple

1 cinnamon stick

5 cloves

1 cup piloncillo (strongly preferred) or dark brown sugar

2 quarts warm water

TEPACHE is a lightly fermented, lightly spiced pineapple drink that is sold by street vendors in Mexico. I didn't become acquainted with this drink in Mexico, however. As a "reduce food waste" kind of cook, I wondered one day during culinary school whether we could do anything with the large amount of pineapple rinds we had from making a pineapple dessert. Although my classmates (and some instructors) looked askance at what admittedly looks a little bit like an aquarium while fermenting, it was love at first sip.

Besides the sweet spices, tepache is sweetened with the caramel flavor of piloncillo, Mexican brown sugar made from sugarcane juice and sold in cone-shaped blocks.

TEPACHE (MEXICAN SPICED FERMENTED PINEAPPLE DRINK)

Serves 8

Thoroughly wash your pineapple, then use a knife to remove top. Then, cut off all its rind (it's okay and preferable to leave a little bit of pulp on; save remaining pulp for enjoying separately).

Place pineapple rind in a 1-gallon container with a lid, add cinnamon stick, cloves, and piloncillo, then pour in water. Water should cover entire pineapple rind; if not, add a little more. Stir to combine, then cover with lid. I like to add a layer of cheesecloth before sealing, to keep away any fruit flies that might be interested in some tepache! Don't worry about dissolving sugar completely; it will dissolve as it sits. Set in a warm place.

After one day, sugar should have dissolved. Stir mixture and cover again.

Check on second day to see whether it's a little bubbly and tastes a little fermented. If it is to your liking, strain through a fine-mesh sieve or cheesecloth and put in refrigerator to chill. If it isn't fermented tasting yet, stir and allow to ferment for another day before straining. Generally speaking, about 3 days is ideal if your house is "room temperature," but 2 days would be enough in a tropical climate.

Serve over ice, diluting with water if desired, and adding Mexican beer if desired. *¡Salud!*

Cinnamon, cloves

Pineapple

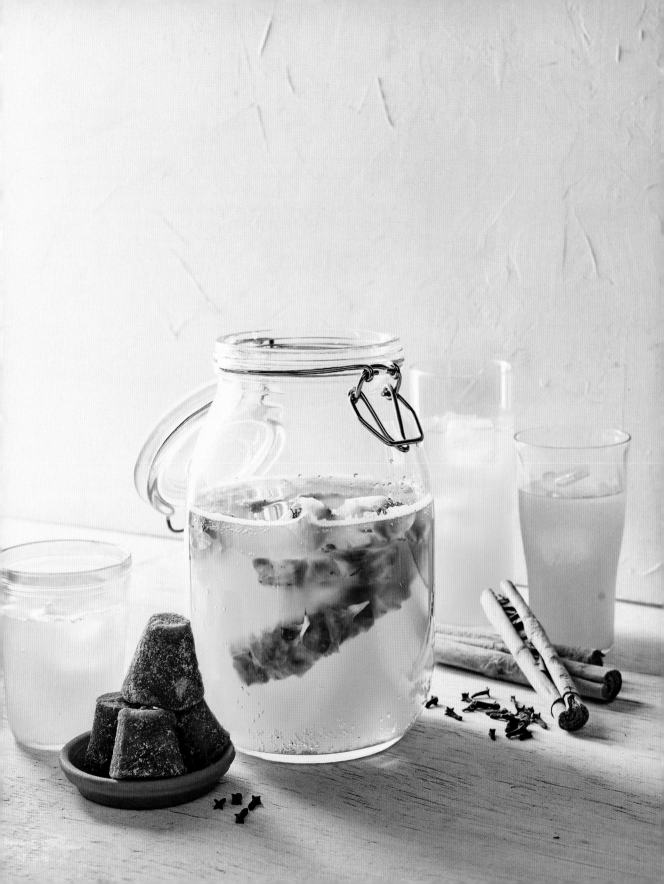

4 cups water, plus 1 cup cold water

½ cup coarsely ground dark roast coffee

¼ cup (2 ounces) piloncillo or dark brown sugar

1 cinnamon stick, ideally Mexican *canela*, about 6 inches long

5 cloves

Peel of ¼ orange, with pith trimmed off

THIS SPICED coffee beverage from Mexico is traditionally prepared in an *olla*, or pot, made of unglazed clay and served in clay mugs as an after-dinner drink. If you can get a clay olla, do so because it will enhance the flavor. But using a regular metal pot will also work. It's a smooth coffee enhanced with the caramel notes of piloncillo, cinnamon, and cloves, and infused with orange. *Note*: Drink this straight up; it's already sweetened and is traditionally not served with milk or cream. This recipe uses about half the sugar of traditional recipes; feel free to adjust to taste.

CAFÉ DE OLLA

Serves 6

Bring 4 cups of water to a boil in an olla or small saucepan.

Add all remaining ingredients, except cold water, reduce heat to a simmer, and stir to melt sugar.

Simmer for 5 minutes, then add cup of cold water, remove from heat, cover, and let stand 5 minutes. Strain and serve.

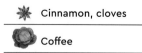

Cinnamon, cloves

Coffee

KALE CHIPS are an excellent introduction to eating this nutritional wonder. They are also a good substitute if you are trying to break your potato chip habit. My basic kale chip recipe simply involves kale roasted with sea salt and olive oil. Most recipes prepare kale chips at higher heat, but I prefer the chewy crispness that lower-temperature baking produces.

KALE CHIPS, WITH GLOBAL VARIATIONS

Makes about 4 cups chips

Preheat oven to 275°F and line two baking sheets with parchment paper (optional, but makes for a crisper chip and easier cleanup).

Wash whole kale leaves, shake out or dry in a salad spinner, then dry thoroughly between two towels.

Once kale leaves are completely dry, tear leaves into bite-size (potato chip–size) pieces. Some people like to remove the central stem before doing this, but I like to keep in the stem for more texture. Place in a large bowl.

Sprinkle with salt and drizzle with olive oil. Toss with tongs or your hands to evenly distribute salt and oil.

Arrange kale leaves in a single layer on prepared baking sheets, with some space around each leaf. (Space is very important to allow air to circulate and allow chips to crisp.) Bake for 20 minutes, turning over leaves at 10-minute point.

Remove from oven and sprinkle with seasoning of your choice, if desired. These are best enjoyed immediately but will maintain some of their crunch for a few days in a tightly covered container.

1 bunch curly green or lacinato kale

Kosher salt

About 2 tablespoons olive oil

Global seasonings of choice (suggestions follow)

GLOBAL FLAVOR SUGGESTIONS

California hippie: nutritional yeast, garlic powder

Mexico: lime juice and cayenne pepper; alternatively, Tajín Clasico seasoning

Japan: furikake

India: curry powder

Italian: oregano, garlic powder

Spain: smoked paprika, garlic powder

Middle East: za'atar

Moroccan: harissa powder

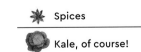

✳ Spices

🥬 Kale, of course!

1 (15-ounce) can low-sodium or no-salt-added chickpeas, drained and rinsed

2 garlic cloves, peeled and minced

½ cup + 2 tablespoons pumpkin puree [½ (15-ounce) can]

¼ cup tahini

¼ cup olive oil

Juice of 1 lemon

1 teaspoon cider vinegar

2 tablespoons water

1 teaspoon fine kosher salt

Garnishes: swirl of olive oil; toasted, raw hulled pumpkin seeds; pomegranate arils; chopped flat-leaf parsley

HUMMUS is a protein and fiber-rich healthy snack. Whereas classic hummus is made of chickpeas and tahini, this pumpkin version is ready for fall and adds additional nutrients and flavor. Use it as a dip or a sandwich spread, or serve with fall crudités, such as broccoli florets, carrot sticks, and whole wheat pita triangles.

PUMPKIN HUMMUS

Makes 3 cups hummus (serving size: 2 tablespoons)

Puree all ingredients, except garnishes, in a food processor until smooth. Add additional water, if needed, to make a loose paste.

Garnish before serving with a swirl of olive oil, toasted pumpkin seeds, pomegranate arils, and chopped parsley.

Garlic

Chickpeas, pumpkin, tahini

2 pounds assorted root vegetables (e.g., potatoes, sweet potatoes, carrots, parsnips, turnips, baby beets), washed thoroughly and dried, peeled if desired, and diced into 2-inch chunks

1 diced onion or shallot (optional)

2 to 3 tablespoons olive oil

Kosher salt

Freshly ground black pepper

ROASTING ROOT VEGETABLES is a great way to bring out their sweetness. The key to roasting is to bake at a high temperature, and to spread vegetables in a single layer with some space between them, so they roast rather than steam.

ROASTED ROOT VEGETABLES

Serves 4

Preheat oven to 425°F.

Place diced vegetables, including onion (if using), in a large bowl. Drizzle with a few tablespoons of olive oil and a few pinches each of salt and freshly ground black pepper, and toss to coat evenly.

Arrange vegetables in a single layer on a baking pan, making sure not to crowd them, or else you'll steam them and they won't be able to brown.

Roast for 15 minutes, then flip vegetables over (add additional olive oil at this point if they are sticking or dried out), and roast for 15 minutes more, or until vegetables are caramelized and fork-tender.

CALIFORNIA

PANTRY: SAUCES, PICKLES, AND SNACKS

✳ Black pepper

Root vegetables are good sources of fiber, especially if their skin is left on.

1 tablespoon olive oil, plus more for drizzling

1 (15.5-ounce) can chickpeas, drained and rinsed

1 teaspoon pimentón (smoked paprika)

1 teaspoon garlic powder

½ to ¾ teaspoon fine kosher salt

THIS IS a very quick pantry recipe that can be made in a minute but has surprisingly good flavor. Use it with pasta and greens for a quick entrée, as a topping for avocado toast or grain bowls, or as a quick side dish.

SMOKY SPANISH CHICKPEAS

Makes 2½ cups chickpeas

Heat a nonstick skillet over high heat and add olive oil.

Add drained chickpeas.

Sprinkle with pimentón, garlic powder, and salt and sauté or stir with spatula to coat evenly.

Continue to cook until chickpeas appear dry and begin to peel, stirring occasionally. This will take about 1 minute. Finish with an additional drizzle of olive oil.

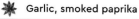 Garlic, smoked paprika

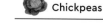 Chickpeas

THIS ALL-PURPOSE creamy topping is an essential and game-changing basic for the plant-based pantry. By simply combining raw, soaked cashews in a high-speed blender until very smooth, nondairy eaters can enjoy this as a whipped topping, heavy cream, or sour cream substitute. You might even prefer it to the original.

1 cup raw cashews, soaked in water for at least 2 hours or overnight in the refrigerator, then drained

Cold water

CASHEW CREAM

Makes 1 cup cashew cream

Place soaked, drained cashews in a high-speed blender.

Add enough cold water to almost cover cashews, ½ to ¾ cup.

Blend on maximum speed, stirring as needed.

Add additional water, as desired, to create a whipped cream consistency. Add seasonings, if desired. Cashew cream will keep for 5 days in a tightly sealed container in refrigerator.

OPTIONAL

For sweet preparations, use the cashew cream as is, as raw cashews are naturally sweet. Or consider adding some pure vanilla extract, about 1 teaspoon.

For a sour cream substitute, add 2 to 3 tablespoons of freshly squeezed lime or lemon juice or 1 to 2 tablespoons of cider vinegar and a pinch of salt, adjusting to taste.

Variation: Cashew Lime Crema

This is a vegan/dairy-free version of Latin American sour cream, or crema. The lime juice complements Latin American flavors well (better than vinegar or lemon juice). Use it as a garnish, as you would sour cream.

Makes about 1 cup crema

Place soaked cashews with remaining ingredients (starting with smaller amount of water) in a blender and blend until completely smooth, adding more water as needed for desired consistency. This will be easiest with a high-speed blender but can be done with any blender.

To serve, transfer into a squeeze-tip bottle or use a small spoon to drizzle or dollop as a garnish. Keeps refrigerated for up to a week.

1 cup raw cashews, soaked for at least 2 hours or overnight in the refrigerator, then drained

½ to ¾ cup water

½ teaspoon salt

Juice of ½ to 1 lime, to taste

 Cashews

1 part vinegar or citrus juice (red wine, sherry, cider, or Champagne vinegars are all great choices; lemon juice is classic, but orange and lime juices are also nice variations)

3 to 4 parts oil (extra-virgin olive oil or other oil—amount needed varies depending on the acidity of the vinegar)

1 teaspoon Dijon mustard per ¼ cup oil

Salt and freshly ground black pepper

SAMPLE RECIPE

1½ tablespoons vinegar or citrus juice

1 teaspoon Dijon mustard

¼ cup olive oil

Salt and freshly ground black pepper

Optional additions: fresh or dried herbs, spices, minced fresh garlic or shallots, citrus zest

AFTER YOU LEARN the basic recipe to make your own salad dressing, you will never buy it again. Store-bought dressings are more expensive and have many additives. Plus, when you make your own, you can customize to your taste. Here, you'll find both a template of the ratio of ingredients to make a vinaigrette, as well as a sample recipe to make a batch of dressing. *A few things to note*: Mustard emulsifies the dressing so that it doesn't separate. You can omit it if you are using the dressing right away. Not sure how your dressing will taste? Dip in a piece of lettuce to sample, then adjust the seasonings further.

CLASSIC VINAIGRETTE

Makes about 6 tablespoons dressing (about 4 servings)

Combine vinegar and mustard in a medium-size bowl and slowly stream in oil, whisking vigorously. Add salt and pepper to taste.

Alternatively, put all ingredients in a jar with a lid and shake vigorously; taste and adjust seasonings. Salad dressing will keep for up to a week in a tightly sealed jar in refrigerator. Bring to room temperature at least 10 minutes before serving.

 Olive oil

8 ounces sliced raw almonds

3 cups cold water to soak, plus more for blending

Special equipment: cheesecloth/nut milk bag

MAKING NUT MILK is as easy as soaking nuts, blending them, and straining the mixture through cheesecloth. But have you ever thought of toasting your nuts first? This brings out a warmth and more "nutty" flavor and is worth the extra step.

TOASTED ALMOND MILK

Makes about 2 quarts almond milk

Toast almonds: Preheat oven to 350°F. Spread almonds in an even layer on a baking sheet. Bake for 5 minutes, then stir to redistribute.

Continue to bake for up to another 10 minutes, checking for doneness (a light golden color) every 3 minutes and stirring to redistribute.

When done, remove from oven and transfer to another plate or baking sheet, so they do not continue to cook. Allow almonds to cool completely, about 20 minutes.

Place cooled, toasted almonds in a jar or container, and cover with cold water.

Soak for at least 4 hours, until completely softened.

Drain soaking water from almonds through a fine-mesh sieve, then place soaked almonds in a blender, and add fresh water to about an inch above level of almonds. Blend until completely smooth. Add additional water, as needed, to reach a liquid consistency.

Transfer blended almonds to cheesecloth or a nut milk bag and squeeze with your hands to extract all of milk. Add additional water, if needed, to reach desired consistency. (Do not skip this step or else you'll have a gritty texture.)

Keep tightly covered in refrigerator. Best if used within 3 days.

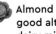 Almond milk is a good alternative to dairy milk.

¼ cup tahini

1 teaspoon pure maple syrup

Juice of 1 large lemon (about 3 tablespoons juice)

½ teaspoon salt

½ teaspoon garlic powder

⅛ teaspoon cayenne pepper

Water to thin, as needed

THIS VERSATILE DRESSING is a great topping for grain bowls and can also be thinned out with more lemon juice or water to make a creamy vegan salad dressing.

LEMON-TAHINI DRESSING

Makes about 1 cup dressing

Whisk together all ingredients in a small bowl.

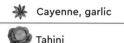 Cayenne, garlic

Tahini

1 jalapeño pepper, stemmed

5 tomatillos, husk removed, quartered

1 garlic clove, peeled and smashed

½ cup fresh cilantro

1 small onion, sliced

1 small or ½ large avocado, peeled and pitted

½ teaspoon salt, or to taste

THIS TOMATILLO-BASED SALSA is very fresh and bright tasting and goes well with seafood or poultry. The avocado adds a nice creaminess, but you can omit it if you want to make a slightly tarter version. The avocado-free version can also be cooked for a slightly different flavor, and this can be the basis of chilaquiles verdes (see page 58 to make your own).

SALSA VERDE

Makes 2½ cups salsa verde

Process all ingredients in a blender or *molcajete*, a Mexican mortar made of volcanic stone, until you have a slightly chunky salsa.

Garlic

Avocado, cilantro, tomatillos

1 fresh pineapple, peeled and sliced into 1-inch pieces

Extra-virgin olive oil, for basting

1 to 2 jalapeño peppers or serrano chiles, seeded if desired, minced (adjust quantity to your heat tolerance level)

½ white onion, chopped

Juice of 1 lime

Kosher salt

¼ cup chopped fresh cilantro

THIS SWEET and spicy salsa is a natural match for fish and other seafood. It's similar to pico de gallo and can also be enjoyed with tortilla chips. (Use the pineapple rind to make Tepache, page 100.)

GRILLED PINEAPPLE SALSA

Makes about 4 cups salsa

Preheat a grill or grill pan over medium-high heat.

Brush pineapple with olive oil and grill until charred on both sides. Set aside to cool, then remove core and chop remainder into bite-size pieces, each about ½ inch.

In a medium-size bowl, mix pineapple with jalapeño, onion, and lime juice. Add salt to taste and garnish with cilantro.

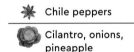

Chile peppers

Cilantro, onions, pineapple

---

1 teaspoon canola oil

1 cup raw hulled pumpkin seeds (pepitas)

Grated zest of 1 orange

½ teaspoon salt

¼ teaspoon sugar

¼ teaspoon cayenne pepper

⅛ teaspoon ground cinnamon

THIS RECIPE is a fantastic way to spice up plain pepitas. They are excellent as a snack or as a spicy-savory addition to trail mix, and can also be used as a garnish for soup, salads, or dips.

ORANGE SPICED PEPITAS

Makes 1 cup pepitas

Heat oil in a small skillet over moderately low heat, then add pumpkin seeds. Toast in heated oil, stirring constantly, until puffed and golden, 8 to 10 minutes.

Combine orange zest, salt, sugar, cayenne, and cinnamon. Toss toasted seeds with spice mixture.

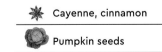

Cayenne, cinnamon

Pumpkin seeds

1 cup water

½ cup cider vinegar

1 tablespoon sugar

1½ teaspoons kosher salt

1 red onion, thinly sliced

IF YOU HAVEN'T HAD much experience with pickling, this is a fun one to start with. This uses the method of "quick pickling," which means exactly what it sounds like—making a pickling brine to submerge raw ingredients, without the time needed for fermentation. Red onion is fun to quick pickle because the color changes quickly and dramatically to a vibrant fuchsia, which will become even more brilliant with time. This is usually used in Mexican food but also is great on grain bowls, sandwiches, salads, and any other dish that could use a pop of color and acidity.

PICKLED RED ONION

Makes about 2 cups pickled onion

Combine all ingredients, except red onion, in a small, nonreactive pan and bring to a boil over high heat until sugar is dissolved.

Place sliced onion in a bowl or jar and pour pickling liquid over it. Place a small plate on top to keep onion submerged. Allow to sit for 1 hour at room temperature.

If not eating immediately, transfer to a tightly sealed jar or container and keep refrigerated for up to 1 month.

 Onions

CALIFORNIA MENUS

SUMMER SALAD MENU

San Francisco Summer
Arugula Salad with
Blackberries, Avocado,
and Cucumber

Summer Peach Burrata
Caprese with Harissa

Lemony Farro Salad with
Avocado and Pistachios

Roasted Sweet Potato
and Corn Salad

Cherry, Plum, and
Nectarine Clafoutis

FALL MENU

Thanksgiving Kale Salad
with Roasted Root
Vegetables

Gateway Brussels Sprouts

Lentil Soup for a Small Planet

Pumpkin Pots de Crème

MEXI-CALI MENU

Mexican Shrimp Ceviche

Pozole Verde

Mexican Corn with
Tomatillos and Green Chiles

Potato and
Mushroom Tacos

Tepache (Mexican Spiced
Fermented Pineapple Drink)

Fresh Fruit:
Pineapple or Mango

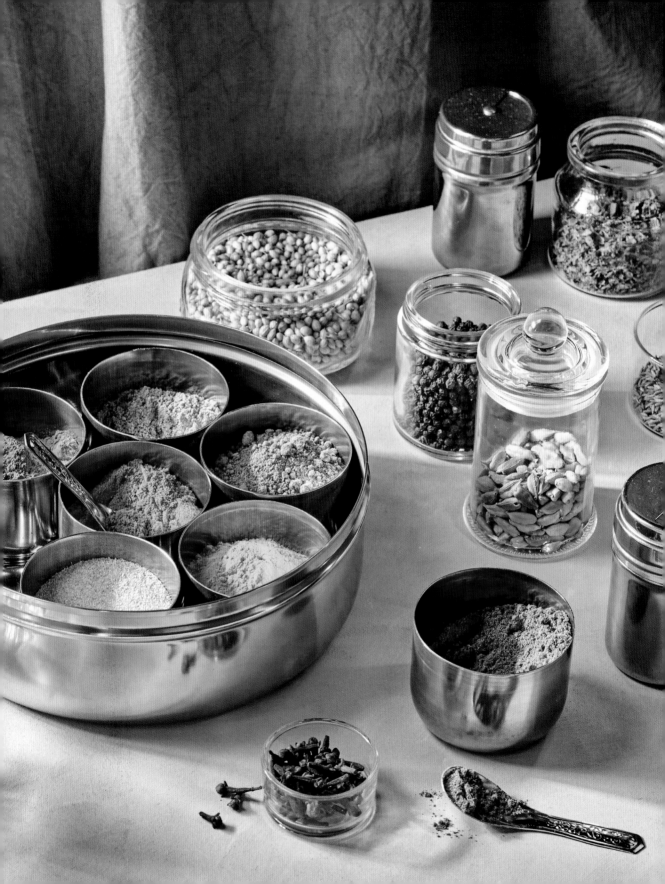

ASIA

spices

chile peppers

cinnamon

cloves

furikake

ginger

gochugaru

dried orange peel

sesame seeds

Sichuan peppercorns

star anise

sauces

Fish sauce, such as Thai *nam pla*, Vietnamese *nuoc mam*, or Filipino *patis*

chili sauce

gochujang

hoisin

mirin

herbs

cilantro

green onions

Thai basil

fats

canola, grapeseed, or peanut oil

coconut oil

toasted sesame oil

acids

rice vinegar

black vinegar

lime

ASIA

F I CLOSE MY EYES, I can imagine myself in Taipei. The humid air, the sounds of the market, the scent of food being cooked by street food vendors, and the taste of pungent and fermented flavors that were once unfamiliar, but I now crave. Asia is a large continent with many distinct countries, cultures, and cuisines, so this section cannot be comprehensive. But I hope to give you a good sampling of the flavors and recipes I most enjoy cooking and eating from the region. Some recipes, I learned from my mother or other family members in Taiwan; others, from time I have spent living, studying, and working in different Asian countries; and still others were inspired by restaurant meals.

My parents immigrated from Taiwan in the mid-1960s as graduate students, and their path as researchers led them to a national laboratory located in semirural eastern Long Island, New York, where I spent a carefree childhood playing in the woods, collecting rocks, and riding my bike. We were the only Asian family in town when I was in elementary school, and there weren't any Asian groceries nearby. In fact, to get the flavors of my parents' homeland, we had to drive two hours to New York City's Chinatown, or fly more than sixteen hours to get to the source. What this meant for my early palate is that I was more familiar with Italian and Jewish food than with any kind of Asian food, and the kind of Chinese food I wanted was egg foo yung and fried chow mein noodles served with sweet duck sauce. What this meant for my mother, who hadn't grown up cooking, was that she had to learn how to cook the foods she missed. And because of where we lived, she simultaneously had to get creative with substitutions, as all immigrants do, such as spaghetti instead of fresh egg noodles, and to learn how to DIY, such as making her own salted duck eggs and chili oil and sprouting her own bean sprouts. When we did make it to New York City, we would stock up on as many shelf-stable staples as we could—dried noodles, short-grain rice, Taiwanese-style pickles, rice vinegar, sesame oil, and dried shrimp.

When I went to college, I had the chance to learn about Asian American culture, as well as the cultures of many other countries from East and South Asia. I joined all the Asian American associations and, for the first time, had a chance to gain some familiarity with the food of countries other than Taiwan, including China, Korea, Japan, India, and Thailand. I studied abroad in Singapore, during which time I also had the chance to visit Thailand, Malaysia, and Indonesia. After college, I worked in Sichuan province in China and was also able to visit other Chinese cities, including Xian and Beijing, and Hong Kong, pre–Chinese control. And while I did this all on a student budget, I ate well and began to understand that a culture's foodways are a great portal to understanding. I learned to appreciate spice and spices, acidity, and the funk of fermentation. I began to love visiting local markets. I married a man from Trinidad whose DNA traces to India, China, and elsewhere and learned how to cook the Trinidadian Indian food he missed. All of these experiences helped me to develop my palate and appreciation for diverse Asian flavors.

I won't claim that these recipes are "authentic" or "traditional"; they are a modern representation of the tastes that have all stayed with me long after I've returned back home. In many cases, I have made plant-based versions of dishes that might be more familiar to you with meat, making them lighter and healthier. As you cook through these recipes, I hope you will feel transported to the different countries and cultures that inspired them. As we say in Taiwan, *chiàh-pñg!* (Literally, "eat rice"; conversationally, "let's eat!")

1 cup dried soybeans

6 cups cold water, plus more for soaking

¼ cup sugar (optional)

JUST A FEW SIMPLE INGREDIENTS—soybeans and flour—form the basis of a satisfying and comforting traditional Taiwanese breakfast. This style of breakfast—soy milk (*dou jiang*) served with scallion pancakes (*cong yu bing*), egg-filled pancakes (*dan bing*), steamed buns (*man tou*), and fried dough (*yu tiao*)—traces its origins to northern China. Making your own fresh soy milk is easy and inexpensive to do at home, and you'll be rewarded with a pure, creamy, and rich beverage to enjoy on its own, or to use as you would regular milk.

FRESH SOY MILK

Makes 2 quarts soy milk

Place soybeans in a large bowl and cover with cold water. Allow to soak for about 3 hours.

Drain and rinse soaked soybeans, and place half of them in a blender. Add 2 cups fresh cold water and blend until smooth.

Skim off foam (using a mesh skimmer) and then pour soybeans into a cheesecloth-lined fine-mesh sieve set over a large pot. Use a spoon to press on slurry to extract soy milk.

Once liquid is all extracted, put solids back into blender with another cup of cold water and blend again. Drain through cheesecloth-lined sieve and do another pressing, then squeeze out remaining liquid through cheesecloth. (You can reserve remaining solids—called *okara*—for composting or for adding hidden fiber into all kinds of baked goods, as my mom likes to do.)

Repeat above steps with remaining soaked soybeans and water.

Once all beans have been pressed, you'll have raw soy milk in your pot. Over medium heat, bring to a boil and then lower heat and simmer for about 20 minutes, stirring every few minutes so that milk doesn't scorch. You'll know it's done when it no longer tastes raw. Add sugar, if desired (adjust to taste). You may drink this soy milk hot or cold. Keep refrigerated; it will last for 7 days.

 Soybeans

1 cup water

1 cup white whole wheat flour

1 cup all-purpose flour, plus more for dusting

¼ cup toasted sesame oil

Salt

2 cups thinly sliced scallions (about 2 bunches)

½ teaspoon crushed Sichuan peppercorns (optional)

Oil, for frying

Accompaniments: Asian Vinaigrette (page 180), Spicy Vegan Peanut Dipping Sauce (page 181), or prepared chili sauce

THE CLASSIC VERSION of Chinese scallion pancakes is made with white flour. To up the nutrition factor while maintaining soft layers and flakiness, I've replaced half the flour with white whole wheat flour. I've also added Sichuan peppercorns, which can be omitted for a simpler version. Pair these with freshly made soy milk (page 119) for a classic Chinese breakfast. *Note*: If you have a thermometer, use it. If not, see instructions below for approximating the correct temperature.

WHOLE WHEAT SCALLION PANCAKES

Makes 4 pancakes

To heat water to the appropriate temperature, boil water and let cool until a thermometer reads 150°F, about 3 minutes. You can also approximate when your water is the right temperature, which is just below simmering. Allow simmering water to cool for 2 to 3 minutes to get to the right temperature.

Sift flours together in a large bowl. Make a well in center of flour mixture, then slowly pour in hot water and mix with a wooden spoon until dough just comes together. Note that 150°F water is hot enough to burn, so you will need to let dough cool slightly before working with it—use only a spoon to incorporate water, not your hands. Do not overmix, or dough will get tough—avoid this!

After dough has cooled to the point where you can comfortably touch it, transfer dough to a floured work surface and knead a few times to form a smooth ball. Cover with a damp, clean towel and let rest for 30 minutes.

Divide rested dough into four equal pieces and roll each into a ball. Work with one ball at a time, keeping others covered. Roll out each ball into an 8-inch circle. Brush or use the back of a teaspoon to spread a thin

Sichuan peppercorns

Whole grains

continued ⟶

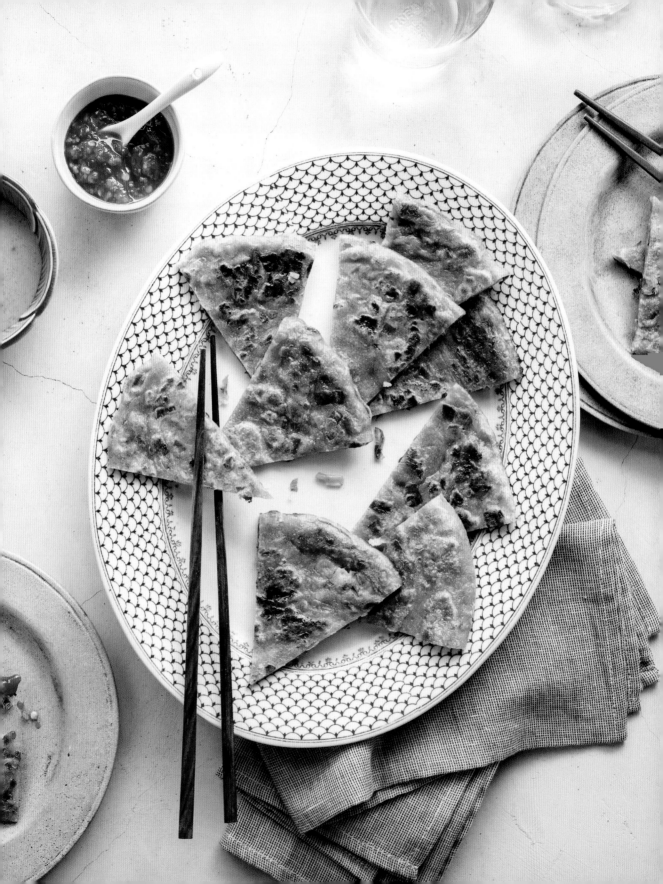

layer of sesame oil on dough's surface, and then roll it up into a log. Next, roll log into a spiral shape, tucking in its end underneath.

Flatten each spiral into an 8-inch disk. Brush with another layer of sesame oil and sprinkle with a pinch of salt, ½ cup of scallions, and ⅛ teaspoon of crushed Sichuan peppercorns (if using). Then, roll into a log, this time pinching ends so the filling doesn't come out, and twist into a spiral, as you did the first time. Repeat with remaining dough balls.

Flatten each filled spiral of dough into an 8-inch disk.

To cook: Heat about 2 tablespoons of oil in a skillet over medium heat until hot. Cook each pancake until golden brown, about 2 minutes per side. Drain on paper towels, sprinkling each with a pinch of salt before it cools.

Serve hot. Cut into eight wedges and serve with dipping sauce, if desired.

WHILE TRINIDADIANS' go-to flatbread is roti, the South Asian flatbread we eat most often in San Francisco is naan, thanks to the many Pakistani restaurants here. Some of these restaurants feature tandoors, clay ovens in which the naan is baked directly on the walls of the oven. This version, which a friend makes as a quick after-school snack for her kids, requires no special equipment and involves just self-rising flour and Greek yogurt, a good introduction to making flatbread.

3 cups self-rising flour
(or make your own: add
4½ teaspoons baking
powder and ¾ teaspoon
salt to 3 cups less a scant
2 tablespoons all-purpose
flour), plus more for dusting

1½ cups Greek yogurt or
nondairy equivalent

2 tablespoons water

Olive oil or melted butter, for
serving (optional)

GARLIC VERSION

Olive oil

3 tablespoons minced fresh
garlic

3 tablespoons roughly
chopped fresh cilantro leaves

Sea salt

NAAN TWO WAYS— PLAIN OR GARLIC

Makes 10 naan

Combine flour and yogurt in a medium-size bowl. Add 1 to 2 tablespoons water, if needed, to help dough come together. Once a dough starts to form, transfer it to a floured surface.

Knead into a smooth ball, then cover with a damp, clean cloth and allow it to rest for 20 minutes.

After dough has rested, roll it into a log shape and then cut it into ten equal pieces. Roll each piece into a smooth ball, then roll each piece out into a 6-inch circle. Keep covered with a clean cloth until ready to cook.

Heat a cast-iron skillet, griddle, or grill pan until very hot. Place each disk, working one at a time, in the hot skillet and cook for 2 minutes, which will cause naan to puff up. Flip it over—you'll see nicely charred spots—and cook the other side.

To make the garlic version: After flipping, drizzle first cooked side, which will now be on top, with olive oil and sprinkle with about ¼ teaspoon each of garlic and cilantro.

When the second side has cooked, flip naan back over so that the garlic side is facing down, and seal garlic onto it by pressing down lightly with a spatula for another couple of seconds. Repeat with remaining pieces.

Serve hot with a drizzle of additional olive oil or melted butter (if using). Extras can be frozen after cooling completely.

✳ Garlic

🥬 Cilantro, Greek yogurt

2 yellow, white, or red potatoes (choose a waxy variety, not russet)

1 fresh red chile, such as Fresno

2 tablespoons canola oil

1 teaspoon Sichuan peppercorns

3 dried chile peppers

2 garlic cloves, minced

1½ teaspoons soy sauce

1½ teaspoons black (Chinkiang) vinegar

Sea salt

Garnishes: 1 scallion, thinly sliced, and fresh cilantro leaves

I FIRST HAD THIS DISH when I worked in Sichuan, China, on a research project. It was served as a cold appetizer. What a revelation! The potatoes taste almost raw—crunchy, not starchy—and were a perfect foil for the *ma la* (numbing and spicy) flavors of Sichuan peppercorn and red chiles. This dish doesn't appear often on Chinese restaurant menus in the US; when I have found it here, it is often served hot, as a stir-fry. This recipe can be used to make either the hot or cold version. (If you want to eat this cold right away, blanch the julienned potatoes instead of stir-frying, then pour the hot, seasoned oil directly on top as a dressing.) The Chinese black (Chinkiang) vinegar is a revelation— savory and sweet with a very smooth acidity. Try to find it if you can; if not, balsamic can substitute.

SICHUANESE SHREDDED POTATOES

Serves 2

Peel and then julienne potatoes. Place in a bowl of cold water and soak for 20 to 30 minutes to rinse off starch. Drain and rinse, then dry on a towel.

Seed and julienne fresh chile.

Heat oil in a wok or skillet over medium heat, then add peppercorns, dried chile peppers, and garlic. Stir-fry for about 30 seconds, making sure peppercorns and peppers do not burn.

Add potatoes and fresh chile and increase heat to high. Stir-fry until potatoes are just barely tender, 30 seconds.

Turn off heat and season with soy sauce, black vinegar, and salt to taste. Garnish with scallions and cilantro. Serve hot or, if desired, cover and refrigerate until cold.

Chile peppers, Sichuan peppercorns

Potatoes

6 large eggs, at room temperature

½ cup dark soy sauce (if unavailable, substitute regular soy sauce)

3 cups water

2 tablespoons sugar

3 pieces star anise

1 cinnamon stick

2 teaspoons jasmine tea leaves (traditionally, black tea leaves are used, but I prefer the fragrance of jasmine-scented green tea)

THESE FRAGRANT and savory hard-boiled eggs remind me of childhood visits to Taiwan. We'd eat these on train journeys, which would transport us from Taipei in the north to the less dense, more tropical, and less hurried southern cities of Kaohsiung and Tainan, passing acres of rural land dotted with Buddhist temples and plantations growing pineapple and bananas. A "tea egg" is a hard-boiled egg cooked in a broth of soy sauce, aromatics, and tea. My version is scented with star anise, cinnamon, and jasmine tea. Cracking the shells of the cooked eggs before placing them in the braise creates a lacy, marbled effect. Enjoy warm or cold.

TAIWANESE TEA EGGS

Makes 6 eggs

Hard-boil eggs: Place eggs in a pot with enough cold water to cover them about an inch, bring water to a boil over high heat, then remove pot from heat, cover, and let stand for 10 minutes exactly. After 10 minutes, drain hot water and replace it with cold or ice water to stop cooking process.

While eggs are cooling, prepare braise by combining other ingredients and bringing to a boil.

Once eggs are cool enough to handle, gently but firmly roll them on a surface to make many little cracks all over each shell. *Do not remove shells.*

Place cracked, hard-boiled eggs in braising liquid and simmer at low heat for 30 minutes.

Turn off heat and allow eggs to steep in braise for at least 2 hours, or overnight in refrigerator. The longer they steep, the darker the color and the stronger the flavor.

When ready to eat, remove eggs from braising liquid and carefully remove eggshells. Braising liquid can be used to make another batch.

SALADS, SOUPS, AND STARTERS

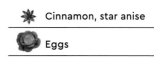

Cinnamon, star anise

Eggs

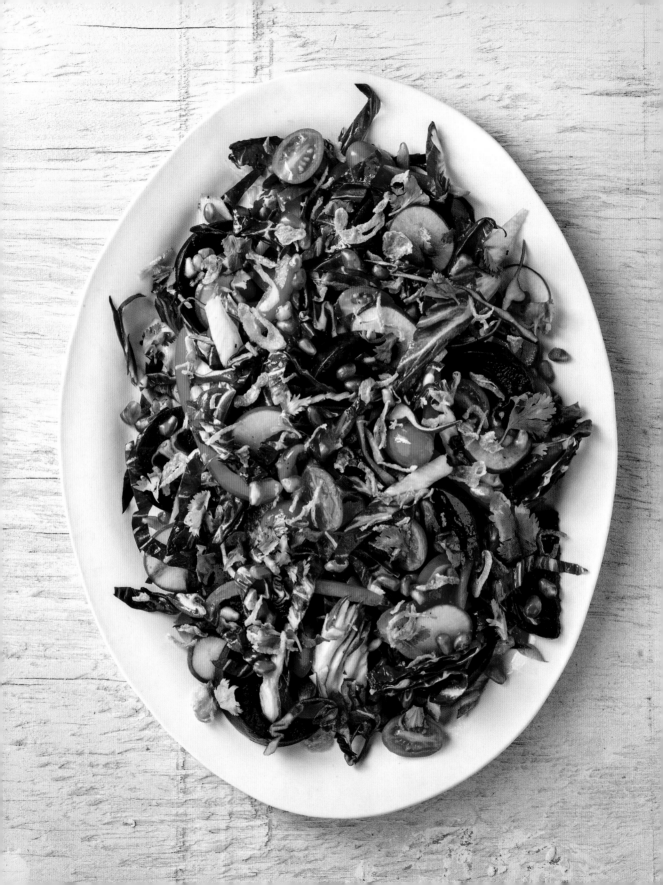

RED IS CONSIDERED the color of good luck, joy, and celebration in Chinese culture. This salad honors that tradition with a festive and dramatic addition to any table. The bite of the radishes, cabbage, and radicchio are mellowed out by the sweetness of the beets and the vinaigrette. Bonus flavor and color come from the crispy fried shallots, cilantro, and pomegranate arils, which were introduced from Iran to China by the trade routes of the Silk Road.

CELEBRATION RED SALAD

Serves 6

Prepare dressing: Whisk together all dressing ingredients in a small bowl or by shaking in a covered jar. Set aside.

Prepare salad: Place all salad ingredients in a large serving bowl. Toss salad ingredients with dressing. Garnish with pomegranate arils, fried shallots, and cilantro just before serving.

DRESSING

1 shallot, peeled and minced

¼ cup balsamic vinegar

1 tablespoon honey

¾ cup olive oil

½ to 1 teaspoon cayenne pepper, to taste

Salt and freshly ground black pepper

SALAD

1 red beet, cooked, peeled, and cut into ½-inch dice (about 1 cup)

1 cup cherry or grape tomatoes, halved

½ cup red or French breakfast radishes, thinly sliced

1 red bell pepper, seeded and julienned

1 cup thinly shredded red cabbage

2 cups thinly shredded radicchio

GARNISHES

½ cup pomegranate arils

¼ cup fried shallots

½ cup fresh cilantro, roughly chopped

Black pepper, cayenne pepper

Beets, cabbage, cilantro, pomegranate, radicchio, tomatoes

1 (14-ounce) package
firm tofu

1 to 2 tablespoons canola or
peanut oil

10 leaves red leaf lettuce,
leaves washed, dried,
separated, and trimmed to
fit within the diameter of the
rice paper

1 small bunch mint

1 large red bell pepper,
seeded and julienned

2 carrots, peeled and
julienned

1 English or 2 Persian
cucumbers, julienned

1 cup thinly shredded red
cabbage

5 cups cooked Vietnamese
rice vermicelli, cooled (2 to
3 uncooked bundles)

10 (12-inch) round sheets
Vietnamese rice paper

Accompaniment: Spicy
Vegan Peanut Dipping
Sauce (page 181)

EVERYONE LOVES Vietnamese fresh spring rolls—pleasantly chewy rice paper rolls filled with vegetables, rice noodles, mint, and usually pork and/or shrimp. Also known as summer rolls, they're a great DIY activity, and they also make a light summer meal: they're served cold (not fried) and filled with fresh crunchy vegetables, making them healthy and wonderfully refreshing. They're also ideal for a picnic and make a great finger food for entertaining.

The rainbow of raw vegetables in this plant-based version provides flavor and texture, and is packed with nutrients.

Tips: Rolling these spring/summer rolls takes a little bit of practice, so you may want to keep a few extra sheets of rice paper handy just in case your rolls tear in your first few attempts.

I would recommend enjoying these immediately, leaving no leftovers; the rice paper tends to harden when refrigerated.

EAT THE RAINBOW
FRESH SPRING ROLLS

Makes 10 spring rolls

Drain tofu, wrap in paper towels, and press for 30 minutes by sandwiching between two cutting boards topped with a heavy object, such as a pan. Cut pressed tofu into ¼ x 1 x ½-inch rectangles.

Once tofu has been pressed, pat dry with a paper towel. (Don't skip this step, or your tofu won't crisp.) Heat oil in a nonstick skillet over medium heat. Add tofu rectangles in a single layer. Fry until golden brown, about 3 minutes per side. Remove from pan and set aside.

Set up your workstation for making rolls: set out all vegetables, cooked and cooled noodles, rice paper, and cooked, sliced tofu. Set aside a large bowl of warm water.

To assemble, dip one sheet of rice paper into water and quickly rotate to moisten entire sheet, just a few seconds. It will appear hard, but it

Tofu; you'll "eat the rainbow" here because different colors correspond to different nutrients, in particular health-promoting antioxidants

continued →

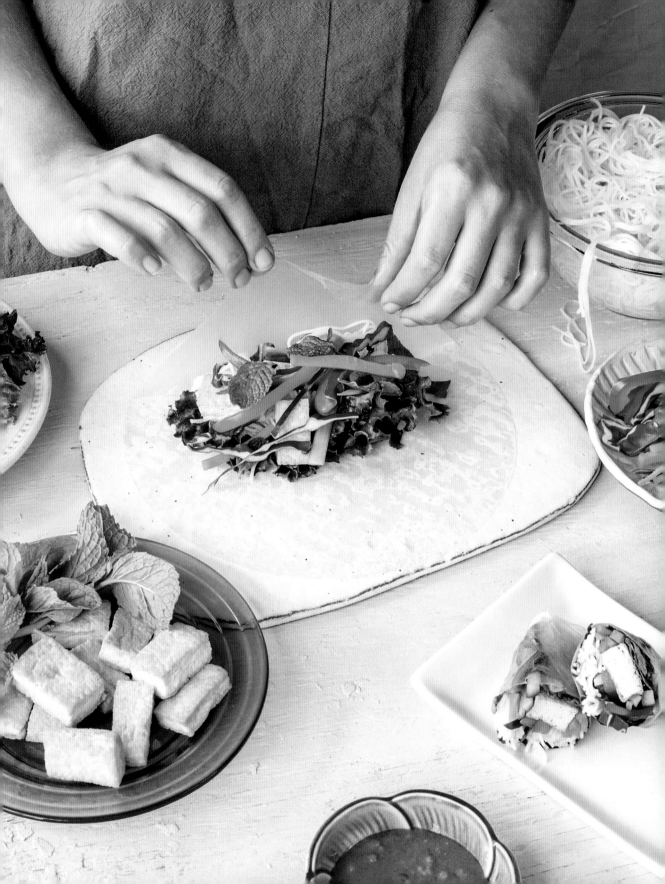

will continue to absorb water as it lays flat. (Do not soak it for more than the time it takes to get it wet, or it will get soggy and break. Trust me on this one.) Lay moistened rice paper on a flat work surface, such as a cutting board or large plate.

Arrange one lettuce leaf over bottom third of moistened rice paper, running your finger along its rib to crack and flatten it. Top with three mint leaves and a thin layer (about ¼ cup) of rice noodles. Add a few slices of tofu and a handful of assorted julienned vegetables. Avoid the temptation to overstuff!

Fold in left and right sides of rice paper, then tightly fold bottom edge up and over filling and roll toward top end, enclosing filling completely and as tightly as you can.

Repeat with remaining ingredients to make additional rolls. To serve, cut each roll crosswise into halves or thirds, and serve with dipping sauce.

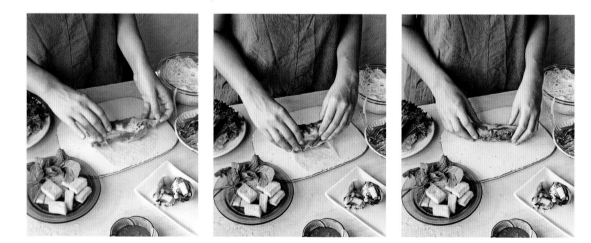

6 cups water

3 tablespoons red or white miso

1 tablespoon mirin (Japanese sweet rice wine)

8 ounces salmon steak or fillet, cut into 4 equal chunks

8 ounces soft or firm tofu, cut into ½-inch cubes

2 cups greens, such as baby bok choy, baby spinach, kale (if not baby, cut roughly into 2-inch pieces)

Steamed brown rice, about ½ cup, cooked, per person, for serving (optional)

8 scallions, sliced into thin rings, for garnish

THIS HEARTY SOUP boasts deep flavor but comes together in about twenty minutes, thanks to miso, the Japanese soybean paste that boasts intense umami due to fermentation. By a quick poach in the simmering broth, this is one of the fastest ways to cook very tender and delicate salmon. This dish is in frequent weeknight rotation in my kitchen.

SALMON MISO SOUP

Serves 4

Combine water, miso, and mirin in a 3-quart pot and bring to a boil. Stir well until miso is completely dissolved.

Add salmon and tofu and bring back to a boil; cook for another 5 minutes.

Add greens, stir well, and turn off heat. (If you continue to boil, greens will discolor. You just want them to wilt.)

Serve in individual bowls. If desired, place ½ cup of cooked brown rice in bottom of each bowl prior to adding soup. Add scallions just before serving.

 Asian greens, miso, salmon, tofu

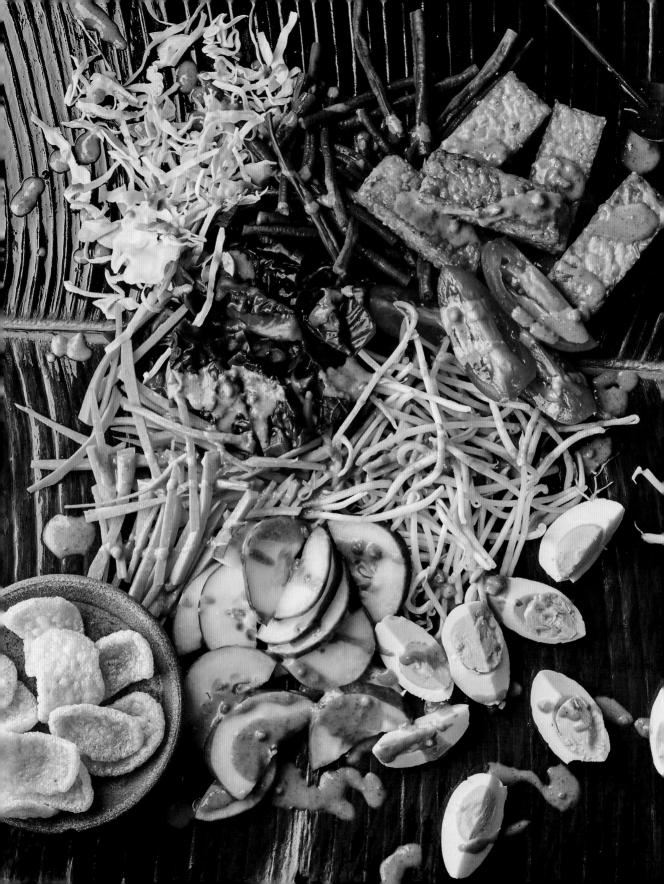

THE NAME of this Indonesian salad translates to "mix-mix." This is more of a template than a recipe—feel free to use whatever vegetables you have and like, some raw and some blanched, plus a protein, such as sliced hard-boiled egg, panfried tofu, or tempeh. Garnish it with *krupuk*, which are shrimp crackers, or small rice crackers. The gingery peanut-coconut sauce brings it all together. I first tried gado gado as an adventurous nineteen-year-old backpacking solo in Indonesia. There were so many new sights, sounds, flavors, and colorful characters offering unsolicited life advice, marriage proposals, and more. This salad is as vibrant as those memories, and as flexible as travel off the beaten track.

BACKPACKER'S GADO GADO

Servings: flexible, depending on the amounts of salad ingredients you use

Whisk all dressing ingredients together in a small bowl until smooth. Add water, if needed, to thin to a pourable consistency.

Place all salad ingredients on a platter with dressing on side.

Use dressing as a dipping sauce or drizzle over your gado gado platter.

SALAD

Mix and match your choice of the following, about 2 cups per serving. Aim for a variety of cooking techniques, colors, and textures.

Steam: green beans, purple cabbage

Panfry: sliced tofu, tempeh

Boil: eggs

Raw: spinach, carrots, tomatoes, cucumbers

Garnish: fried shallots, krupuk

DRESSING (MAKES 2 CUPS)

¾ cup light coconut milk

⅔ cup natural crunchy peanut butter, at room temperature

¼ cup freshly squeezed lime juice

2 tablespoons low-sodium soy sauce

2 tablespoons sugar

1 tablespoon grated fresh ginger

✳ Ginger

 Peanut butter, tempeh, tofu; you'll "eat the rainbow" here because different colors correspond to different nutrients, in particular health-promoting antioxidants

2 tablespoons cooking oil

¼ cup small-diced onion

3 garlic cloves, minced

2 Roma tomatoes, 1 cut into large dice, the other quartered

1 tablespoon bagoong (see headnote) or fish sauce, or vegan versions of either

8 ounces kabocha squash (about ½ small kabocha), or butternut or delicata squash, peeled and seeded, cut into 2-inch cubes

1 cup water

1 bitter melon (about 4 ounces), halved lengthwise, seeded, cut into quarters, and soaked in salted water for 20 minutes and rinsed before use (this decreases bitterness)

8 ounces long beans or string beans, trimmed and cut to 2-inch lengths

8 ounces Chinese eggplant or small Asian eggplants, cut diagonally into ½-inch-thick slices

6 whole okra, trimmed at both ends

Pinch of salt

Garnish: fried shallots (optional)

❋ Garlic

🥬 Bitter melon, eggplant, winter squash (kabocha)

SEVERAL YEARS AGO, I had the opportunity to have a private, all-day cooking class in Manila. Chef Pam Obieta taught me how to make several classic vegetable-forward Filipino dishes, including this vegetable stew, which uses the antioxidant-rich *ampalaya* (bitter melon). Widely available in Asian markets, and prized in these cuisines for its health benefits, this light green fruit has a taste that is almost entirely bitter. Its bitterness is reduced by soaking briefly in salted water, and tempered by spices and other ingredients. It adds a characteristic flavor to this dish.

Pinakbet, also called *pakbet*, originated in the northern part of the Philippines. Traditionally, the vegetables are left to stew, without stirring, in an earthen pot called a *banga*. Although pinakbet usually includes pork and *bagoong* (fermented fish or shrimp paste), it's delicious without meat, and vegan substitutions for bagoong are available: there's a very good vegan shrimp paste made by Red Lotus, available online; or you can substitute Chinese fermented bean paste, fermented tofu (mashed into a paste), Chinese salted black beans, or soy sauce.

PINAKBET (FILIPINO VEGETABLE STEW)

Serves 4 to 6

Preheat a 3-quart Dutch oven or sauté pan with a lid over medium-high heat and add oil. Add onion, garlic, and diced tomato. Add bagoong and fry for 15 seconds, or until fragrant.

Add squash and water and stir. Bring to a boil and cook, uncovered, for about 10 minutes, until just tender.

Add remaining vegetables in layers on top of squash in order of cooking time: bitter melon, long beans, eggplant, okra, and tomato wedges. Season with a pinch of salt. Lower heat to a simmer and cover.

Allow to simmer for 10 minutes, covered, without stirring. After 10 minutes, check to see that most of liquid has evaporated and vegetables are tender when pierced, but not falling apart. Garnish, if desired, with fried shallots.

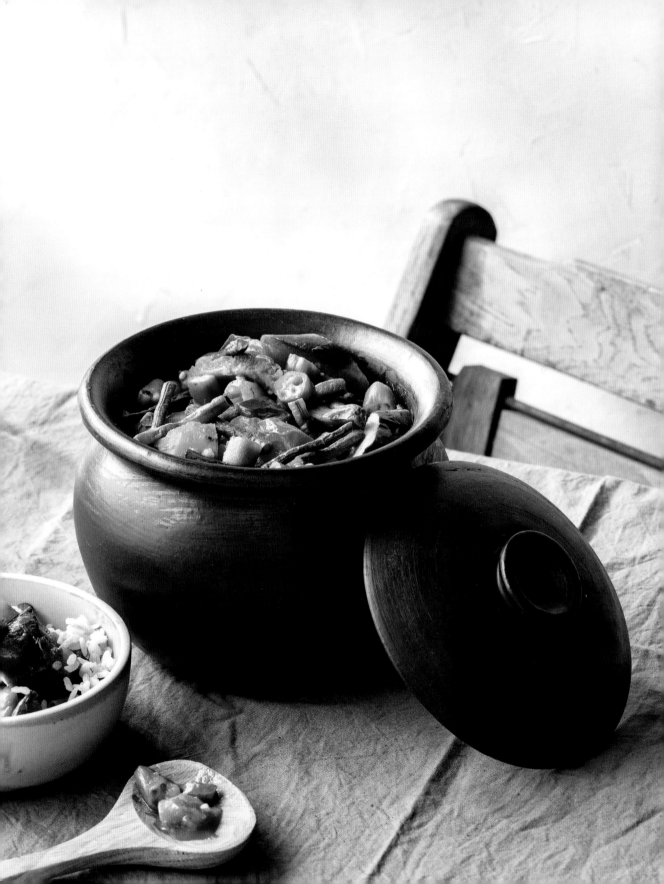

SOUP

2 cups buttermilk

4 cups frozen green peas

Salt

10 fresh mint leaves, plus more sprigs for garnish

Freshly ground black pepper

Fresh peas, for garnish

INDIAN-SPICED OIL

1 tablespoon cumin seeds

1 cup olive oil

4 garlic cloves, peeled and crushed

2 quarter-size slices fresh ginger, slightly crushed

2 tablespoons minced onion

2 Thai green or 1 serrano chile, minced

2 tablespoons cilantro, minced

DANIEL PATTERSON, the founding chef at Coi in San Francisco, created a lovely chilled minted pea soup, which inspired this recipe. Its sweetness is tempered by the tang of buttermilk, which gives it both a richness and silkiness that elevate it from its simple origins.

I've adapted Chef Patterson's recipe, which reminded me of the classic English dish of mushy peas, by garnishing it with a swirl of an Indian spice–infused oil, with a nod to the mint chutneys that I ate with samosas, papadums, and kebabs while traveling in London.

CHILLED MINTED PEA SOUP WITH INDIAN SPICES

Serves 4

Prepare soup: In a medium-size saucepan, bring buttermilk to a simmer and add peas and a large pinch of salt. Simmer for 1 to 2 minutes over medium heat, stirring often so that buttermilk does not boil over. Peas should not be fully cooked, just warmed—you want them to remain brilliant green.

Transfer peas and liquid immediately to a blender along with mint leaves and, starting on low speed, carefully blend (holding lid on firmly with a dishcloth), working up to high speed for 60 seconds.

To preserve the vibrant color and flavor of the peas, the soup must be cooled immediately. Pass through a fine-mesh sieve into a bowl set into an ice bath. Stir continuously until soup is cool. Adjust seasoning with salt and black pepper. Refrigerate until cold.

While soup is chilling, make Indian-spiced oil: Heat a dry skillet over medium heat. Add cumin seeds and lightly toast for a few seconds, until aromatic, being careful not to burn them. Remove toasted seeds from pan.

Black pepper, chile peppers, cumin, garlic, ginger

Mint, peas

Add olive oil to pan and heat over medium heat.

Add garlic, ginger, onion, chiles, and cilantro and sauté for a few minutes, or until onion is translucent.

Remove from heat and pour over half the toasted cumin seeds, reserving the other half of seeds for garnish. Allow oil mixture to sit for at least an hour for flavors to infuse.

Strain infused oil and transfer oil to a squeeze-tip bottle.

To serve, ladle soup into bowls or shot glasses. Use a squeeze bottle to swirl a stream of infused oil on top, and garnish with fresh peas, mint sprig, a pinch of toasted cumin seeds, and black pepper.

3 dried whole chiles

½ teaspoon cumin seeds

¼ teaspoon coriander seeds

¼ teaspoon black peppercorns

2 teaspoons tamarind pulp

3½ cups hot water

1 cup mango pulp

2 teaspoons salt, or to taste

2 teaspoons canola oil

¼ teaspoon black mustard seeds

2 green Thai bird chiles or 1 serrano chile, stemmed and slit

6 to 8 curry leaves

¼ teaspoon asafetida

¼ teaspoon cayenne pepper

¼ cup fresh cilantro, chopped, plus more for garnish

I'VE NAMED this vibrantly flavored mango-tamarind broth "magical" after the main character in Chitra Banerjee Divakaruni's novel *Mistress of Spices*. She is described as a priestess of the magical powers of spices. One taste of the complex spice blend in this *rasam* and you'll be a believer. A rasam is a savory sweet-sour-spicy broth that is served in Indian cooking like an aperitif, to stimulate the appetite. The combination of flavors, from the sweet mango, sour tamarind, fiery chiles, and fragrant curry leaves combine synergistically to do just that. I used prepared mango pulp for its smoothness in this broth; canned versions are widely available in Indian groceries. If you cannot find canned mango pulp, you can make your own by boiling a peeled mango, pureeing, and then straining it.

MAGICAL MANGO-TAMARIND RASAM

Serves 6

Prepare rasam spice blend: Place dried chiles, cumin seeds, coriander seeds, and peppercorns in a spice grinder and grind into a coarse powder.

Place tamarind pulp in hot water. Stir until it is all dissolved, then pour into a medium-size saucepan and add spice blend, mango pulp, and salt. Stir, bring to a boil, and lower heat to a simmer.

Make a tempering oil (this is where the magic happens!): Pour oil into a small skillet, add mustard seeds and green chiles, and heat over medium heat for a few minutes, until mustard seeds begin to pop. Then, add curry leaves and asafetida, stir until combined, and remove from heat. Add cayenne and cilantro and stir again.

Add finished oil to soup. Serve hot or warm, with additional cilantro for garnish.

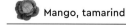

Asafetida, black pepper, chile peppers, coriander, cumin, mustard seeds

Mango, tamarind

1 pound Roma tomatoes (about 6, or any slightly firm, but very ripe, tomatoes will do), cut into ¼-inch dice

Pinch of salt

2 tablespoons toasted sesame oil, or to taste

2 scallions, thinly sliced

Garnish: furikake

POKE IS ALL THE RAGE NOW: the delicious raw fish (often tuna or salmon) salad dressed in Japanese flavors with sesame oil, soy sauce, and sometimes furikake (the Japanese seasoning blend of toasted seaweed, sesame seeds, salt, sugar, and occasionally other flavors, such as wasabi and bonito). Furikake is widely available in supermarkets that carry Asian ingredients, but if you don't have access, you could also crush some roasted seaweed, add some toasted sesame seeds with a pinch of salt and sugar, and make your own. I was inspired to create this vegan variation by a bounty of delicious summer tomatoes.

HAWAIIAN-STYLE TOMATO POKE

Makes 3 to 4 cups poke

Place diced tomato in a small bowl.

Sprinkle with salt, drizzle with sesame oil, and toss to coat. Adjust sesame oil to taste. Stir in scallions. Transfer to a serving bowl or plate.

Sprinkle with desired amount of furikake. This should be sprinkled evenly on top as a garnish.

Eat on its own, or if you want to enjoy it one of the ways poke is savored in Hawaii, make a poke bowl by serving over steamed rice.

✳	Furikake
🥬	Seaweed (in furikake), tomato

3 tablespoons low-sodium
soy sauce

2 teaspoons rice vinegar

1 teaspoon sesame oil

3 tablespoons canola oil

4 large eggs, beaten

2 garlic cloves, minced

1 (1-inch) knob fresh ginger,
peeled and minced

2 cups chopped or sliced
slow-cooking (hard) *Brassica*
vegetables, such as kohlrabi
and green cabbage (1-inch
pieces)

2 cups torn or sliced quick-
cooking (leafy) *Brassica*
vegetables, such as kale,
collards, and mustard greens

4 cups cold, cooked short-
grain brown rice

4 green onions, thinly sliced
into rings

Garnishes: fresh cilantro,
Chinese chives, or other
herbs

WHEN MY KIDS were in elementary school, they were both lucky to
have a few teachers who enjoyed cooking and seamlessly worked in
cooking with lessons in math, science, and more. One of the recipes
that they came home with was for "Brassica Fried Rice," from the
former Education Outside, a nonprofit that provided experiential
science and environmental education with school gardens in San
Francisco public schools. At the time, I didn't even know what *Brassica*
meant! I've adapted the recipe to use hearty short-grain brown rice for
added nutrition and toothsomeness, and specified the greens that I
think taste best. Feel free to substitute your favorites, but please include
kohlrabi, which really makes the flavor in this recipe.

EAT YOUR GREENS!
FRIED RICE

Serves 8

Combine soy sauce, vinegar, and sesame oil in a small bowl. Set aside.

Heat a wok or large skillet over high heat. Add 2 tablespoons of oil.

Add eggs and scramble until medium firm. Break into small pieces with
a wooden spoon. Remove from skillet and set aside.

Remove pan from heat and wipe it out with a paper towel. Heat again
over high heat. Add remaining tablespoon of oil.

Add garlic and ginger and stir-fry until fragrant, about 5 seconds.

Add kohlrabi and other slow-cooking vegetables and stir-fry until
al dente, about a minute or two.

Add quick-cooking vegetables and stir-fry until wilted, about
30 seconds.

Garlic, ginger

Brassica vegetables,
herbs, brown rice
(whole grains)

Add rice, and use a spatula or wooden spoon to break up clumps. Stir-fry for about 5 minutes, or until grains are separate and interspersed with vegetables.

Lower heat to medium, add sauce mixture, and stir-fry until rice is coated, another 1 to 2 minutes.

Add eggs and green onions.

Remove from skillet and garnish with herbs.

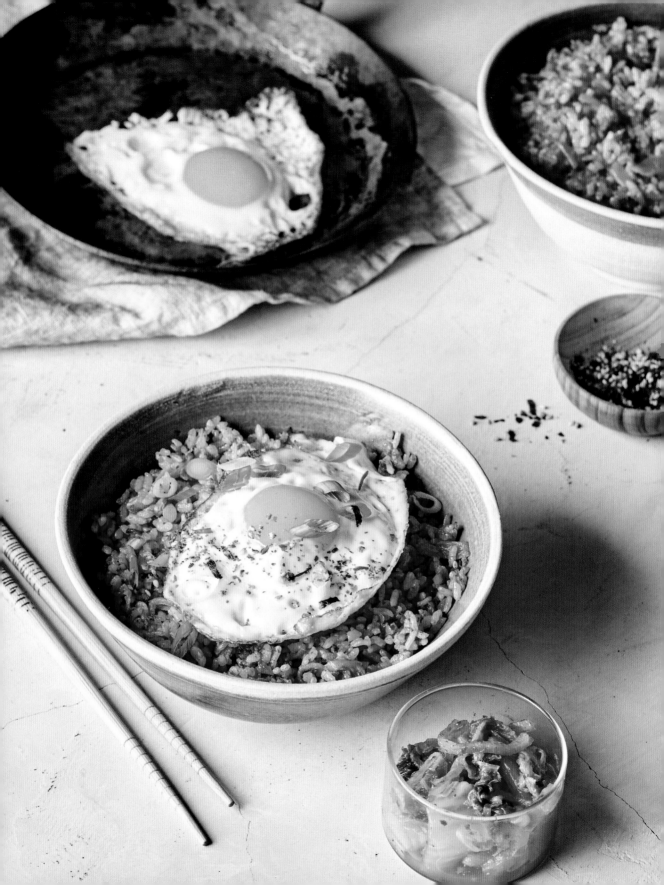

1 to 2 tablespoons canola oil

2 cups diced kimchi, 2 to
4 tablespoons kimchi juice
reserved

4 cups cold cooked brown
sushi or Calrose rice

1 large egg per person
(optional)

1 tablespoon unsalted butter

2 teaspoons sesame oil

Salt

Garnishes: toasted sesame
seeds, or furikake and sliced
scallions

THIS POPULAR home recipe makes use of leftover rice and the intense
flavor of kimchi, the traditional Korean pickle of napa cabbage leaves
fermented in bright red chile pepper and garlic. I use brown rice, which
not only adds nutrition but also has a more toothsome texture that
works perfectly in this dish—it really soaks up the flavor of the kimchi
juice. Make sure to use brown sushi or Calrose rice, not a long-grain,
for the ideal texture. Using cold, leftover rice is key—hot rice will get
too mushy. Finally, the butter at the end is a Korean American touch,
but it really brings it all together. This recipe serves four people, but
consider this a template. The ratio is 1 part kimchi to 2 parts rice, with
the optional addition of a runny-yolked fried egg on top.

KIMCHI FRIED RICE

Serves 4

Heat canola oil in a large skillet or wok over medium heat. Add kimchi
and cook for several minutes until it is hot and starting to caramelize.

Increase heat to high and add rice, using a spatula or wooden spoon
to break up clumps. Add reserved kimchi juice and stir-fry for several
minutes, until rice is hot and evenly coated with kimchi.

Meanwhile, if desired, fry some sunny-side up eggs in another pan.

Just before serving, stir in butter and sesame oil, and season with salt to
taste. Divide among four bowls and top each with a fried egg (if using).
Garnish with sesame seeds or furikake and scallions.

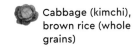
Cabbage (kimchi),
brown rice (whole
grains)

DRESSING

⅔ cup freshly squeezed lime juice (from 2 large or 6 small limes)

1½ teaspoons grated fresh ginger

2 teaspoons sugar

2 teaspoons fish sauce (if unavailable or for a vegan version, substitute ½ teaspoon salt or 2 teaspoons soy sauce)

2 teaspoons water

4 Thai bird chiles, thinly sliced (or equivalent amount of other fresh red chile)

SALAD

1 large or 2 small Granny Smith apples (for about 2 cups julienned)

½ small red onion or 1 large shallot, thinly sliced

1 celery stalk, finely chopped

Garnish: 2 to 4 tablespoons roasted peanuts, crushed

THIS RECIPE was inspired by a long-ago trip to Ubud, Bali. Ubud, in the central rainforest of the Indonesian island, attracts artists and seekers of enlightenment. I found myself drawn to our hotel's freshly prepared juice blends, each promising some form of revitalization and rejuvenation. I chose a blend of green apple, celery, and ginger, which promised cleansing, invigoration, and, perhaps, enlightenment. This slaw draws on those flavors and brings in the traditional lime juice and fish sauce found in Southeast Asian dressings served with barbecued meats.

BALINESE GREEN APPLE SALAD

Serves 4

Make dressing first so flavors have time to blend: Place all dressing ingredients in a bowl and stir well. Set aside.

Core and julienne green apples and immediately combine with dressing to prevent apples from turning brown. Add onion and celery, toss to coat, and allow to sit for 10 minutes or more before serving. (If using salt, adjust to taste.)

Crush peanuts. I find it easiest to use a mortar and pestle. Alternatively, place peanuts in a resealable plastic bag, seal, and roll with a rolling pin until coarsely crushed.

Just before serving, sprinkle crushed peanuts on top. Serve as an appetizer or as an accompaniment for grilled food.

Chile peppers, ginger

Apple (They say an apple a day keeps the doctor away, and I'm okay with that!), celery

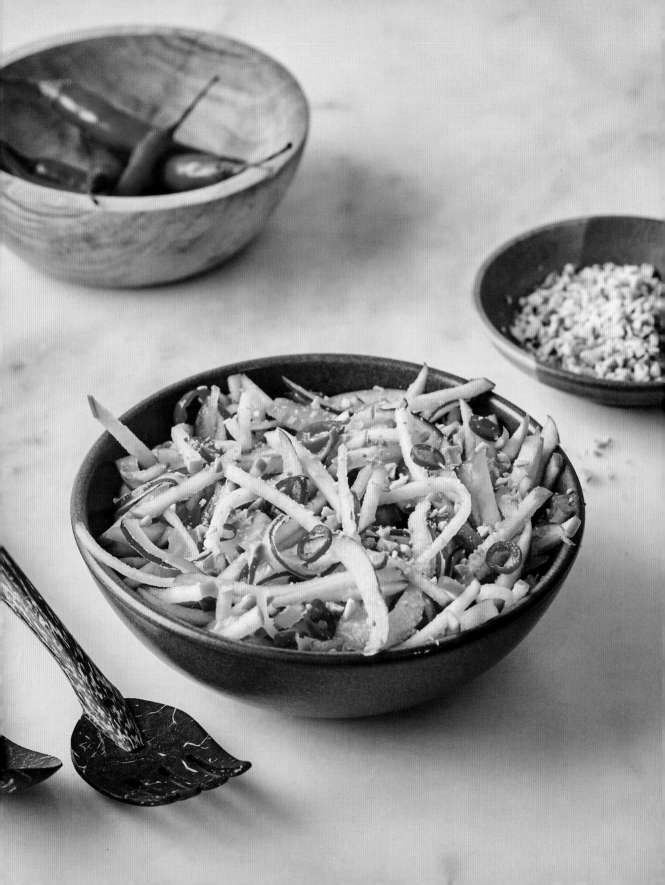

1 tablespoon coconut oil

1 onion, finely chopped

1 (1-inch) piece fresh ginger, peeled and minced

6 garlic cloves, peeled and minced

1 teaspoon ground coriander

1 teaspoon garam masala

½ teaspoon ground cumin

¼ teaspoon ground turmeric

6 cups packed coarsely chopped kale, stem included

2 pinches of salt

2 pinches of freshly ground black pepper

Steamed rice or naan (see page 123 to make your own), for serving

IF YOU'VE EATEN in an Indian restaurant, you've probably had *palak paneer*, the warmly spiced spinach and cheese dish. This vegan version is a lighter dish that evokes the flavors of that Indian restaurant favorite, without the cheese, and cooked briefly, for a firmer texture.

INDIAN SPICED KALE WITH COCONUT AND TURMERIC

<u>Serves 4</u>

Heat oil in a large sauté pan over medium heat.

Add onion. Cook, stirring frequently, for about 8 minutes, or until onion becomes translucent. Add ginger and garlic and stir in.

Add coriander, garam masala, cumin, and turmeric and stir well for several seconds.

Add kale along with salt and pepper. Cook over medium heat for 5 minutes or so, or until its stems are softened but kale remains bright green. Add a tablespoon or 2 of water, if needed, to prevent sticking. I prefer this lightly cooked, but you can cook longer if you prefer a softer texture. Serve with rice or naan.

❋ Black pepper, coriander, cumin, garam masala, garlic, ginger, turmeric

Kale

1 to 2 tablespoons canola oil

3 to 4 garlic cloves, peeled, smashed, and coarsely chopped

1 pound Chinese green vegetables (such as bok choy, napa cabbage, kale, or spinach), roughly chopped in bite-size pieces

Pinch of salt

2 tablespoons water

2 tablespoons low-sodium soy sauce

2 teaspoons sesame oil

ALTHOUGH MANY Chinese-American restaurants serve stir-fried mixed vegetables in a thick, starchy sauce, this simpler preparation is much more likely what you'll find in Chinese homes. Simple green vegetables, often slightly bitter, are cut into bite-size pieces and quickly stir-fried with chopped garlic to tenderize slightly but maintain their structure. A bit of soy sauce is all the flavor you need, with a taste of toasted sesame oil stirred in for a finishing touch. Make sure to keep the garlic chunky, so it doesn't burn.

CHINESE STIR-FRIED GREENS

Serves 4 to 6

Heat canola oil in a wok or skillet over high heat. Add garlic and stir-fry until fragrant, 15 to 20 seconds.

Add leafy greens, salt, and water and stir-fry for about 3 minutes, or until just tender. Then, add soy sauce and stir-fry until vegetables are coated, another 5 seconds.

Plate and drizzle with sesame oil.

 Garlic

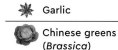 Chinese greens (*Brassica*)

4 Chinese eggplants

Salt

2 tablespoons black
(Chinkiang) vinegar

2 tablespoons soy sauce

2 teaspoons chili sauce

Canola oil, for frying

2 tablespoons minced fresh
ginger

2 tablespoons minced fresh
garlic

¼ cup fresh Thai basil leaves

2 scallions, thinly sliced

THIS IS A LIGHTER VERSION of the Sichuanese classic dish known as Fish Fragrant Eggplant (a misleading name, so called for the flavorings, which are also used to season fish, not for any fishiness). I love the slightly spicy, sweet, and sour flavors of the original dish but sometimes find it too heavy. Instead of deep-frying the eggplant, I lightly panfry it. The sauce, too, is lightened up here without using any starch, and I've brightened it with Thai basil, which is how this dish is often served in Taiwan.

CHINESE EGGPLANT WITH BLACK VINEGAR AND THAI BASIL

Serves 4 as a side dish

Cut eggplants crosswise into 3-inch lengths, then cut each segment lengthwise into four pieces, to get sticks.

Place cut eggplant in a colander and salt evenly. Allow to sit for about 10 minutes, until eggplant begins to "sweat." Rinse with cool water, then gently squeeze each piece to crush slightly. This will get rid of excess water, to allow it to better soak up sauce, and also tenderizes the eggplant.

Combine vinegar, soy sauce, and chili sauce in a small bowl.

Heat a skillet over medium-high heat and add 1 to 2 tablespoons canola oil. Add minced ginger and garlic and stir-fry for 30 seconds.

Add eggplant to pan and stir-fry for a minute.

Add sauce mixture and toss or stir to coat evenly. Cook for another minute or two, or until sauce has reduced slightly and eggplant is glazed. You should still have a little sauce in pan. Stir in basil so it wilts.

Transfer to a serving plate and garnish with scallions.

Chile pepper, garlic, ginger

Basil, eggplant

1 pound Chinese eggplant

Salt

1 tablespoon (about 3 cubes) fermented tofu, mashed into a paste

1 tablespoon Chinese rice wine

3 to 4 tablespoons water

1½ teaspoons low-sodium soy sauce

1 teaspoon sugar

½ teaspoon sesame oil

2 tablespoons canola oil

1 teaspoon minced fresh ginger

2 scallions, thinly sliced

THIS RECIPE was inspired by a dish my mother-in-law cooked for us, just once, twenty years ago. Mommy was born in rural Taishan County, in Guangdong Province in China, then spent her early adulthood managing a jewelry factory in Hong Kong. She married my late father-in-law, a half-Chinese, quarter-Scottish, and quarter-Indian man from Trinidad, while they were in their late teens. When he had to return to run the family business in Trinidad and couldn't afford to bring them, she then raised their daughter as a single mom for a few decades. This is all to say, she's one tough cookie. Mommy probably doesn't remember making this dish for me. I am happy to say that I was able to faithfully re-create the flavors, based upon that long-ago taste memory. The funky fermented tofu, which can be bought jarred in Chinese groceries and has a fragrance and flavor similar to blue cheese, mellows out when mashed into a sauce, becoming almost like miso with a creamy undertone.

CHINESE EGGPLANT WITH FERMENTED TOFU

Serves 4

Cut eggplant crosswise into 2½-inch lengths, then cut each segment lengthwise into four pieces, to get sticks.

Place cut eggplant in a colander and sprinkle evenly with salt. Allow to sit for about 10 minutes until eggplant begins to "sweat." Rinse with cool water, then gently squeeze each piece to crush slightly. This will get rid of excess water, allowing it to absorb sauce better, and also tenderize the eggplant. This is key to getting a tender yet firm, not mushy, texture.

Meanwhile, prepare sauce by mashing fermented tofu with rice wine, water, soy sauce, sugar, and sesame oil in a bowl. Set aside.

Heat canola oil in a medium-size skillet over medium-high heat, then add ginger and fry until fragrant, about 30 seconds. Add eggplant, cut side down. Cook, stirring a few times, until tender but not mushy, and slightly golden, 3 to 4 minutes.

Lower heat to low, add sauce mixture, stir to coat eggplant evenly, and cook to reduce sauce slightly, another 2 minutes. Add additional water if pan is dry, so that there is some sauce. Garnish with scallions.

✳ Garlic, ginger

🥬 Eggplant, fermented tofu

2 tablespoons canola oil

2 to 3 Roma or other small tomatoes, as ripe as possible, sliced into quarters

½ teaspoon sugar

1 tablespoon soy sauce

6 large eggs, beaten

2 scallions, cut on the diagonal into 2-inch pieces

Steamed rice, for serving

THIS IS ONE of the first dishes I learned to cook, a classic comfort food in every Chinese home. It's the meal we eat when we return home from our travels, or after a run of overly rich meals. Served with some steamed rice, it's a tasty and comforting dinner. The key to this is to cook the tomatoes first and long enough so that there's a sauce into which you add the beaten eggs, which you then want to cook slowly and gently so that they end up creamy and custardy.

TAIWANESE TOMATO EGGS

Serves 2 or 3

Heat oil in a medium-size skillet over medium heat, then add tomato wedges. Cook for about 5 minutes, turning over and pressing with a spatula to gently crush and release juices. When tomatoes are soft and their juices have created some sauce, add sugar and soy sauce and cook for another minute.

Add beaten eggs and scallions and lower heat to low. Allow to cook, occasionally stirring (making softly scrambled eggs).

Serve over steamed rice.

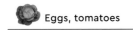 Eggs, tomatoes

2 tablespoons canola oil

2 teaspoons minced fresh ginger

½ onion, cut into small dice

2 teaspoons minced fresh garlic

1 teaspoon sugar

2 tablespoons low-sodium soy sauce

1 teaspoon ground white pepper

5 cups frozen vegetables (to include shelled edamame or green peas, diced carrots, corn)

2 large eggs, beaten

¼ cup packed fresh basil leaves

THIS HOME-STYLE Taiwanese dish is one of the first that I learned to make independently—probably by third grade, standing on a stool in front of the avocado green electric range in my childhood home. I made it again decades later for my Taiwanese cousin, and he teased me that I cooked like a Taiwanese housewife. That's one fine compliment! So, from this Taiwanese housewife's kitchen to yours, here's my recipe for a comfort food dish that reminds me of my childhood. This version substitutes edamame for the ground pork that is usually used but is otherwise reminiscent in flavor and texture to the original. I've named it "picadillo" for its similarity to the ground meat dish that has origins in Spain, made there with capers and olives, and similar dishes in the former Spanish colonies of Puerto Rico, Cuba, and other parts of Latin America, where it's cooked with olives and raisins, and the Philippines, where it's made with tomatoes, potatoes, and carrots.

TAIWANESE "PICADILLO"

Serves 6

Heat oil in a wok or skillet over high heat. When oil is shimmery, add ginger and onion and stir-fry for about 30 seconds.

Add garlic and stir for about 5 seconds, add sugar, soy sauce, and white pepper, then stir to mix seasonings evenly into mixture.

Add frozen vegetables and stir-fry for a few minutes until tender but not soft.

Pour in beaten eggs, allow to set for a minute, then scramble into rest of mixture.

Remove from heat and stir in basil leaves to wilt.

We eat this with rice, but you could also try it in lettuce cups or even in tortillas, for Taiwanese tacos.

✳ Garlic, ginger, white pepper

🥬 Basil, edamame

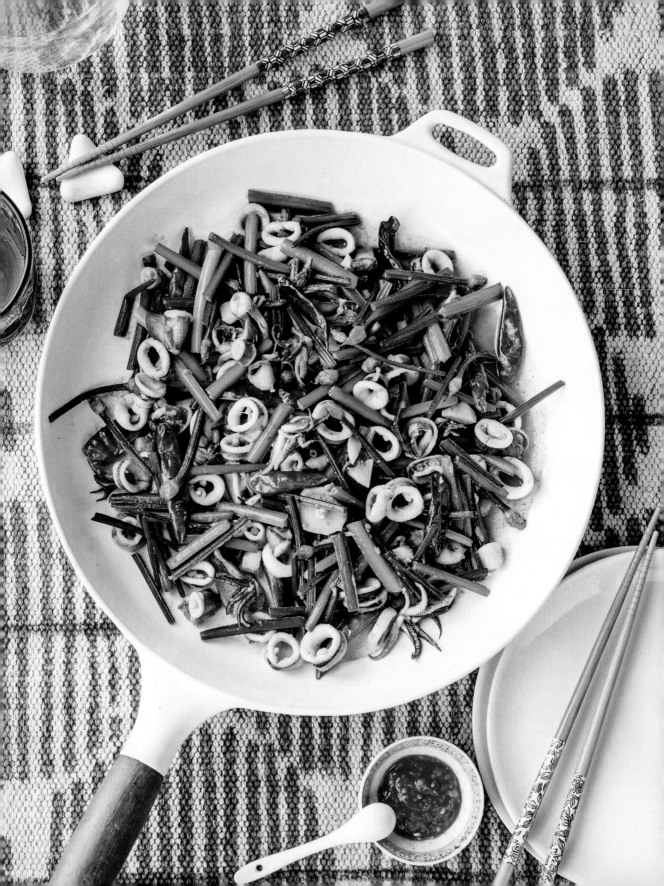

1 pound squid

1 pound Chinese chive flowers or chives (also known as garlic chives, *jiu cai* in Mandarin and *kú chhài* in Taiwanese)

Canola or vegetable oil, for frying

2 to 3 garlic cloves, peeled, crushed, and coarsely chopped

2 quarter-size slices fresh ginger, smashed slightly

4 dried red chiles

Salt

THIS IS A FRESH and fragrant and very speedy way to serve squid. The brininess and chewiness of the squid pairs well with the sweetness and slight crunch of the Chinese chives, complemented by garlic and ginger and a little heat from dried chiles. If you're not sure about cleaning squid on your own, you can ask your fishmonger to clean it for you, and you can also find precleaned squid in the frozen seafood section of many supermarkets. One of the main seafood lessons I learned from culinary school was, when cooking squid, either cook it very briefly or for a very long time, anything in between will make it rubbery. Take note!

STIR-FRIED SQUID WITH CHINESE CHIVES

Serves 4

If using cleaned squid, cut into ¼-inch-thick rings plus tentacles. If starting with whole squid, begin by preparing squid. To clean, lay each squid flat onto a cutting board. Cut off tentacles right above the eye, and remove hard beak from center. Next, pull off the head and pull out plasticlike spine and all innards. If desired, you can slip off purple skin, but I like to leave it on. Rinse tentacles and body and then cut body into ¼-inch-thick rings.

Cut chives into 2-inch lengths.

Heat about 1 tablespoon oil in a skillet over medium heat, then add garlic, ginger, and chiles. Stir-fry until fragrant, 30 to 60 seconds.

Add squid, increase heat to medium-high, and stir-fry until it turns pink and opaque, about a minute.

Add chives and stir-fry for another 30 seconds.

Add a pinch or two of salt to taste—you won't need much with the brininess of squid.

Chile peppers, garlic, ginger

Garlic chives, squid

1 tablespoon Chinese rice wine

1 tablespoon soy sauce

1½ tablespoons ketchup

¼ teaspoon ground white pepper

1 teaspoon sugar

½ cup warm vegetable stock or water

2 tablespoons canola oil

2 tablespoons minced garlic (from about 6 cloves)

3 tablespoons peeled and minced fresh ginger (from about a 3-inch length)

2 scallions, thinly sliced, whites and greens separated

1 pound medium shrimp, shells on, deveined (frozen is fine if defrosted before cooking)

Cooked rice, for serving

THIS HOME-STYLE Chinese dish has a surprising ingredient: ketchup. Not so surprising if you know that the word *ketchup* has Asian roots, in the late seventeenth century: from the Chinese Hokkien dialect's *kê-chiap* "brine of pickled fish or shellfish," perhaps partly via Malay *kecap* or *kicap*, "soy sauce." This sauce is simple but sophisticated, with Chinese rice wine and soy sauce and other sources of umami added to the ketchup. This savory dish comes together in minutes, making this an easy pantry/freezer weeknight meal.

Note: It is essential to use shrimp with the shells still on for optimal flavor and texture. Yes, eating will be messy (which is what makes it home-style) but worth it. To eat, first suck the flavor and sauce off the shell, then shell the shrimp before eating. In Taiwan, restaurants typically provide wet wipes instead of napkins for this reason.

SHRIMP IN CHINESE RICE WINE AND TOMATO SAUCE

Serves 4

Mix together rice wine, soy sauce, ketchup, white pepper, sugar, and stock in a small bowl and set aside.

In a wok or sauté pan, heat oil over medium heat and fry garlic, ginger, and scallion whites for 15 seconds, or until fragrant.

Increase heat to high, then add shrimp and cook until pink, 1 to 2 minutes.

Add sauce mixture and stir to coat. Continue to cook until sauce has reduced by about half, another minute.

Garnish with scallion greens and serve with rice.

Garlic, ginger, white pepper

Shrimp

1 pound salmon steak or fillet, skin on or off, your choice

Pinch of salt

1 tablespoon canola oil

1 teaspoon sugar

1 tablespoon soy sauce

2 garlic cloves, peeled and smashed

2 scallions, cut on the diagonal into 2-inch lengths

PEOPLE who are not accustomed to cooking fish think that it's complicated, but it's actually one of the simplest and fastest things to cook. I make this dish for my family once or twice a week, and it is modeled after the way my mother has always cooked salmon, a one-pot meal that's a simple riff on teriyaki. You can use either salmon steaks or salmon fillets for this. When I buy salmon, I try to buy two portions, cook one fresh, and keep one in the freezer, which can be defrosted overnight in the refrigerator for another quick pantry/freezer meal.

TEN-MINUTE TERIYAKI SALMON

Serves 4

If you're using a salmon fillet and like a crispy skin, follow these steps:

- Pat skin dry with a paper towel. Season both sides with a pinch of salt.
- Heat a medium-size nonstick skillet over medium-high heat, then add oil.
- Place fillet, skin side down, in the pan and leave it to cook until its skin has crisped up and releases easily with a spatula, 3 to 5 minutes. If it doesn't release easily, it's not ready to flip yet. Continue to cook until you can easily slip a spatula under the skin.
- Sprinkle sugar on top, lower heat to low, then flip the fillet over so that the skinless side is facing down.
- Add soy sauce to the pan, swirling so that it goes under the fish, then add smashed garlic and scallions on the side. Cook for an additional 3 to 5 minutes, depending on the thickness of your fillet, until it is opaque, turning garlic and scallions occasionally so they don't burn. By now, the sugar and soy sauce should have formed a nice glaze.

If you're cooking a salmon steak or a skinless fillet, heat a medium-size skillet over medium heat, add oil and garlic, and then add salmon. Cook for about 4 minutes on first side, then turn over. Once you flip salmon, sprinkle with sugar, pour soy sauce on top, and add scallions. Continue to cook, lowering heat to medium-low, for another 5 minutes, then turn salmon over to original side and continue to cook for another 1 to 2 minutes, or until both sides are glazed and browned, and flesh begins to flake apart when pierced with a fork or tip of a paring knife.

🌼 Garlic

🌸 Salmon

Cooking spray

1 tablespoon sesame seeds

2 tablespoons white miso paste, reduced-sodium if available

2 tablespoons mirin (Japanese sweet rice wine)

1 tablespoon reduced-sodium soy sauce, or tamari

½ teaspoon grated fresh ginger

1 tablespoon water, if needed to thin glaze to a pourable consistency

1 pound skin-on, center-cut salmon fillet, cut into 4 portions

2 tablespoons thinly sliced scallion

THIS IS A SIMPLE and quick way to prepare very flavorful salmon. Extra glaze can be stored, tightly covered, in the refrigerator indefinitely and also be used to glaze tofu, eggplant, and other vegetables.

MISO-GLAZED SALMON

Serves 4

Position oven rack in upper third of oven; preheat broiler.

Line a small baking sheet with foil. Coat foil with cooking spray.

Toast sesame seeds in a small, dry skillet over low heat, stirring constantly, until fragrant, 3 to 5 minutes. Set aside.

Whisk together miso, mirin, soy sauce, and ginger in a small bowl until smooth. Thin with water as needed; glaze should be thick but pourable.

Place salmon fillets, skin side down, on prepared baking sheet. Brush with miso mixture.

Broil salmon, 3 to 4 inches from heat source, until opaque in center, 6 to 8 minutes.

Transfer salmon to serving plates and garnish with toasted sesame seeds and sliced scallion.

Ginger

Miso, salmon, sesame seeds

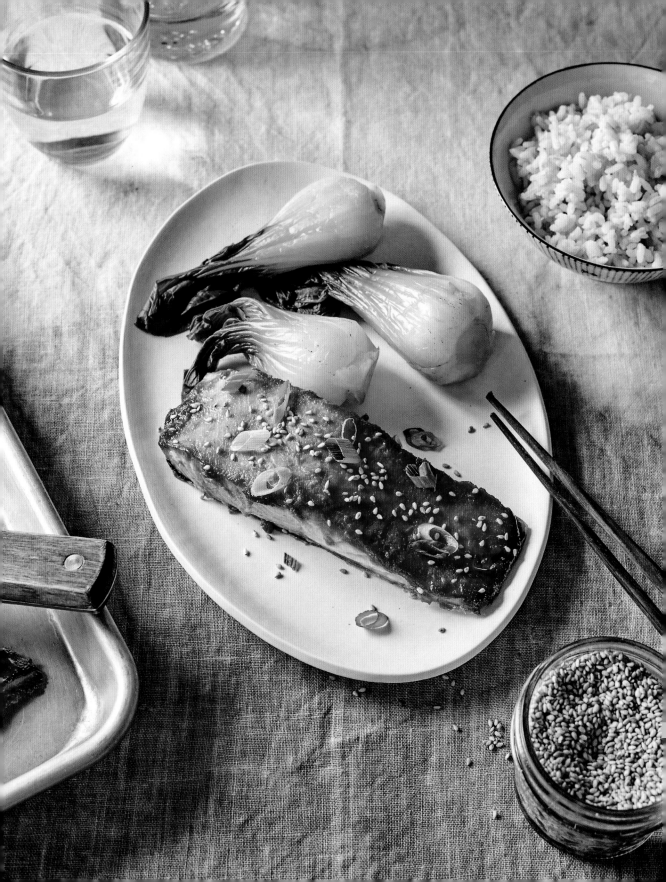

TOFU

1 (14-ounce) package
firm tofu

2 tablespoons canola oil

6 dried red chiles

1 teaspoon Sichuan
peppercorns

3 scallions, dark green
and white parts separated,
thinly sliced

1 red serrano chile, sliced

1 (1-inch) piece fresh ginger,
peeled and finely chopped

2 garlic cloves, sliced

½ cup unsalted, roasted
peanuts

KUNG PAO SAUCE

2 teaspoons low-sodium
soy sauce

1 tablespoon Chinese black
vinegar or balsamic vinegar

2 teaspoons hoisin sauce

1 teaspoon toasted
sesame oil

———

Steamed rice, for serving

Chile peppers, garlic,
ginger, Sichuan
peppercorn

Peanuts, tofu

KUNG PAO CHICKEN, a Chinese takeout favorite, originated in Sichuan Province during the Qing Dynasty and is named for the word meaning "palace guardian." The original recipe contained only chicken, leeks, and peanuts, seasoned with chiles and Sichuan peppercorn, but the Chinese American version typically has celery and other vegetables as well. In this chickenless vegetarian version, I've kept all the spicy, tangy flavor of the original but lightened it up, which actually enhances the flavors.

KUNG PAO TOFU

Serves 4 to 6

Drain tofu and wrap in two layers of paper towel. Sandwich wrapped tofu between two cutting boards, place a heavy pot on top, and press for 30 minutes.

Meanwhile, make Kung Pao sauce: Stir together soy sauce, vinegar, hoisin sauce, and sesame oil in a small bowl and set aside.

Once pressed, slice tofu into bite-size pieces (¼ x 1 x 2-inch rectangles).

Heat a tablespoon of canola oil in a nonstick or cast-iron skillet over medium-high heat, and swirl to distribute oil evenly on pan. Add sliced tofu and fry, undisturbed, until top and bottom are golden brown, 5 to 7 minutes on each side. Transfer to a plate.

Add dried chiles and peppercorns to pan and cook, tossing, just until fragrant (be careful not to burn), about 30 seconds. Transfer chiles and peppercorns to a plate.

Add remaining tablespoon of oil to pan and increase heat to high. Add white parts of scallions, serrano chile, ginger, and garlic and stir-fry until fragrant, about 30 seconds. Then, add fried tofu and prepared Kung Pao sauce and cook, stirring often, until sauce is fragrant and coats tofu evenly. Add peppercorn mixture and peanuts and stir-fry until well combined, about 1 minute.

Transfer to a serving dish and top with scallion greens. Serve with rice.

1 (14-ounce) package
firm tofu

2 tablespoons low-sodium
soy sauce

2 tablespoons sugar

1 to 2 tablespoons canola oil

Nori sheets

3 cups cooked haiga rice
(preferred), brown sushi rice,
or mixed rice

Furikake

Special equipment: musubi
maker/sushi press (available
in Japanese supermarkets or
online); you may also shape
by hand

IF YOU'VE VISITED the Hawaiian Islands, you've probably encountered Spam musubi, which might best be described as Spam sushi. Spam was a main course for the troops during WWII, and the large military presence in Hawaii led to Spam's widespread local adoption as an inexpensive, shelf-stable form of meat. A Japanese American woman, Barbara Funamura, reportedly created Spam musubi in the 1980s, by placing teriyaki-glazed slices of Spam on top of a block of compressed rice and wrapping the whole thing in a strip of nori (the roasted seaweed used for sushi), to make a portable snack. For a similar taste and appearance, I've created this teriyaki-glazed tofu version for a snack that is a pretty good facsimile of the original, with much better nutrition.

TERIYAKI TOFU MUSUBI

Makes 8 to 10 musubi

Drain tofu and wrap in two layers of paper towel. Sandwich wrapped tofu between two cutting boards, place a heavy pot on top, and press for 30 minutes. Then, slice into ¼-inch-thick pieces that are the size of your musubi maker, about 2 x 3 inches.

Mix together soy sauce and sugar in a small bowl and stir to dissolve.

Heat a large skillet over medium-high heat, then add oil. Add sliced tofu and cook for 2 minutes on each side. Then, pour sauce mixture over tofu. Cook for another 2 minutes on each side, or until crispy and caramelized. Remove from heat and set aside.

To shape with a musubi maker (if using): Cut nori sheets into 1-inch-wide strips and lay them on a flat surface, such as a cutting board. Center musubi maker over nori strip, add about ½ cup of rice to center, and press firmly. Remove press and sprinkle furikake on top, then add a prepared slice of tofu. Wrap nori around rice and tofu and seal ends with a dab of water, if needed. Repeat until you have used up all rice and tofu.

continued ⟶

Furikake

Haiga rice, seaweed, tofu

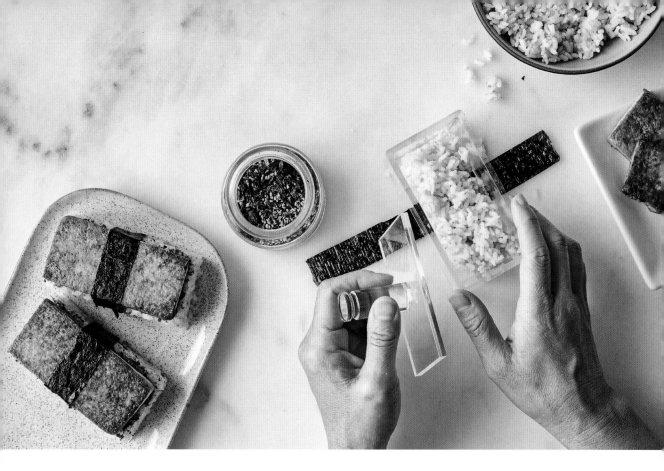

To shape by hand: Cut nori sheets into 1-inch wide strips and lay them on a flat surface, such as a cutting board. Top with about ½ cup of rice and press firmly to shape into a 2 x 3-inch rectangle. Sprinkle furikake on top, then add a prepared slice of tofu. Wrap nori around rice and tofu and seal ends with a dab of water, if needed. Repeat until you have used up all rice and tofu.

Eat immediately or wrap tightly in plastic wrap for a portable snack.

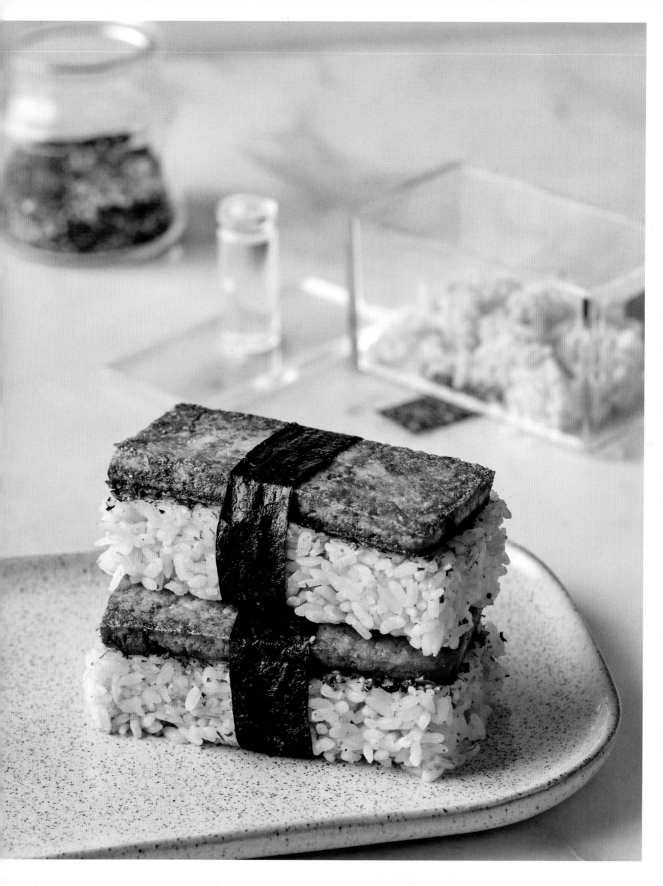

1 tablespoon neutral oil (such as canola)

6 garlic cloves, smashed

1 cup chopped kimchi

4 cups low-sodium vegetable stock

1½ tablespoons gochujang (Korean hot pepper paste)

14 ounces silken tofu, sliced into 10 slabs

4 ounces enoki or bunapi mushrooms (1 standard package); or any sliced mushrooms

6 scallions, white and light green parts, sliced

Steamed rice, for serving

1 large egg (optional)

THIS WARMING Korean stew is perfect for a cold, rainy night. It traditionally includes pork belly or seafood, but you won't miss it in this vegan version. Depth of flavor comes from the umami in the fermented ingredients (kimchi and gochujang), as well as the mushrooms. Traditionally, this is cooked in a stone pot, but any heavy pot (such as a Dutch oven) will work well. The finishing touch is usually a raw egg, added and stirred in to cook in the bubbling stew just before serving.

KIMCHI JJIGAE (VEGAN KOREAN SOFT TOFU AND KIMCHI STEW)

Serves 4 to 6

Heat oil in a 3-quart saucepan or small Dutch oven over medium heat. Add garlic and kimchi and cook for 1 minute.

In a bowl, whisk together stock and gochujang until smooth, then add to pot. Bring to a boil.

Once kimchi is tender and slightly translucent, carefully add tofu in a single layer (it's delicate, so you don't want to stir and break it), then add mushrooms. Lower heat, cover, and simmer for 15 to 30 minutes to allow flavors to develop.

Just before serving, top stew with scallions. Increase heat to bring to a rapid and vigorous boil, then remove from heat and serve immediately.

Serve over rice and stir in raw egg, if desired.

✳ Chile peppers (gochujang), garlic

 Kimchi, mushrooms, tofu

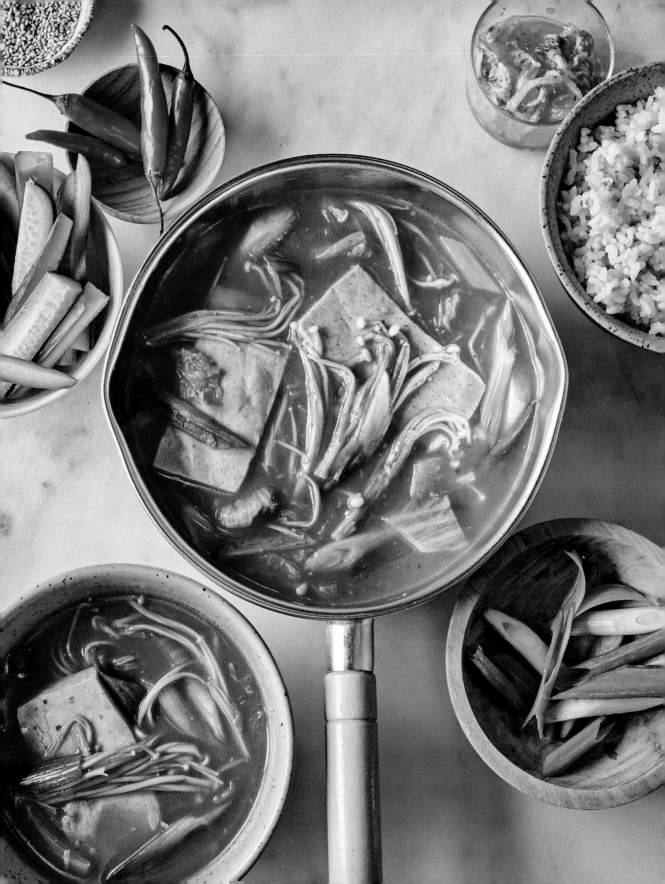

1 (14-ounce) firm tofu

3 tablespoons canola oil

1 medium-size yellow onion, cut into medium dice

1 teaspoon fine kosher salt

4 medium-size garlic cloves, finely chopped

1 tablespoon peeled and finely chopped fresh ginger (from about a 1½-inch piece)

2 tablespoons Thai red curry paste

1 cup unsweetened regular coconut milk

1 cup water, plus more if needed

½ medium-size kabocha squash or butternut squash (about 1 pound total), peeled, seeded, and cut into 1-inch cubes

1 medium-size green bell pepper, stem, seeds, and ribs removed; halved crosswise; then sliced into ¼-inch-wide strips

1 medium-size red bell pepper, stem, seeds, and ribs removed; halved crosswise; then sliced into ¼-inch-wide strips

Juice of ½ lime

8 to 12 leaves basil (preferably Thai basil)

Steamed brown jasmine rice, for serving

🌟 Curry paste (includes turmeric)

🥬 Bell pepper, kabocha squash (winter squash), tofu

THIS IS A TRADITIONAL Thai curry, with bright, herbaceous flavors of makrut lime leaf, lemongrass, turmeric, and galangal. Using prepared curry paste makes this an easy weeknight meal that tastes as if you've been cooking for hours. Adding the peppers and basil at the end preserves their vibrant colors.

THAI RED CURRY WITH KABOCHA SQUASH AND TOFU

Serves 8

Drain tofu and wrap in two layers of paper towel. Sandwich wrapped tofu between two cutting boards, place a heavy pot on top, and press for 30 minutes. Once pressed, dry surface and slice into ¼ x 1 x 2-inch rectangles.

Heat 2 tablespoons oil in a large, nonstick pan over medium-high heat. Add tofu in a single layer and fry on each side until golden, about 5 minutes per side. Set aside.

Heat remaining 1 tablespoon of oil in a large sauté pan with a lid or medium-size Dutch oven over medium heat until shimmering. Add onion, sprinkle with salt, and cook, stirring occasionally, until onion has softened, about 5 minutes. Add garlic and ginger, stir to combine, and cook until fragrant, about 1 minute.

Add curry paste, stir to coat onion mixture, and cook until fragrant, about 1 minute. Add coconut milk and water, stir to combine, and bring to a low boil.

Stir in squash and prepared tofu and add water, if needed, to cover all ingredients in a thin sauce. Bring back to a low boil, then lower heat to medium-low and continue to simmer, covered, stirring occasionally, until squash is fork-tender but still holds its shape, about 20 minutes. Add bell peppers and cook, uncovered, until tender, about 5 more minutes. Remove pan from heat and stir in lime juice. Taste and season with salt as needed. Add basil and serve with steamed rice.

12 dried shiitake mushrooms

1 (1-pound) package
Taiwanese rice vermicelli
(Hsinchu rice noodles)

1 pound kabocha squash

Salt

1 to 2 large carrots (about
8 ounces)

12 ounces napa cabbage

2 to 3 tablespoons canola oil

1 onion, sliced (about 2 cups)

½ cup plus 1 tablespoon
low-sodium soy sauce

3½ teaspoons ground white
pepper

1 (10-ounce) package
Chinese five-spice tofu,
sliced into ¼-inch-thick,
2-inch-long pieces

Up to 1 cup vegetable stock
or water, if needed

Garnishes: 3 scallions, thinly
sliced into rings; ground
white pepper, chili sauce

THE TASTE MEMORY of this dish is such a strong one that I almost
didn't want to learn how to make it myself. But as my mom has started
cooking less, I thought I should finally learn how to make her recipe.
She's varied her recipe over the years, and now I've done that as well.
The main difference is that I've made it completely plant based, adding
more mushrooms and mushroom broth for umami, and swapping in
sliced five-spice tofu, available in Asian markets. I also like to add in
some kabocha squash. I recommend serving this with your favorite chili
sauce, such as chili-garlic sauce or sriracha. *Ingredient note*: Look for rice
noodles from Taiwan, or labeled "Hsinchu rice noodles." If unavailable,
get the thinnest rice vermicelli you can find. Besides being thin, the
Taiwanese variety has the texture of "Q," or bouncy chewiness, that
is especially adored in Taiwan. The other key ingredient to make this
taste Taiwanese is the white, not black, pepper.

MAMA'S CHHÁ BÍ-HÚN —
TAIWANESE STIR-FRIED
RICE NOODLES

Serves 6 to 8

Rinse shiitake mushrooms with water to remove grit, then soak in
2 cups of hot water for 20 to 30 minutes, or until softened, keeping a
plate or other object on top to keep them submerged. When softened,
remove mushrooms, squeeze out all water, remove and discard stems,
and slice caps thinly. Strain remaining mushroom broth through a fine-
mesh strainer lined with a coffee filter or paper towel. Reserve broth.

While mushrooms soak, use scissors to cut rice noodle bundles in half,
then cover with cold water and soak for about 10 minutes, or until
softened. Drain and set aside.

Also while mushrooms soak, peel and seed kabocha and cut into
½-inch-thick, 2-inch-wide wedges. Place in a saucepan and cover with
an inch of water, add ¼ teaspoon salt, and bring to boil over high heat.

continued ⟶

Five-spice, white
pepper

Cabbage, carrots,
kabocha squash
(winter squash),
mushrooms, tofu

MAINS

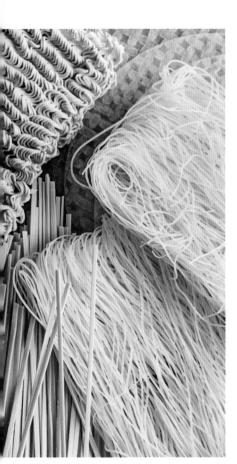

Lower heat to a simmer, cover, and cook until tender but not falling apart, 10 to 15 minutes, then drain and set aside.

Julienne carrots and shred cabbage; set both aside.

Heat a large wok or sauté pan over high heat and add 2 tablespoons oil. When shimmery, add onion and stir-fry for a minute, or until just beginning to become translucent but still firm.

Add mushrooms and stir for 30 seconds. Add carrots, cabbage, soy sauce, and white pepper and stir until well combined. Add reserved mushroom broth and lower heat to low.

Gradually add softened rice noodles in a few batches, stirring after each addition to combine with vegetable mixture. (Long chopsticks or tongs work best for this. This can be a little tricky! If your pan is too small, you might want to divide between two pans at this point, for easier stirring.) If noodles seem dry, add vegetable stock or water. Adjust seasoning and gently stir in cooked kabocha and sliced tofu until well distributed.

Garnish with scallions, additional white pepper, and chili sauce, if desired.

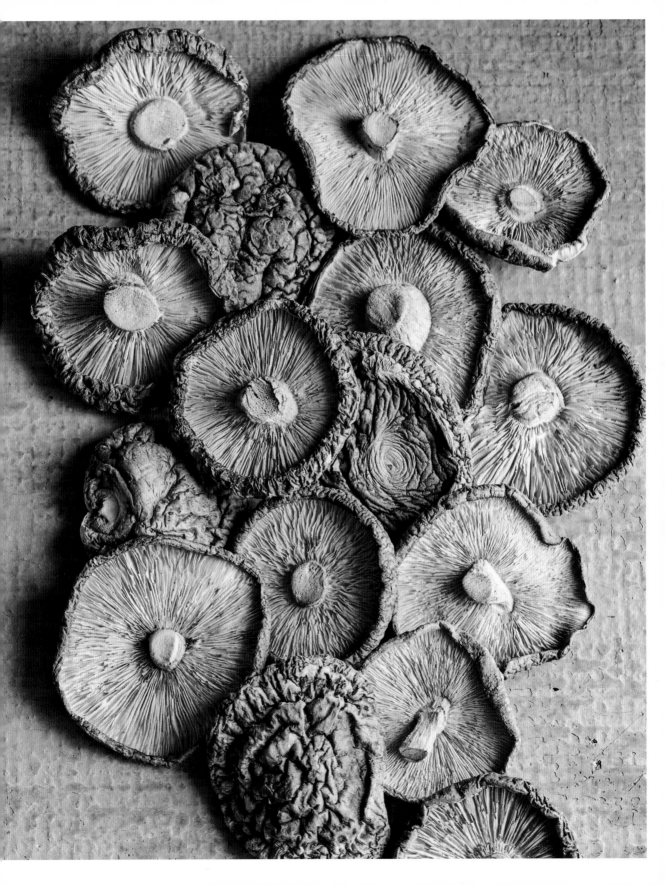

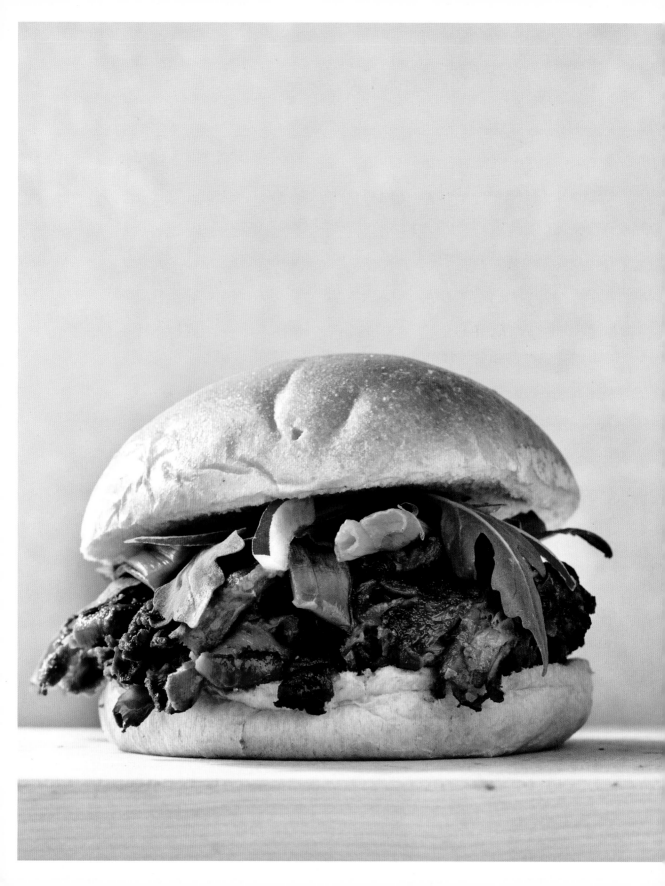

2 tablespoons unsalted
butter

1 pound maitake mushrooms,
cleaned and divided
into 4 clusters, or oyster
mushrooms

6 scallions, cut into 2-inch
lengths

Salt and freshly ground black
pepper

1 tablespoon miso thinned
with 2 tablespoons water

4 soft burger buns, ideally
potato or brioche

1 cup grated Swiss cheese

½ cup thinly sliced red onion

2 cups arugula

I'M NOT A FAN of most veggie burgers—too bready—but I am a fan of "meaty" vegetables in buns. This is my version of a veggie burger—using the meatiness of seared clusters of maitake (hen of the woods) mushrooms gives an additional layer of umami with a miso glaze. The mushrooms pair well with Swiss cheese, complemented by the bite of sliced red onions and arugula. You can substitute oyster mushrooms.

MISO-GLAZED MAITAKE MUSHROOM BURGERS

Makes 4 burgers

Melt butter in a medium-size skillet over medium-high heat, then add mushrooms and cook for about 3 minutes on each side, or until golden and slightly crisped. Press down with a spatula to maximize browning.

Add scallions to pan and cook for a minute, until wilted and slightly charred. Add salt and some black pepper to taste.

Pour miso mixture over mushrooms, and turn over until evenly coated and absorbed.

Toast buns, then assemble burger:

· Place bottom half of each bun on a plate.
· Sprinkle each with ¼ cup of grated Swiss cheese.
· Place hot mushrooms and scallions on top of cheese layer.
· Top with sliced red onion and arugula.

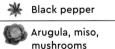

Black pepper

Arugula, miso,
mushrooms

1 (13.5-ounce) can light coconut milk

3 tablespoons chia seeds

1 tablespoon matcha powder

1½ tablespoons honey

¼ teaspoon pure vanilla extract

THE PRACTICE of milling tea leaves into a fine powder and then whisking in water originated in China around the tenth century but is most associated these days with Japan, where matcha, as it's known there, is the staple ingredient upon which traditional Japanese tea ceremonies were developed in the twelfth century. This matcha pudding was inspired by bubble, or boba, tea. Chia seeds become like boba pearls when soaked in liquid. The coconut milk complements the natural bitterness of the matcha to make a smooth, creamy, light dessert.

MATCHA COCONUT CHIA PUDDING

Serves 4

Mix all ingredients together in a bowl until smooth. Keep tightly sealed in a jar or container with a lid and refrigerate overnight.

Stir well before serving. Thin with additional water, if desired.

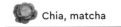 Chia, matcha

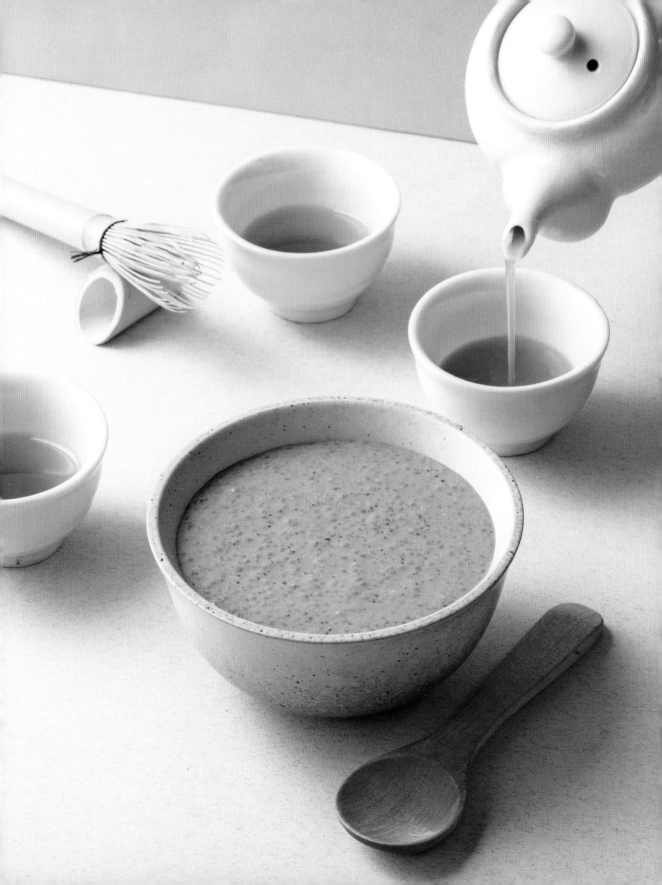

1 large papaya

1½ cups milk (any kind, though whole milk is traditional)

¼ cup sugar, or to taste (depends on ripeness of your papaya)

Ice

LONG BEFORE BUBBLE TEA stole the spotlight, papaya milk was a popular fruit drink in Taiwan. It's such a popular taste in Taiwan that you can buy it in grocery and convenience stores, similar to how chocolate and strawberry milk are sold in North America. I'll drink that in a pinch, but whenever I can get my hands on a ripe papaya, I'd rather blend my own. If you're not familiar with this tropical fruit, it tastes most similar to cantaloupe. If you can get them, use a fresh papaya and make sure it is ripe, which you'll know when the skin changes from green to yellowish, and you begin to smell its sweet, fruity scent. The more common variety of papayas you'll find are the big, red-orange fleshed Mexican papayas, which are closer in taste to the ones in Taiwan than the small papayas from Hawaii. You may also be able to find frozen, cut papaya in supermarkets.

TAIWANESE PAPAYA MILK

Serves 2

Wash papaya, cut it in half, and scoop out seeds with a spoon. Peel off skin with a knife. Cut papaya into 1-inch cubes. Use 1 cup of cubes for this recipe. Extra may be frozen for later use.

Place cubed papaya in a blender, add milk and sugar, and blend until smooth. Serve over ice.

 Papaya

½ cup uncooked basmati rice

4½ cups 2% milk, or your favorite creamy-tasting alternative milk, such as coconut, hemp, oat, or cashew milk

3 green cardamom pods, lightly crushed

2 tablespoons sugar

¼ teaspoon salt

¼ cup unsweetened flaked coconut

¼ cup golden raisins

Garnishes: 2 tablespoons finely chopped pistachios, ground cardamom

MANY INDIAN SWEETS are heavy with cream, ghee, and sugar. Kheer is an exception, a mildly flavored dessert that highlights the cardamom. I make mine even lighter than most versions, using 2% milk and taking advantage of the natural sweetness of golden raisins to cut back on the amount of sugar.

KHEER (INDIAN RICE PUDDING)

Serves 6

Place rice, milk, and cardamom in a saucepan and heat over medium heat, stirring occasionally so milk does not scald. When it begins to simmer, lower heat to low, stir again, and cook, partially covered, stirring occasionally, until rice is tender and pudding has thickened, 20 to 30 minutes.

Turn off heat and add sugar, salt, coconut, and raisins. Adjust sweetness, if desired.

May be served warm or chilled. If pudding has become too thick, loosen with a little more milk. Garnish with a sprinkle of chopped pistachios and ground cardamom just before serving.

 Cardamom

1 cup rice vinegar

⅓ cup sugar

1½ cups water

1 teaspoon plus 1 tablespoon salt

4 garlic cloves, peeled and lightly crushed

1 to 2 star anise

½ teaspoon Sichuan peppercorns

6 dried red chiles

1 pound green cabbage (about ½ head)

Equipment: 1 quart-size jar or two 3-cup jars

IN RESTAURANTS in Taiwan, you'll be given small plates of pickled cabbage along with small plates of peanuts as soon as you're seated, to be nibbled on with chopsticks while you're perusing the menu. This Taiwanese-style pickled cabbage is the perfect appetizer dish to complement any meal. This is a quick pickle, not requiring fermentation, so you can eat it as soon as an hour after preparation, but for best results, allow it to sit overnight before consumption. This will keep, refrigerated, for several weeks.

TAIWANESE PICKLED CABBAGE

Makes 2 to 3 cups pickled cabbage

Combine rice vinegar, sugar, water, and 1 teaspoon salt in a nonreactive saucepan and bring to a boil. Stir and simmer until sugar is fully dissolved, about 5 minutes, then add garlic, star anise, Sichuan peppercorns, and dried chiles and remove from heat. Allow to cool to room temperature, about 1 hour.

Cut cabbage into 2 x 3-inch pieces, place in a large bowl, and toss with remaining salt. Allow to sit for about an hour, while pickling liquid is cooling. Then, rinse off salt completely, drain, and use your hands to wring out as much liquid as possible.

Transfer cabbage leaves to jar(s), packing them in tightly. Then, pour pickling liquid over leaves, seal tightly, and allow to sit for a minimum of an hour in the refrigerator before serving.

Note: After you've consumed your pickled cabbage, remaining pickling liquid can be reused to make another batch.

✳ Chile peppers, Sichuan peppercorns, star anise

🌹 Cabbage

1 medium-size cucumber

2 garlic cloves, thinly sliced

½ teaspoon sugar

2 teaspoons sesame oil

2 teaspoons low-sodium soy sauce

1 tablespoon rice vinegar

1 Fresno or red Thai bird chile, seeded and thinly sliced (optional)

THESE QUICK PICKLES, inspired by my mother's recipe, add zesty flavor and crunch to any meal, and make a frequent appearance at our table. This is a flavorful side to anything you might grill and also makes an excellent accompaniment to Japanese or Chinese meals along with steamed rice.

TAIWANESE CUCUMBER QUICK PICKLE

Makes 2 cups quick pickle

Peel cucumber, leaving on some strips of skin for color.

Slice peeled cucumber into 1-inch-thick disks, then slice each disk into quarters, to get chunks.

Place sliced cucumbers in a bowl, add all other ingredients, including chile (if using), and stir until well combined.

Allow to sit at room temperature for at least 10 minutes before serving.

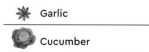

Garlic

Cucumber

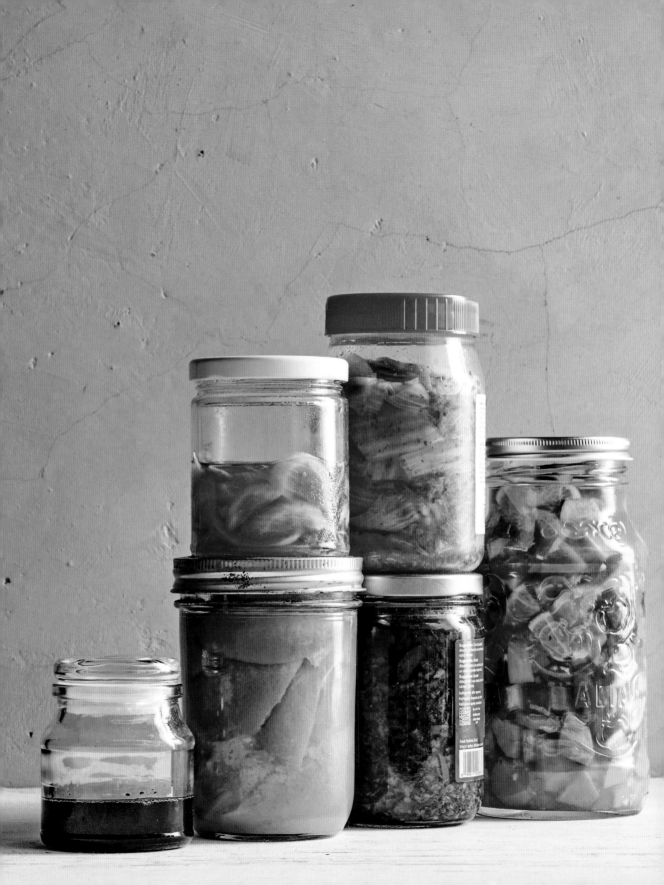

1 medium-size napa cabbage
(about 2 pounds)

¼ cup fine kosher salt

2 tablespoons grated garlic
(about 6 cloves)

1 tablespoon peeled and
grated fresh ginger

1 teaspoon sugar

2 tablespoons fish sauce

3 tablespoons water

¼ cup gochugaru (Korean
red pepper flakes) or Aleppo
chile flakes, or 2 tablespoons
crushed red pepper flakes,
smashed in a mortar and
pestle or ground in a spice
grinder into finer flakes

8 ounces daikon radish,
peeled and cut into 1-inch-
long matchsticks

1 bunch scallions, cut into
2-inch lengths

KIMCHI IS AN ICON of Korean cuisine, eaten both as an accompaniment to pretty much anything, or as an ingredient to add tremendous flavor to such things as fried rice, kimchi jjigae (kimchi stew), and more. The traditional method of making kimchi is laborious and time-consuming (and the recipes are tightly held family secrets). This version is a slightly streamlined recipe (the brining time is shorter, the cabbage leaves are cut before fermenting, and fish sauce is used rather than whole seafood), but I think you'll find it better than many versions you can buy. For a vegan version, use a vegetarian fish sauce or substitute ¾ teaspoon kelp powder mixed in 2 tablespoons water.

QUICK KIMCHI

Makes 2 quarts kimchi

Cut cabbage into quarters lengthwise, remove core, and then cut crosswise into 2-inch-wide strips. Place in a large bowl and sprinkle evenly with salt, using your hands to work salt evenly through leaves. Add enough cold water to just cover cabbage, then place a heavy plate or pan on top to weight it down. Allow to sit for 2 hours or overnight until wilted and water has been released.

To make the spice paste, combine garlic, ginger, sugar, fish sauce, water, and gochugaru in a small bowl.

Once cabbage has wilted, drain brining liquid, then rinse thoroughly with cold running water, twice. After draining thoroughly in a colander, squeeze out as much liquid as you can. (This will allow for more intense flavor.)

Place cabbage back in its large bowl and add daikon and scallions, then put on a pair of gloves and work the spice paste into the vegetables, making sure all vegetables are evenly coated.

Place in glass jars, packing tightly so that kimchi is submerged in its own liquid (there may not be too much liquid at first, but it will develop

continued →

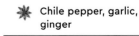

※ Chile pepper, garlic, ginger

🥬 Cabbage

within a few hours). Seal jars and place on a plate to catch any overflow of juices as kimchi ferments. You can eat it immediately, but it won't be fermented yet.

Check daily to see when it is at your desired level of fermentation. You'll start to notice bubbling by second day, increasing as fermentation continues. Days 3 through 5 are the sweet spot for me, but any time from day 3 to 7 will yield a deliciously funky product. Use a clean spoon daily to keep cabbage leaves submerged in their liquid.

Once kimchi is ready, keep refrigerated.

⅔ cup sugar

⅔ cup water

⅔ cup rice vinegar

2 teaspoons salt

1 pound daikon radish

THIS QUICK PICKLE is served as *banchan*, the many little side dishes that accompany a Korean meal. This is a crunchy and refreshing palate cleanser that goes especially well with fried or spicy food.

KOREAN PICKLED DAIKON

Makes about 3 cups pickled daikon

Combine sugar, water, vinegar, and salt in a nonreactive pot and heat over medium-high heat. Stir until sugar fully dissolves, 2 to 3 minutes. Remove from heat and allow to fully cool.

Meanwhile, peel daikon radish and cut into ½-inch-diameter disks. Cut each disk into ½-inch cubes.

Place cubed radish in a quart-size jar and pour cooled pickling liquid over it. Seal and place in refrigerator for at least 30 minutes, or overnight, shaking occasionally to evenly coat daikon. Enjoy cold!

 Daikon

2 tablespoons grated garlic
(about 6 cloves)

1 tablespoon peeled and
grated fresh ginger

1 teaspoon sugar

¼ cup gochugaru (Korean
red pepper flakes) or Aleppo
chile flakes, or 2 tablespoons
crushed red pepper flakes,
smashed in a mortar and
pestle or ground in a spice
grinder into finer flakes

2 tablespoons fish sauce
(vegan options are available
from online sources)

3 tablespoons water

1 ripe pineapple, peeled and
cut into 1-inch cubes (core
included)

I FIRST MADE pineapple kimchi when we were celebrating
Thanksgiving in Hawaii. I wanted side dishes to make our turkey
dinner taste more "local" and came up with the idea of combining
chunks of sweet local pineapple with kimchi, to use in place of
cranberry sauce. If you have robustly flavored kimchi, such as the
version in this cookbook, or a flavorful store-bought version (no watery
kimchi, please!), you can do as I did the first time and mix 2 parts
kimchi to 1 part cubed pineapple and allow to sit for thirty minutes.
If you want to have pineapple kimchi alone, you can use the same
spice paste used for the Quick Kimchi (page 177). Feel free to increase
amounts of gochugaru and fish sauce to taste.

ALOHA PINEAPPLE KIMCHI

Makes 1 quart kimchi

Place garlic, ginger, sugar, gochugaru, fish sauce, and water in a blender
or food processor and blend until smooth.

Combine spice mixture with pineapple in a bowl and allow to sit
at room temperature for 30 minutes. Enjoy immediately and store
remainder in refrigerator.

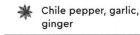 Chile pepper, garlic,
ginger

Pineapple

½ cup chopped Asian pear (about ¼ Asian pear)

½ cup coarsely ground gochugaru (Korean red pepper flakes) or Aleppo chile flakes, or ¼ cup crushed red pepper flakes, smashed in a mortar and pestle or ground in a spice grinder into finer flakes

¼ cup fish sauce or vegan fish sauce (available online)

3 garlic cloves, minced

½ cup sugar

2 teaspoons minced fresh ginger

WHEN I WAS DEVELOPING the kimchi recipes for this book, I accidentally added too much sugar to one batch of the spice paste. I tasted it, of course, and found that it tasted, first of all, really good but also reminiscent of gochujang, the Korean chili paste. Traditional gochujang is made through a complex process involving chili powder in addition to glutinous rice, barley, and soybeans, and ferments for months or even years. This version, while not at all traditional, makes a quick, homemade substitute, with fish sauce adding a bit of fermented flavor, and unlike many versions sold in Asian groceries, is made without corn syrup.

ACCIDENTAL GOCHUJANG

Makes 1 cup gochujang

Combine all ingredients in a blender and blend until smooth, adding a little water if needed to process.

Enjoy immediately and store remainder in a tightly sealed jar in the refrigerator; it will keep for up to a month.

✳ Chile pepper, garlic, ginger

🥬 Asian pear

---

1 garlic clove, minced

1 green onion, chopped

1 teaspoon gochugaru (Korean red pepper flakes) or Aleppo chile flakes, or ½ teaspoon crushed red pepper flakes

1 teaspoon sugar

2 tablespoons low-sodium soy sauce

2 teaspoons sesame oil

1 teaspoon rice vinegar

1 teaspoon toasted sesame seeds

THIS VERSATILE SAUCE can be used as a dipping sauce for fried tofu, as a dressing for an Asian-style grain bowl, or as a stir-fry sauce.

ASIAN VINAIGRETTE OR DIPPING SAUCE

Makes ½ cup sauce

Combine all ingredients in a bowl, using a spoon, or by shaking in a jar. This will keep in fridge for up to a week.

✳ Chile peppers, garlic

🥬 Sesame seeds

¼ cup creamy natural peanut butter (made with only peanuts)

Juice of 2 limes

2 tablespoons low-sodium soy sauce

2 teaspoons sugar

2 to 4 tablespoons water, to thin out the sauce, if necessary

3 garlic cloves, minced

1 tablespoon chili-garlic sauce, or red pepper flakes, or to taste

I DEVELOPED this peanut sauce to accompany the Eat the Rainbow Fresh Spring Rolls (page 128), but it is also excellent when used as a dressing for grain bowls, or drizzled onto steamed or roasted vegetables. It's important to use only natural peanut butter, without added emulsifiers or sweeteners, or else you won't get the correct consistency or flavor.

SPICY VEGAN PEANUT DIPPING SAUCE

Makes about 2 cups dipping sauce

Stir together all ingredients in a bowl until well combined. This will keep in the refrigerator for up to a week.

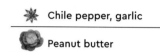

※ Chile pepper, garlic

Peanut butter

½ cup plain whole-milk yogurt or plant-based plain yogurt (not Greek style)

½ medium-size cucumber, peeled, seeded, and diced into ¼-inch pieces

2 tablespoons finely diced red onion

¼ teaspoon salt

½ teaspoon cumin seeds

A COOLING yogurt-based condiment that pairs well with spicy curries, raita also tastes great over basmati rice.

RAITA

Makes 1 cup raita

Stir all ingredients together.

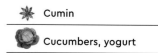

※ Cumin

Cucumbers, yogurt

Leaves from 1 bunch mint

Leaves from 1 bunch cilantro

Juice of 1 lemon

½ onion

1 (1-inch) piece fresh ginger, peeled and grated

½ medium-size green apple

½ teaspoon salt

½ teaspoon smoked cumin

1 teaspoon amchur

Pinch of garam masala

Chiles (optional)

OUR FRIEND NALIN is part of Spicebox Supperclub, which is made up of a group of our friends. Nalin describes this green chutney as ubiquitous in Indian food. "The classic type is the 'pudina' or mint chutney variant. It's a blended mixture of herb (mint), onion, lemon, garlic, ginger, and green chili if spiciness is desired. Its flavor comes from salt, sugar, cumin, and amchur (or amchoor), a seasoning agent from India made from powdered, dried green mangoes, used to tenderize proteins or as a souring agent (amchur is available from Indian groceries or online). Most people use cilantro along with mint to balance the flavors." Rather than including brown sugar, Nalin uses apple to add a mild degree of sweetness and to thicken.

NALIN'S MINT-CILANTRO CHUTNEY

Makes about ¾ cup chutney

Combine all ingredients in a blender, including chiles to taste, and blend, adding water as needed to thin.

Allow to sit overnight in the refrigerator for flavors to meld. Chutney will keep in the fridge for up to a week.

 Amchur, cumin, garam masala, ginger

Apple, cilantro, mint

1 cup frozen shelled
edamame (green soybeans)

¼ cup tahini

¼ cup water

½ teaspoon freshly grated
lemon zest

Juice of 1 lemon (about
3 tablespoons)

1 garlic clove, peeled and
smashed

¾ teaspoon kosher salt

3 tablespoons extra-virgin
olive oil

GARNISHES

¼ teaspoon ground cumin

¼ teaspoon ground
coriander

½ teaspoon pimentón
(smoked paprika)

¼ teaspoon salt

Drizzle of extra-virgin olive oil

1 tablespoon chopped fresh
flat-leaf parsley

THE LOVELY PALE GREEN HUE of this hummus makes it perfect for springtime. Like all hummus, this makes a great dip for an appetizer or snack—serve with crudités (sliced carrots, Persian cucumbers, radishes) and whole wheat pita. It can also be used as a spread on bread to make a base for a vegetable sandwich.

EDAMAME HUMMUS

Makes 1¼ cups hummus

Bring 4 cups of salted water to a boil, then add edamame and cook for 5 minutes. Drain and rinse under cold water until cool.

Combine cooked, cooled edamame and remaining ingredients, except garnishes, in a food processor and process until smooth. Add water, if needed to thin to desired consistency.

Prepare garnish: Combine all garnish ingredients, except oil and parsley, in a small bowl.

Transfer hummus to a serving bowl and garnish with spice mixture, a drizzle of olive oil, and parsley.

May be refrigerated, covered, up to 3 days.

※ Coriander, cumin,
smoked paprika

 Edamame, tahini

1 cup peeled and chopped taro (2-inch chunks)

¼ cup tahini

¼ cup water

Juice of 1 lemon (about 3 tablespoons)

2 garlic cloves, peeled and smashed

¾ teaspoon kosher salt

2 tablespoons extra-virgin olive oil

I'VE LONG BEEN captivated by the Hawaiian Islands, which are distinct geographically and culturally from the mainland US, including its food culture, which is multicultural, but still retains much of traditional Native Hawaiian ingredients. A staple of the Polynesian diet for over a thousand years, taro is a beloved root vegetable, or tuber, that has a special place in Hawaiian cuisine. Most commonly enjoyed as fermented poi, this is a nonfermented way to enjoy taro, which makes for a delicious version of the Mediterranean dip, hummus. Enjoy this with raw vegetable crudités, flatbread, or pita chips for a healthy snack. Taro is available in Asian and Latin American markets.

TARO HUMMUS

Makes 1¼ cups hummus

Put taro chunks in a saucepan and cover with cold water. Bring to boil, uncovered, then lower heat and cover and cook until tender, about 10 minutes. Rinse in cool running water until cool.

Combine cooked, cooled taro and remaining ingredients in a food processor and process until smooth. Add more water, if needed, to thin to desired consistency.

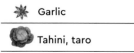

✳ Garlic

Tahini, taro

ASIA MENUS

CHINESE MENU

Taiwanese
Pickled Cabbage

Sichuanese
Shredded Potatoes

Stir-Fried Squid
with Chinese
Chives

Kung Pao Tofu

Chinese Stir-Fried
Greens

Seasonal Fruit

INDIAN MENU

Garlic Naan

Magical Mango-
Tamarind Rasam

Indian Spiced Kale
with Coconut and
Turmeric

Nalin's Mint-
Cilantro Chutney

Raita

Kheer (Indian
Rice Pudding)

SOUTHEAST ASIAN SUMMER MENU

Celebration
Red Salad

Balinese Green
Apple Salad

Backpacker's
Gado Gado

Eat the Rainbow
Fresh Spring Rolls

Matcha Coconut
Chia Pudding

HAWAIIAN BEACH PICNIC MENU

Edamame
Hummus, Taro
Hummus, and
Crudités

Hawaiian-Style
Tomato Poke

Teriyaki Tofu
Musubi

Ten-Minute Teriyaki
Salmon

Aloha Pineapple
Kimchi

Fresh Tropical Fruit

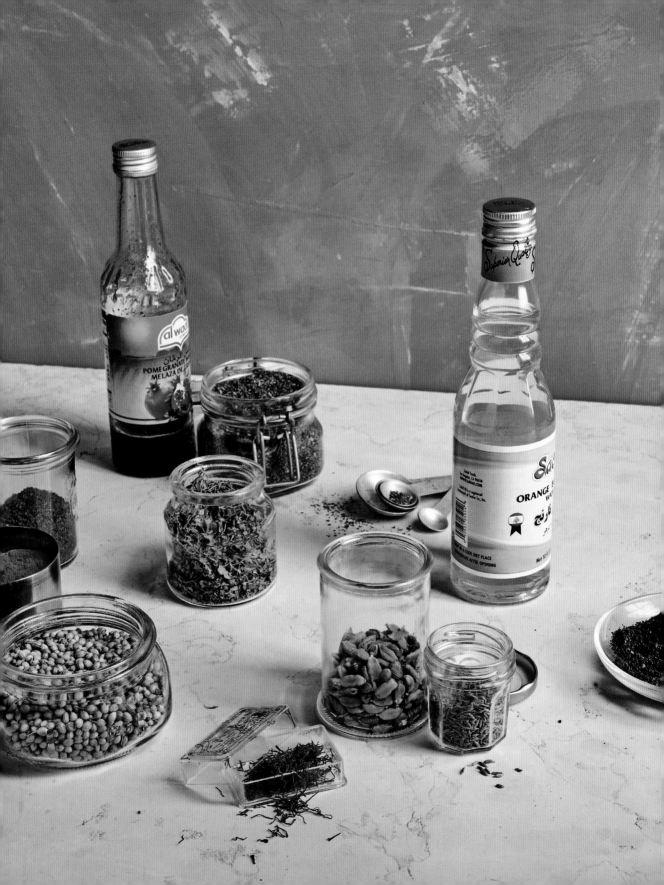

MEDITERRANEAN AND THE MIDDLE EAST

MEDITERRANEAN AND THE MIDDLE EAST PANTRY

spices

cayenne

cinnamon

cumin

fenugreek

garlic

harissa

oregano

pimentón

saffron

turmeric

za'atar

fruit extracts

orange flower water

pomegranate molasses

preserved lemon

herbs

basil

oregano

parsley

tarragon

thyme

fats

olive oil

acids

lemon

balsamic vinegar

red wine vinegar

MEDITERRANEAN AND THE MIDDLE EAST

A LITTLE BIT SWEET, a little bit spicy, bright with acidity, and vibrantly fresh with herbs, the flavors of the Mediterranean have wide appeal. Mediterranean cuisine includes many cultures, including the Maghrebi culture of North Africa (Algeria, Libya, Morocco, Tunisia, and Mauritania), the Levant (countries of the eastern Mediterranean, including modern-day Syria, Lebanon, Palestine, Israel, Jordan, and Cyprus), Egypt, Turkey, Greece, Italy, France, and Spain. In addition to highlighting some favorite recipes from these cuisines, I am also including a few recipes from neighboring Iran, whose rich cuisine uses many ingredients in common with the cuisines of the eastern Mediterranean, linked by the trade routes of the Silk Road. While the region is vast and encompasses many cultures, you'll find a lot of overlap in the flavors.

This varied cuisine shares health benefits too. The Mediterranean diet is one of the dietary patterns for which there is the most positive scientific evidence; it has been shown to lower risk of type 2 diabetes, heart disease, certain cancers, and death from all causes, and more recent studies have also shown benefits for brain health, including memory, and mood disorders, such as depression and anxiety.

Prior to culinary school, my experience with Mediterranean cuisine was mostly with the cuisines of Italy, France, and Spain. But once I was introduced to the food of Morocco through Paula Wolfert's recipes, my curiosity and taste buds were piqued. One of my contributions to our culinary school's restaurant week menu was one of Wolfert's tagines, a sweet and savory stew of lamb, prunes, almonds, and cinnamon. I finished my culinary school program with the tremendous opportunity of doing an externship in the kitchen of San Francisco's Michelin-starred Moroccan restaurant Mourad. There, I was surrounded by counter-to-ceiling jars of colorful and fragrant spices ranging from the familiar—turmeric, curry, cinnamon—to ones I had barely heard of—ras el hanout, harissa, *zhug*, *urfa*, long pepper, and my favorite name, grains of paradise. This was my playground. I celebrated my culinary school graduation by making a pilgrimage to Morocco, in search of spices.

We spent most of our trip in Marrakesh, in a *riad* (a traditional home built around an interior courtyard) just outside the medina, the ancient walled city that is home to the *souk*, the lively and varied marketplace selling food, spices, and dry goods. We started each morning at a table next to the dipping pool of our riad, with a bounteous and graciously served Moroccan breakfast of bread and jam, sometimes the crumpetlike crepe called *baghrir*, and endless glasses of Moroccan mint tea. For me the most magical part of the trip was a pilgrimage to the spice markets to purchase ras el hanout—the blend of more than a dozen sweet and fiery spices whose name translates as "head of the shop," harissa, and other spices. Following the tip of a local, I asked for a special blend of ras el hanout used for spicing coffee. It was almost like giving a secret password. I was led to the back room of a spice shop where the vendor pulled out a jar of the blend, and told me that it had more than thirty spices, including ginseng. Afterward, still excitedly clutching my special spices, we had dinner at a rooftop restaurant, where we had incredible views of the sun setting over the Jemaa el-Fnaa (the main market square), which transformed from mundane daytime market stalls to a lively nocturnal world of drummers, dancers, monkeys, and snake charmers as the backdrop for food stalls selling traditional dishes ranging from tagines, grilled meats, and snails braised in a richly spiced broth.

My trip to Morocco was what I hope to be the first of many, and I hope to be able to explore more of the Mediterranean soon. For now, I am content to journey there through my taste buds, and bring you along with me through these recipes. A word on the organization of this section: You'll notice that there's a higher proportion of starters in here relative to the number of mains. This is because many of the cuisines in this region serve a large number of salads and spreads with the meal, and in fact, sometimes make a meal of small plates, whether it's tapas in Spain or meze in the Middle East.

1½ cups semolina

¼ cup all-purpose flour

1½ teaspoons instant yeast

½ teaspoon salt

2 cups warm water, about 110°F

1 tablespoon baking powder

Unsalted butter, for pan

ONE OF THE SPECIAL ITEMS at our Moroccan breakfasts were these crepes, which are typically served with butter and honey. They are made with semolina (ground durum wheat), which brings a slight, pleasant crunchiness to the batter, and because they are yeasted, they have many tiny holes that soak up whatever you top them with. To bring in one of my favorite sweet flavors from Morocco, I combined these elements with orange flower water in a syrup. This seems slightly decadent as a breakfast, and wouldn't be wrong as dessert.

BAGHRIR (MOROCCAN "1,000 HOLE" CREPES) WITH ORANGE FLOWER WATER HONEY SYRUP

Makes 15 crepes

Place all ingredients, except butter, in a blender and blend until smooth, about 1 minute. Keep covered and allow to rest for 30 minutes.

After resting, blend batter for another second before cooking.

Heat an 8-inch nonstick, lightly buttered skillet (use an omelet pan, if you have one) over medium-low heat. Pour ¼ cup of batter into pan— it should spread immediately into a circle almost fitting the diameter of the pan. Cook until the surface is covered in holes, about 30 seconds. Cook only one side. Err on the side of underdone—if the sides start to curl up, you've overcooked the baghrir and it will be tough. Its underside should be at most lightly golden. Keep warm on a plate covered with a clean, dry towel until ready to serve. Repeat with remaining batter.

Serve hot with butter and honey or jam, or Orange Flower Water Honey Syrup (recipe follows).

continued ⟼

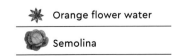

✺ Orange flower water

🌸 Semolina

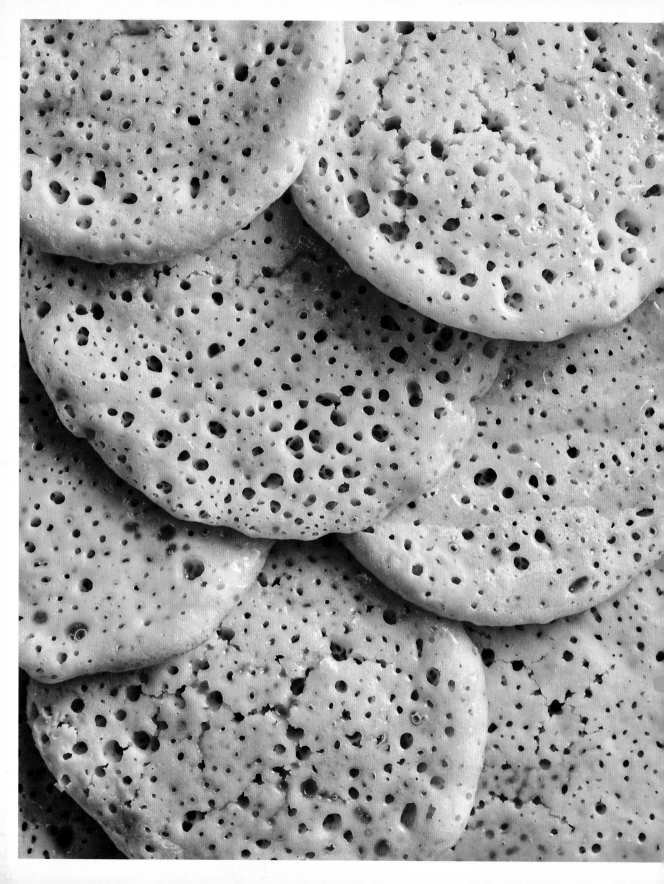

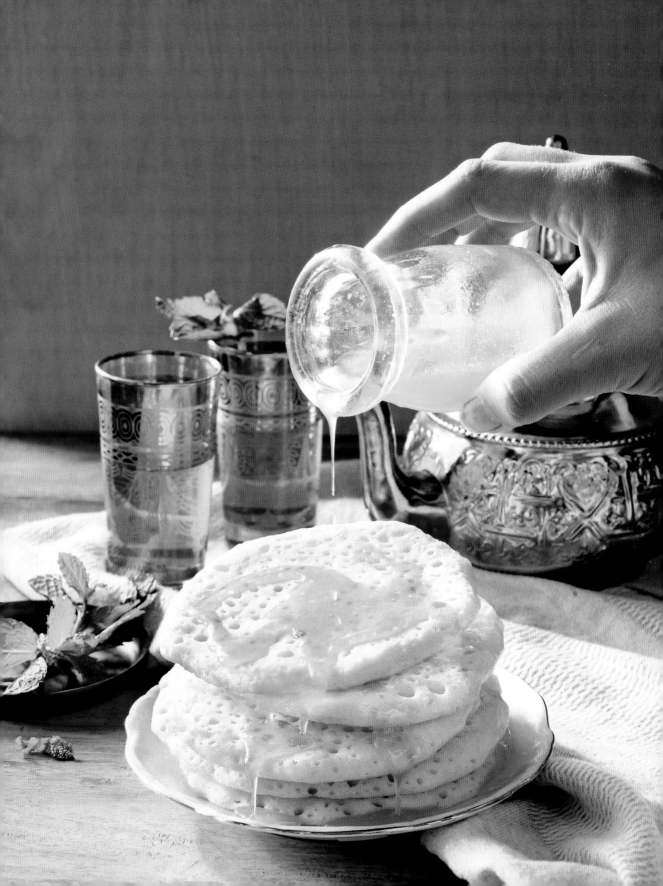

Orange Flower Water Honey Syrup

Makes about 1½ cups syrup

8 tablespoons (1 stick) unsalted butter

¾ cup honey

½ to 1 teaspoon kosher salt

2 to 4 teaspoons orange flower water, to taste

Melt together first three ingredients in a small saucepan over low heat and whisk until smooth.

Stir in orange flower water and serve warm.

THE INGREDIENTS in this Turkish breakfast dish look, at first glance, like a western omelet, minus the ham. But a few seasonings and cooking technique differentiate this egg dish and make *menemen* taste entirely different from its Rocky Mountain doppelgänger. Using smoked hot paprika, oregano, and slightly spicy green chiles plants this firmly in the eastern Mediterranean. And by cooking the vegetables until very soft and gently cooking the eggs until creamy, this is very different from an American-style scramble. The texture, in fact, reminds me of Taiwanese-style tomato eggs. This would be a perfect candidate for breakfast for dinner.

3 tablespoons extra-virgin olive oil

1 yellow onion, finely diced

½ teaspoon pimentón (smoked paprika), preferably hot

½ teaspoon dried oregano

1 cup seeded and finely diced slightly spicy green pepper, such as Anaheim or Hatch chile, or shishito or Italian sweet pepper

2 very ripe summer tomatoes, diced, or if not in season, ½ cup drained, canned diced tomatoes

Salt and freshly ground pepper

4 large eggs

MENEMEN (TURKISH SCRAMBLED EGGS WITH TOMATOES AND PEPPERS)

Serves 2 or 3

Heat olive oil in a nonstick skillet over medium heat, then add onion and cook, stirring frequently, until soft and translucent, 5 to 7 minutes.

Add pimentón and oregano and stir to coat onion.

Add green peppers and tomatoes, and season to taste with salt and black pepper. Cook, stirring often, until very soft, about 10 minutes.

Add beaten eggs, swirling to mingle with vegetables, and cook over low heat until just set, about 5 minutes, stirring gently with a spatula just a few times. When very softly set, remove from heat.

Serve immediately with crusty bread (olive bread would be a great choice).

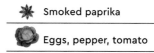

Smoked paprika

Eggs, pepper, tomato

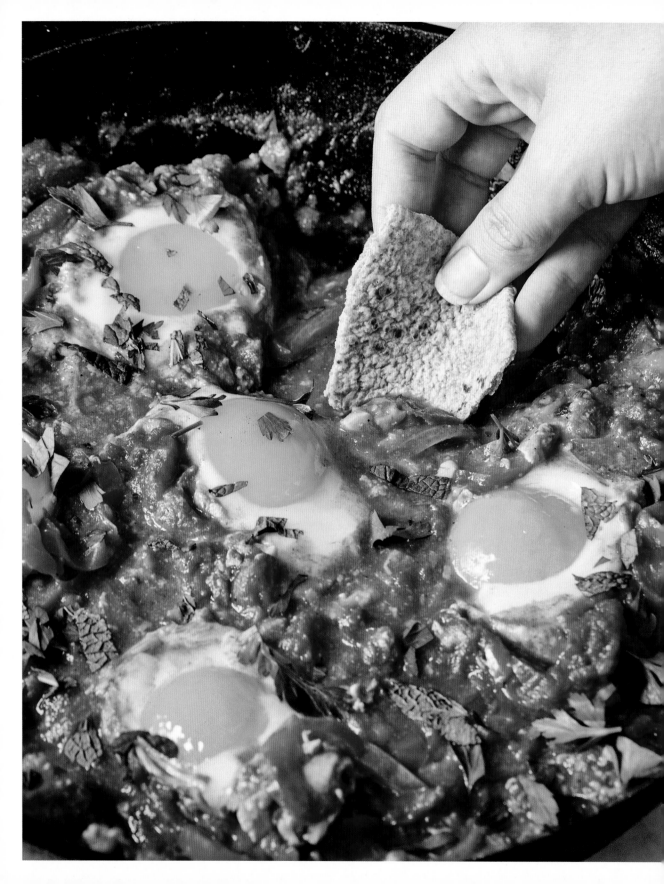

THIS DISH OF EGGS baked in a spiced tomato and pepper sauce is popular throughout the Middle East. I've used some of my favorite flavors from the spice market in Marrakesh, Morocco—including harissa, cumin, and preserved lemon. Shakshuka is traditionally served at breakfast but can be enjoyed at any time of day.

SHAKSHUKA

Serves 4 to 6

Heat olive oil in a cast-iron skillet or sauté pan with a lid over high heat. When oil is shimmery, add onion and bell pepper with a pinch of salt and sauté, stirring occasionally, for 10 minutes, or until vegetables are soft. Add garlic and cook for 30 seconds, or until fragrant. Add pimentón, cumin seeds, harissa, and cayenne and cook until fragrant, another 30 seconds, then add tomatoes. Lower heat to a simmer and cook, covered, for another 10 minutes. Add water, if needed, to get the consistency of pasta sauce. Stir in preserved lemon rind, then add salt and black pepper to taste.

Use a spoon to make a well in the sauce near the edge of the pan and crack one egg directly into well. Continue around pan, repeating the process for the remaining five eggs, with an inch or so between each egg. Cover, and continue to cook over low heat for 5 minutes, or until whites are set but yolks are still runny.

Garnish with chopped parsley and mint and serve immediately with wedges of warm pita or crusty bread (it's excellent with olive bread).

Remaining sauce can be used to cook another set of eggs, if desired.

2 tablespoons extra-virgin olive oil, plus more for garnish

1 onion, thinly sliced

1 red bell pepper, thinly sliced

Salt

3 garlic cloves, peeled and smashed

1 tablespoon pimentón (smoked paprika)

1 tablespoon cumin seeds

1 tablespoon harissa powder

¼ teaspoon cayenne pepper

1 (28-ounce) can whole peeled tomatoes, chopped

2 tablespoons minced preserved lemon rind

Freshly ground black pepper

6 large eggs

½ cup chopped fresh flat-leaf parsley leaves

½ cup chopped fresh mint leaves

❋ Cayenne, cumin, garlic, harissa, smoked paprika

 Bell pepper, eggs, lemon, herbs, tomato

2 pounds ripe tomatoes, roughly chopped

1 medium-size red bell pepper, roughly chopped

½ medium-size cucumber, peeled and roughly chopped

½ red onion, roughly chopped

⅓ cup extra-virgin olive oil, plus more for garnish (optional)

1 (½-inch-thick) slice white bread, torn into 1-inch pieces

3 tablespoons red wine vinegar

1 medium-size jalapeño pepper, seeded and roughly chopped

2 garlic cloves

½ teaspoon salt

Freshly ground black pepper

GAZPACHO is a classic Spanish tomato-based cold soup that dates back to ancient times. It was originally a peasant food and a good way to use up leftover bread and vegetables. The vinegar and garlic provide a lot of flavor with minimal added salt. This is meant to be a thick soup—if it is too thick to blend, add a bit of water, not tomato juice, which is a commonly made error that will alter the intended flavor. Think of this as a blended salad; it's refreshing on a hot day and comes together in minutes. *¡Salud!*

CLASSIC GAZPACHO

Serves 8

Reserving a few tablespoons each of bell pepper, cucumber, and red onion for garnish, combine tomatoes, bell pepper, cucumber, onion, olive oil, bread, vinegar, jalapeño, and garlic in a blender. Blend until smooth, adding up to ½ cup of water if necessary. (Work in batches if all ingredients can't fit in your blender at once.) Season with salt and black pepper to taste. Transfer to a pitcher.

Refrigerate for up to a few hours before serving or serve immediately, garnishing with reserved diced vegetables and a swirl of olive oil, if desired.

SPICEBOX KITCHEN

 Black pepper, chile pepper, garlic

Bell pepper, cucumber, tomato

2 navel oranges, or 1 navel and 2 blood oranges, plus ½ navel orange, for juicing

4 to 6 large fresh mint leaves, torn

2 tablespoons Marcona almonds, coarsely chopped

12 green pitted Spanish olives, halved lengthwise

GARNISHES

1 tablespoon extra-virgin olive oil

Flaky sea salt, such as Maldon

Aleppo or Calabrian pepper flakes, or crushed red pepper flakes

THIS SIMPLE and refreshing salad is a slightly unusual combination of ingredients and is visually stunning. The citrus and brininess of the olives really complement each other, with the crunch of the almonds adding texture (as well as richness). Most of the salty flavor comes from the olives, so you might not need to add much salt—something to keep in mind when you are using salty ingredients in a recipe.

SPANISH ORANGE AND OLIVE SALAD

Serves 4

Cut away peel and pith from all oranges, except the extra ½ orange, using a paring knife. Try to cut to preserve the round shape of each orange. Then, cut peeled oranges into ¼-inch-thick disks. Arrange orange slices on a small serving platter.

Scatter with mint, almonds, and olives, then squeeze juice of remaining ½ orange over the salad.

Garnish with a drizzle of olive oil and a sprinkle of sea salt and pepper flakes just before serving.

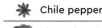 Chile pepper

Almonds, mint, olives, oranges

1 loaf crusty sourdough bread
or ciabatta

2 large, very ripe tomatoes
(any variety except Roma)

Olive oil

Salt and freshly ground black
pepper

OPTIONAL ACCOMPANIMENTS

2 hard-boiled eggs, sliced
crosswise

1 (5-ounce) can Italian tuna or
anchovies in olive oil, drained

½ cup cooked cannellini
beans

Your favorite olives, sliced

Thinly sliced red onion

Fresh mint and basil leaves

Pickled vegetables of your
choosing

FOR THE FIRST SEVERAL YEARS that we lived next door to Mario, a retired San Francisco police officer, I avoided him whenever I heard him come into his yard. Even in his eighties, Mario still had a commanding presence, with a ramrod-stiff posture and stern countenance. But when my kids were born, I saw a soft side of Mario. He started to hand all manner of presents for the kids over the fence; "Hello, girls!" he'd say, in a gentle voice. I relaxed a bit after realizing that Mario was a softie. Then, I started to get presents too. And I daresay that mine were even better than the kids': Mario's homegrown, vine-ripened tomatoes—some of the best tomatoes I've had. Mario traces his heritage to Malta, the tiny Mediterranean island nation off the coast of Italy. In honor of Mario's roots, here is a classic Maltese dish that relies upon the vine-ripened tomatoes of summer. This sandwich combines the Spanish *pan con tomate* with fillings reminiscent of the French salade niçoise. It turns out to be a perfect San Francisco meal—sourdough bread and vine-ripened, sun-kissed tomatoes lovingly handed over the fence by my Maltese neighbor.

MALTESE BREAD AND TOMATO SANDWICH

Serves 4 to 6

Slice bread into four sections, then slice each section in half.

Lightly toast sliced bread.

Halve tomatoes, then rub each slice of bread with a sliced tomato half, so that bread soaks up juice.

Drizzle with olive oil, and sprinkle with salt and pepper to taste. Stop here, if desired.

If you want to dress it up further, serve on a plate alongside an assortment of remaining ingredients, or layer into a sandwich.

✳ Black pepper

🌸 When all ingredients are used, this sandwich contains most of the elements of the Mediterranean diet— omega-3 fish, fiber-rich vegetables, and beans, and olives and olive oil.

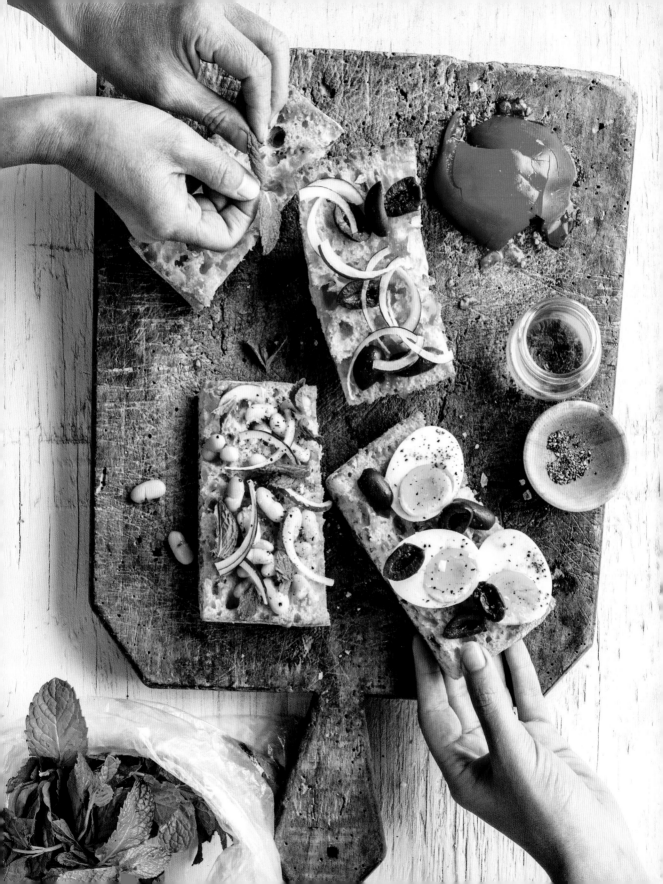

TOPPING (MAKES 2 CUPS)

2 teaspoons olive oil

1 medium-size yellow onion, chopped

Salt and freshly ground black pepper

3 garlic cloves, minced

2 tablespoons pine nuts

16 small pitted black or green olives, thinly sliced

¼ cup golden raisins or currants, soaked for 10 minutes in hot water and drained

1 bunch rainbow or red chard, leaves cut into ribbons, stems finely chopped

½ teaspoon crushed red pepper flakes

POLENTA ROUNDS

Olive oil, for pan

2 (18-ounce) tubes prepared polenta, each sliced into about 12 disks

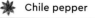

✳ Chile pepper

🌺 Polenta (cornmeal), rainbow chard

THIS RECIPE COMBINES a traditional chard dish served in Italy over Christmas and makes it into a festive appetizer. It also makes a lovely vegan entrée. The greens are cooked until delicately tender, with a savory and sweet taste and a texture that combines the chewiness of the raisins and the crunch of the pine nuts. I couldn't resist calling this "Eat the Rainbow" as a reminder of the best and simplest nutrition advice to ensure getting a variety of nutrients in your diet. You can substitute regular Swiss chard or other dark leafy greens, including kale or collards.

EAT THE RAINBOW CHARD POLENTA ROUNDS

Makes 24 rounds

Prepare topping: Heat oil in a medium-size skillet over medium heat. Add onion along with a pinch of salt and black pepper and sauté until softened. Add garlic and pine nuts and stir for a minute, or until slightly browned.

Add olives, raisins, and chard and sauté for 6 minutes, or until greens are tender.

Add red pepper flakes and stir for 2 more minutes.

Adjust salt to taste. Set aside.

Prepare polenta rounds: Heat a small amount of olive oil (just enough oil to thinly coat bottom) in a large, nonstick skillet and fry polenta disks over medium-high heat, about 5 minutes per side, until golden brown and lightly crisp on each side. (Do not use excess oil, or else polenta will get soggy and sticky.)

Top each round with a few spoonfuls of chard mixture. Serve hot or warm.

2 to 3 eggplants (about 2 pounds total)

4 garlic cloves, minced

Kosher salt

Juice of 1 to 2 lemons, to taste

¼ cup tahini

¼ cup extra-virgin olive oil, plus more for serving

¼ teaspoon pimentón (smoked paprika)

½ cup chopped fresh parsley leaves

BABA GHANOUJ (also spelled baba ghanoush) has origins in Lebanon. It is one of my favorite dips, with the great contrast of the smokiness of the eggplant with the creaminess of the tahini. Traditionally, the eggplant is cooked directly on a fire, which infuses it with smoky flavor. I add a little pimentón to ensure the smokiness of this version whether you cook it on the grill directly or use your broiler.

BABA GHANOUJ

Serves 6 as an appetizer

Roast eggplants: You'll get the best, smokiest flavor if you cook directly on a gas or charcoal grill. Cook until eggplants are completely tender (almost like a deflated balloon) and evenly charred on all sides, rotating occasionally with tongs. This will take 30 to 40 minutes. When done, wrap in foil and allow to rest for 15 minutes.

Alternatively, use the broiler. Preheat broiler to HIGH. Place eggplants on a foil-lined baking sheet and broil for about an hour, rotating occasionally with tongs, until they are completely tender and their skin is evenly charred, as above. Wrap, using the same foil, and allow to rest for 15 minutes.

After eggplants rest, open foil, cut each eggplant in half lengthwise, and place on a collapsible metal steamer basket or colander placed over a bowl. Allow juices to drain for at least 15 minutes, collapsing steamer basket or using a spoon to press and squeeze out liquid. (Liquid is bitter, so you want to drain as much as you can.)

Meanwhile, make a garlic paste by placing minced garlic in a mortar, adding a sprinkle of salt, and working it in with the pestle, or by using the side of a chef's knife to rub the garlic against salt.

Use a spoon to carefully scoop flesh from eggplant skins, being careful not to include skin, and place in a medium-size bowl.

Add garlic paste, lemon juice, tahini, olive oil, and pimentón to eggplant and stir vigorously to create a chunky paste. It should look light and creamy. (Alternatively, pulse a few times in a food processor.) Adjust salt to taste. Garnish with parsley and a drizzle of olive oil, if desired, and serve with pita bread and crudités.

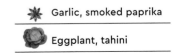

Garlic, smoked paprika

Eggplant, tahini

2 red bell peppers, or
1 (7-ounce) jar roasted red
peppers, drained

1 cup walnuts

3 garlic cloves, minced

Juice of 1 lemon

2 tablespoons pomegranate
molasses

1 teaspoon ground cumin

1 teaspoon red pepper flakes

2 tablespoons extra-virgin
olive oil

Salt

 Chile pepper, cumin,
garlic

Bell peppers,
pomegranate, walnuts

I FIRST CAME UPON a recipe for *muhammara* when I was asked to bring three dips to a Thanksgiving potluck. I remember wanting to impress, as my hosts were sophisticated cooks who also happened to have published several cookbooks. (No pressure there!) Although I had never had muhammara before, when I saw a recipe for it, I knew it would be a winner. With its base of red bell peppers, muhammara gets its creaminess from walnuts, and a little bit of sweetness and tanginess from pomegranate molasses (if you can't find it store-bought, see page 251 to make your own).

MUHAMMARA (LEBANESE RED PEPPER, WALNUT, AND POMEGRANATE MOLASSES DIP)

Makes 2 cups dip

Roast bell peppers, if using fresh: Preheat oven to 450°F. Place whole bell peppers in a baking dish and bake for about 30 minutes, rotating once or twice for evenness, until their skin has blackened and peppers are soft to touch. Remove from oven and put right away into a small resealable plastic bag and seal tightly. Let rest for about 5 minutes, then remove from bag and quickly peel off skin (be careful, peppers will still be quite hot). Remove seeds, then cut peppers into long strips and set aside until ready to use.

Toast walnuts: Preheat oven to 350°F. Spread walnuts on a baking sheet and toast in oven for 10 to 15 minutes, or until golden and aromatic. Alternatively, toast in a dry skillet over low heat, tossing frequently. Allow to cool before finely chopping and combining with other ingredients.

Combine roasted peppers, walnuts, garlic, lemon juice, pomegranate molasses, cumin, and red pepper flakes in a food processor and process until mixture is smooth. Then with motor running, add oil gradually so it can emulsify rather than separate. Transfer muhammara to a bowl and add salt to taste. Serve at room temperature with pita.

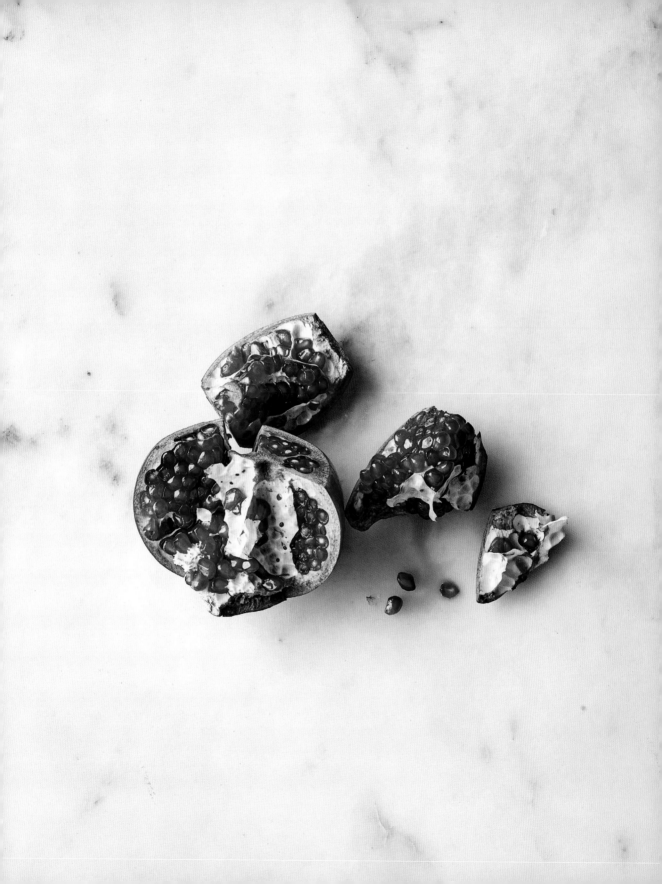

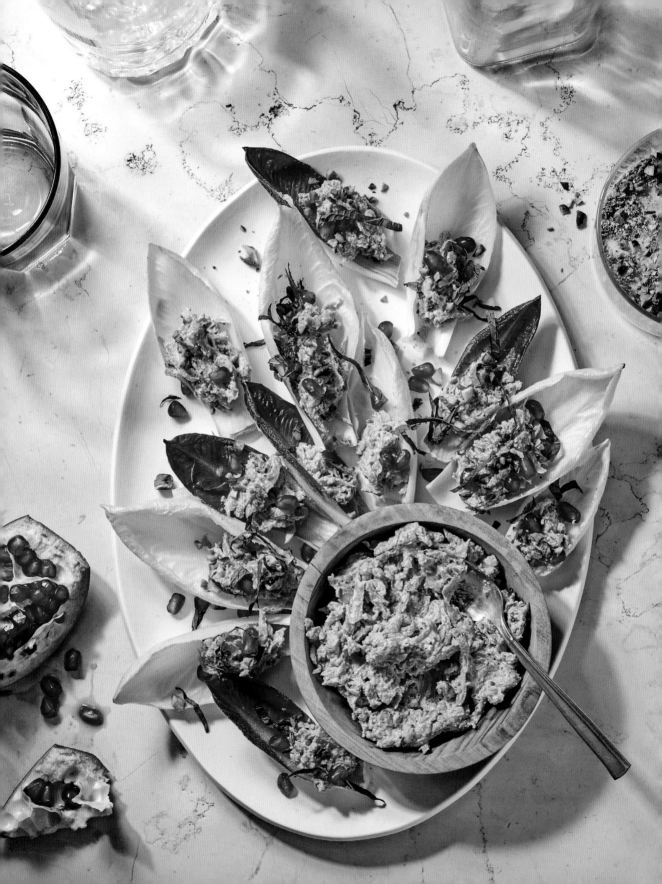

NEW TO ENDIVE? These pale green or purple-tinged leaves were made for filling for easy and elegant appetizers. Some find endive to be bitter, so choosing a filling that balances the bitterness is key. The creaminess of the yogurt, sweetness of the carrots, and slight heat of the harissa are a perfect complement.

The yogurt dip was inspired by Turkish Carrot Yogurt Dip in *The Vegetable Butcher* by Cara Mangini (New York: Workman, 2016).

ENDIVE LEAVES WITH HARISSA CARROT YOGURT

Makes about 36 leaves

Prepare dip: Heat olive oil in a medium-size skillet over medium heat until shimmering. Add carrots and cook, stirring frequently, for 3 to 5 minutes, or until they start to soften.

Add pistachios and salt, then cook for an additional 3 to 4 minutes, stirring constantly, until carrots start to brown. Add garlic and cook for another minute, or until fragrant. Remove from heat and allow to cool for 5 minutes.

Put yogurt in a medium-size bowl, then add cooled carrot mixture and harissa. Stir together and adjust seasoning to taste.

To fill endive leaves: Hold each leaf in one hand, facing upward like a boat. Add a teaspoon-size dollop to bottom/root end (only) of each endive leaf. Arrange prettily on a platter, then garnish each filled leaf with a few pomegranate arils, minced herbs, a few chopped pistachios, and a pinch of salt.

YOGURT DIP

¼ cup extra-virgin olive oil

12 ounces carrots (3 to 5 carrots), peeled and grated coarsely

⅓ cup unsalted pistachios, chopped, plus more for garnish

1 teaspoon fine kosher salt

4 medium-size garlic cloves, peeled and minced

2 cups plain Greek yogurt

1 teaspoon harissa (if unavailable, use paprika and Aleppo or cayenne pepper to taste)

———

6 heads endive, carefully separated into leaves; choose the largest/crispest

GARNISHES

Pomegranate arils

Minced carrot greens, fresh parsley, or fresh mint

Flaky salt

Garlic, harissa

Carrots, endive, pomegranate, pistachios, yogurt

2 pounds eggplant

1 tablespoon olive oil, plus more for brushing eggplant and finishing salad

Salt

3 garlic cloves, crushed

1½ teaspoons sweet paprika

1½ teaspoons ground cumin

1 teaspoon ground cinnamon

¼ teaspoon crushed red pepper flakes, or more to taste

2 cups peeled and chopped tomatoes

½ cup water

1 teaspoon salt

Freshly ground black pepper

1 bay leaf

1 lemon

¼ to ½ cup fresh cilantro (a large handful), chopped

THIS WARM SALAD combines roasted eggplant, tomatoes, and warm spices and can be enjoyed as a side or alone with lots of bread. It's one of the more common salads you'll be served to start a meal in Morocco. The cinnamon is not typical, but I added it because this was the magic touch in my favorite version of this dish. It was prepared this way at Café la Tolérance, located in Essaouira, an ancient seaport on Morocco's west coast, where we enjoyed a live performance of *gnaoua* music, a mystical Sufi musical tradition from North and West Africa, and had a fascinating conversation with the owner about the culture and politics of Morocco and North Africa.

ZAALOUK (MOROCCAN ROASTED EGGPLANT SALAD)

Serves 4 to 6

Preheat oven to 450°F. Line a large baking sheet with parchment.

Peel eggplant, leaving a few strips of skin for color and structure, and slice lengthwise into ½-inch-thick slices. Brush both sides with olive oil, arrange in a single layer on prepared baking sheet, sprinkle with a pinch of salt, and roast in oven until slices are soft and browned, around 35 minutes.

Heat 1 tablespoon of olive oil in a large sauté pan with a lid over medium-high heat, add garlic, and cook for around 30 seconds. Add paprika, cumin, cinnamon, and red pepper flakes and bloom spices in hot oil for 10 seconds before adding chopped tomatoes, water, salt, black pepper to taste, and bay leaf. Let sauce simmer for 5 minutes.

While sauce is simmering, slice roasted eggplant into bite-size pieces. Add them to sauté pan, stirring to combine. Lower heat to medium-low, cover, and let simmer for another 5 minutes. Eggplant should now be fully cooked and tender but should still maintain its shape. Remove from heat, squeeze in lemon juice to taste, and sprinkle with chopped cilantro. Adjust seasoning to taste. Serve hot, or at room temperature, with a drizzle of olive oil and another squeeze of lemon juice.

Cinnamon, chile pepper, cumin, garlic, paprika

Eggplant, tomatoes

6 Roma tomatoes

Salt

½ cup coarsely chopped
fresh flat-leaf parsley

1 serrano chile, seeded and
minced

1 teaspoon ground cumin

1 tablespoon white vinegar

1 tablespoon olive oil

Freshly ground black pepper

ONE OF THE HIGHLIGHTS of my trip to Morocco was a guided tour
to the Atlas Mountains, which included a stop for a camel ride. My
camel, a five-year-old named Shakira, was as gentle as she could be,
but I still found myself higher up than expected, with a bit of a rocky
ride. Our tour guide, Bachir, came from a line of Berber nomads in the
Sahara known as the Tuaregs or Blue Men, so named for the color of
their turbans. Tuaregs rely on camels for transportation, for milk, and
sometimes for meat, and Bachir waxed poetically about the camels
he had known and cared for in his lifetime. At the end of our tour of
the Berber villages in the Atlas Mountains, we stopped for a leisurely
traditional lunch, prepared by an elderly woman named Habiba. She
made the best food we had on our entire trip. It was quite traditional,
beginning with bread and olives and several salads, including this
classic tomato salad, followed by a few tagines. This salad resembles
Mexican pico de gallo in appearance, but with a very different flavor
profile, with parsley instead of cilantro, vinegar instead of lime juice,
and the Moroccan accents of olive oil and cumin. Salting the tomatoes
to concentrate their flavor is a key step; do not skip it.

SALADE MAROCAINE
(MOROCCAN TOMATO SALAD)

Serves 4 to 6

Dice tomatoes into ¼-inch pieces and place in a colander. Sprinkle
with salt, toss gently, and allow to drain for 30 minutes. This will drain
off excess liquid and concentrate tomato flavor, as well as tenderize
tomatoes.

Combine parsley, serrano chile, cumin, white vinegar, and olive oil in
a medium-size bowl. Season with salt and black pepper to taste. Add
tomatoes, mix thoroughly, and serve at room temperature.

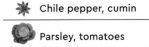

Chile pepper, cumin

Parsley, tomatoes

1 acorn squash or delicata, or any other winter squash

2 tablespoons extra-virgin olive oil

Salt and freshly ground black pepper

Harissa powder

10 to 12 dates, pitted and thinly sliced

GARNISHES

Lemon-Tahini Dressing (page 110)

Handful of fresh mint leaves, torn or coarsely chopped

Pomegranate arils

THIS IS A COLORFUL fall salad that would make a lovely addition to a Thanksgiving spread. The recipe came about when I was doing an inventory of my pantry and refrigerator and wanted to do something different with my lemon-tahini dressing. I use acorn squash wedges, but you can substitute any variety of winter squash in any shape you like, or consider substituting other roasted root vegetables the next time you're doing meal prep.

ROASTED ACORN SQUASH SALAD WITH DATES AND POMEGRANATE

Serves 4

Preheat oven to 400°F. Line a rimmed baking sheet with foil or parchment.

Wash and scrub acorn squash and dry. Cut in half lengthwise, then scoop out seeds and stringy parts with a spoon. Place squash halves cut side down and cut each half into wedges about 1 inch thick. Put squash wedges into a large bowl, drizzle with olive oil, and sprinkle with a few pinches of salt, pepper, and harissa powder. Toss until evenly coated.

Place squash wedges on prepared baking sheet and bake for about 20 minutes, turning wedges over at about 10-minute point, or until tender but still holding their shape. If the tip of a paring knife or a fork can't pierce flesh easily, roast for another 5 to 10 minutes. Remove from oven and allow to cool.

Once squash has cooled, arrange onto a platter and scatter with sliced dates. Drizzle desired amount of dressing, and garnish extravagantly with torn mint and pomegranate arils.

 Harissa

Acorn squash (winter squash), dates

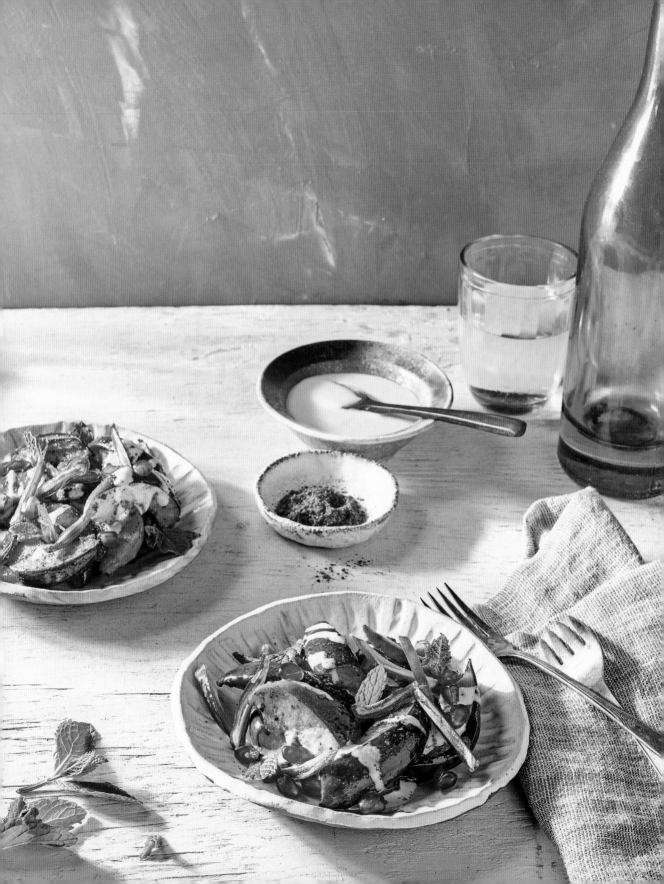

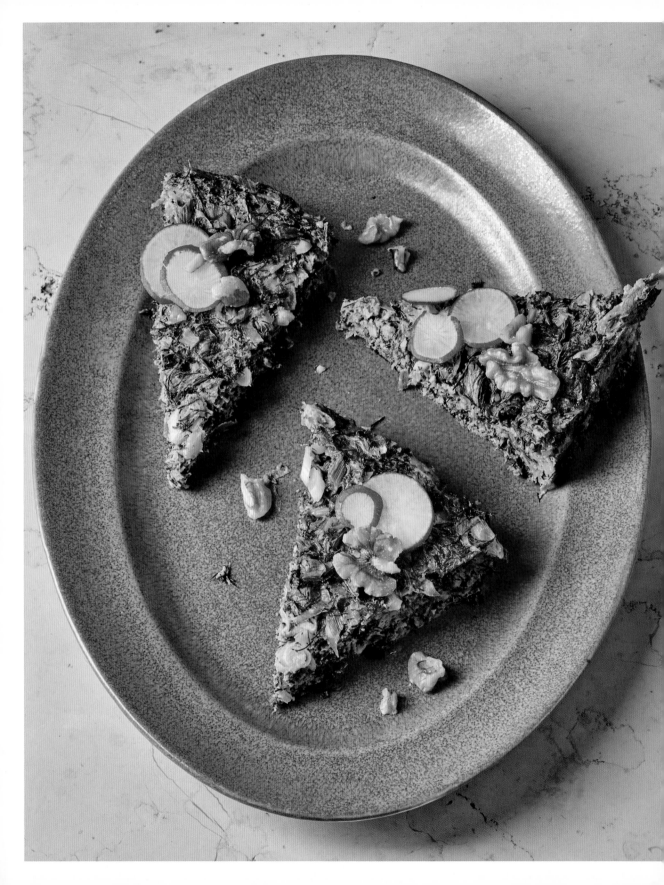

I TEACH THIS RECIPE in my cooking classes not only because it's delicious, but to illustrate the idea of using herbs for more than garnish, to enjoy them as you might eat green leafy vegetables. Meals in Iran, where herbs are used generously, start with *sabzi khordan*, a plate of fresh herbs, lavash, walnuts, radishes, and feta. *Kuku sabzi* is an everyday meal but is also one of the dishes made during Nowruz (Persian New Year) because the green herbs symbolize rebirth, and the eggs, fertility and happiness for the year to come. Walnuts and barberries are optional. *Zereshk*, the Persian name for dried fruit barberries, are tart berries available online or in Middle Eastern markets. They can be replaced with unsweetened dried cranberries, currants, or chopped sour cherries.

KUKU SABZI (PERSIAN HERB FRITTATA)

Serves 8

Whisk together eggs, fenugreek, baking powder, salt, pepper, and turmeric in a large bowl. Fold in scallions, chopped herbs, walnuts, and barberries or other berries, if using.

Heat 2 to 4 tablespoons oil (enough to cover bottom of pan) in an 8- or 10-inch nonstick, ovenproof skillet with a lid over low heat; cast iron is great for this recipe. Pour in egg mixture, then flatten top with a spatula to distribute herbs evenly. Cook, covered, for 5 to 10 minutes, or until bottom of kuku is set (check by lifting edge with a spatula).

Continue to cook on stovetop or use a broiler. If finishing on stovetop, when bottom is set, run spatula around perimeter of pan to loosen kuku. Invert kuku by placing a plate or baking sheet slightly larger than pan on top, then flipping covered pan over. Remove pan, then slide inverted kuku, cooked side up, back into pan to cook other side. Cook for another 5 to 10 minutes, uncovered, or until kuku is cooked through. Alternatively, once bottom is set, kuku can be placed (without flipping) under a broiler for a few minutes until just set. This is my preferred method, as it will give it a more vibrant green top.

Cut into wedges and place on a serving platter. Garnish with (more!) fresh herbs, radishes, barberries, and walnuts.

5 large eggs

1 tablespoon dried fenugreek leaves, crushed

1 teaspoon baking powder

½ teaspoon fine kosher salt

1 teaspoon freshly ground black pepper

½ teaspoon ground turmeric

1 bunch scallions, thinly sliced

1½ cups fresh parsley, leaves and small stems, finely chopped

1½ cups fresh cilantro, leaves and small stems, finely chopped

1½ cups fresh dill or mint leaves, finely chopped

⅓ cup walnuts, toasted and finely chopped

1 to 2 tablespoons dried barberries, unsweetened dried cranberries, currants or chopped dried sour cherries, soaked in water until soft, then drained

Canola or other vegetable oil, for frying

Optional garnishes: fresh herbs, sliced radishes, additional barberries, walnuts

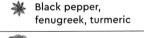

✴ Black pepper, fenugreek, turmeric

🥬 Eggs, herbs, walnuts

2 red beets

1 (15-ounce) can low-sodium
or no-salt-added chickpeas,
drained and rinsed

2½ tablespoons tahini

2 garlic cloves

Juice of ½ lemon

1 teaspoon kosher salt

½ teaspoon ground cumin

1 teaspoon ground coriander

¼ cup olive oil

Garnishes: olive oil, chopped
fresh parsley, and dukkah or
za'atar (see pages 252 and
253 to make your own)

THIS BEET-BASED HUMMUS is a festive fuchsia-hued version of the familiar chickpea and tahini spread. The sweet earthiness of beets is mellowed by the creaminess of chickpeas, nuttiness of tahini, and acidity of the lemon juice. Adds a pop of color to your meze platter!

ROASTED BEET HUMMUS

Makes 2½ cups hummus

Preheat oven to 400°F.

Remove greens from beets, reserving for another purpose, then wash and dry unpeeled beets. Wrap each beet in foil, making individual packets. Make sure to leave a little room around each beet and then seal tightly, so that they can steam inside their foil wrappers.

Place wrapped beets on a baking sheet and roast in oven for 45 to 60 minutes, or until tender. (Check for tenderness with a fork.) Remove from oven and allow to cool for about an hour.

Wearing disposable gloves, peel cooled, roasted beets. Their skins should slip off easily by rubbing with your fingers. Cut beets into large chunks.

Place beets with remaining ingredients in a food processor and process until you have a smooth paste, adding water if needed. Adjust lemon juice and salt to taste.

Serve in a wide bowl. Use a spoon to create a well, and garnish with a drizzle of olive oil, and scatter with parsley and dukkah or za'atar.

Coriander, cumin,
garlic

Beets, chickpeas,
tahini

1 bunch asparagus

Olive oil

Salt and freshly ground black pepper

Gremolata (page 247)

ONE OF MY FAVORITE WAYS to enjoy asparagus is quickly grilled. Just a few minutes of direct heat brings out its succulence and sweetness. A drizzle of olive oil and a sprinkling of salt and pepper are already delicious, but for something a little more special, top with freshly made gremolata, an Italian herb condiment, for a perfect summer backyard grilling treat.

GRILLED ASPARAGUS WITH GREMOLATA

Serves 4

Preheat grill for high heat.

Lightly coat asparagus spears with olive oil. Season with salt and pepper to taste.

Grill over high heat for 2 to 3 minutes, turning once, to desired tenderness.

Transfer to a platter and sprinkle with gremolata. Serve hot or at room temperature.

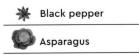

✳ Black pepper

🌹 Asparagus

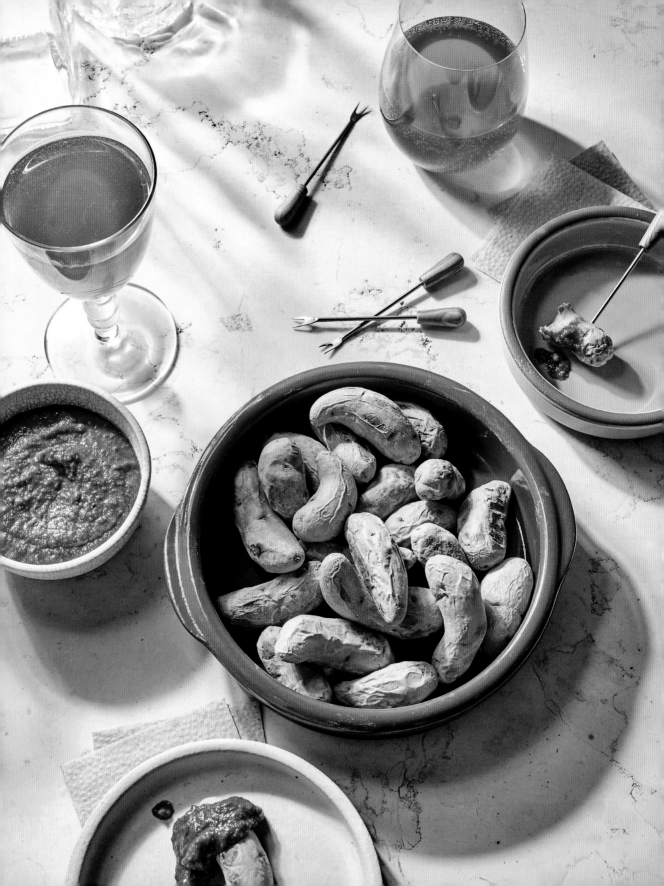

1 pound fingerling potatoes, well scrubbed

¾ cup kosher salt

1 recipe Romesco (page 246)

THE CANARY ISLANDS, hundreds of miles from Spain near the northwest coast of Africa, has its own cuisine, influenced by its tropical climate and location near Africa. When Spain colonized the islands, it also brought over New World foods from its trade routes, including potatoes. This dish is a classic of Canary Island cuisine, served as a starter or a side to most foods. These potatoes were traditionally boiled in sea water. This stovetop version uses a large amount of salt to replicate that taste. Don't worry; the potatoes do not absorb the salt, due the barrier of the potato skin, but instead will taste of the sea, with a creamy interior.

CANARY ISLAND WRINKLED POTATOES (PAPAS ARRUGADAS) WITH ROMESCO

Serves 4 as a side dish

Place potatoes in a pot and add enough water to cover.

Add salt and stir to dissolve.

Bring to a boil, then lower heat to medium and cook, partially covered, until tender when pierced with a fork, about 8 minutes.

Once tender, pour out water and put pot over low heat, stirring or shaking periodically until skins have "wrinkled" on all sides, about 10 minutes.

Serve with romesco.

Potatoes

1¾ cups water

1 cup uncooked bulgur

1 teaspoon salt

2 tablespoons unsalted
butter or vegan butter
(I recommend Miyoko's)

2 carrots, peeled and
julienned

½ onion, thinly sliced

¼ cup sultanas (golden
raisins)

3 pitted dates, sliced into
¼-inch slivers

¼ cup toasted whole
almonds, skin on

¼ teaspoon ground
cinnamon

⅛ teaspoon cayenne pepper

Garnish: chopped fresh
flat-leaf parsley

THIS RECIPE MAKES an excellent sweet and savory accompaniment
to grilled fish, meats, or roasted vegetables. It can also be used as a
stuffing for roasted acorn squash for a hearty vegetarian main dish. Its
base is bulgur, a cracked whole wheat that cooks quickly, maintains
a pleasantly firm texture, and has a nutty, hearty taste that is really
complemented by the sweetness of the fruits.

TURKISH BULGUR PILAF WITH SPICED ALMONDS, DATES, AND SULTANAS

Serves 6

Bring water to a boil in a small saucepan, add bulgur and ¾ teaspoon
salt, stir, and bring back to a boil. Lower heat to a simmer, cover, and
cook until all water is absorbed, checking after 10 minutes. Then,
fluff with a spoon and cover for at least 5 minutes, until all moisture
has been absorbed. Keep covered until ready to add to remaining
ingredients.

Meanwhile, melt butter in a large skillet over low heat. Then, add
carrots, onion, sultanas, and dates with remaining ¼ teaspoon of salt
and cook until softened, about 3 minutes, stirring occasionally. Stir in
almonds, cinnamon, and cayenne and continue to cook until fragrant,
another minute or two.

Add cooked bulgur to carrot mixture and stir until evenly distributed.
Adjust salt to taste, then garnish with parsley and serve immediately.

 Cayenne, cinnamon

Almonds, bulgur, carrots

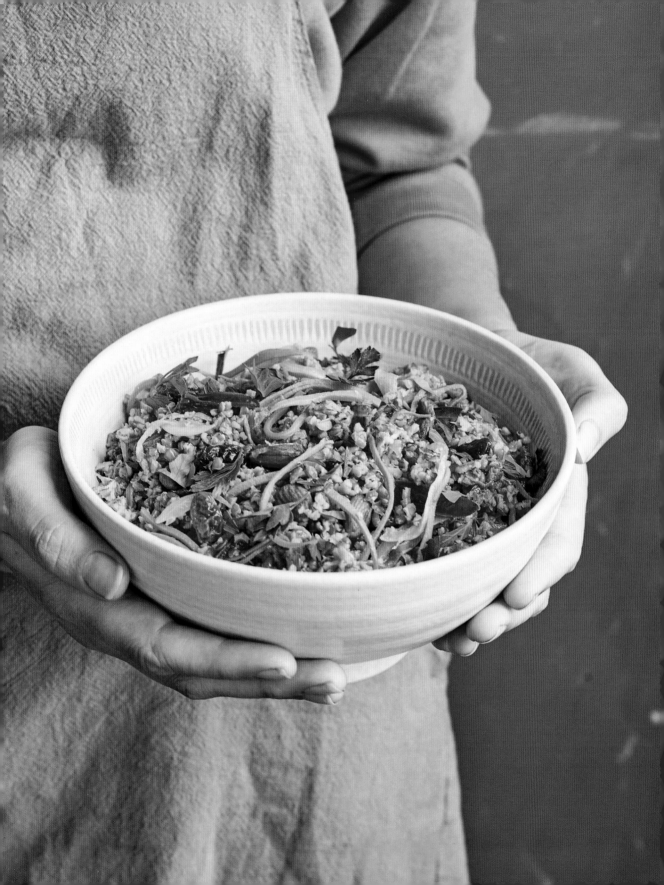

4 cups unsalted vegetable stock

3 cups water

1 pound red beets

2 tablespoons olive oil

1 tablespoon unsalted butter or vegan butter (I recommend Miyoko's)

1 medium-size onion, finely chopped

2 teaspoons kosher salt

Freshly ground black pepper

1½ cups Arborio rice

¼ cup white wine

2 tablespoons fresh dill, chopped, plus additional fronds for garnish

Juice of 1 lemon

THIS IS A DRAMATICALLY HUED RISOTTO—scarlet red—with a robust flavor that combines that of borscht with a classic risotto. I developed this recipe for a cooking class featuring heart-healthy beets, which was held in February, both American Heart Month and the month of Valentine's Day, hence the red beets. Although the combination may be surprising, it works well. The salty, savory, creamy risotto base tones down the earthy sweetness of beets, and the grated beets cook down into a similar texture to the rice grains. *Note*: Although Arborio rice is not whole grain, I would not substitute whole-grain rice as it won't give the same creaminess. The added nutrition from the beets, which includes fiber, balances out some of what is nutritionally missing from this refined rice.

BEET RISOTTO

Serves 4 to 6

Combine stock and water in a large pot and bring to a boil over high heat, then lower heat to low and keep covered, simmering as you prepare other risotto ingredients.

Meanwhile, peel beets, then coarsely shred with large holes of a box grater. I recommend wearing gloves! (*Tip*: If you don't wear gloves, you can use lemon juice to remove incriminating beet stains from your hands.)

Heat oil in a Dutch oven or wide sauté pan over medium-high heat. Melt 1½ teaspoons of butter in oil, stirring occasionally, until butter melts. Add onion and sauté until softened and translucent, about 5 minutes. Add beets, 1 teaspoon of salt, and ½ teaspoon of pepper and sauté until beets are softened, about 10 minutes.

Add rice and stir until coated completely with beet mixture. Add wine and stir constantly, about 2 minutes, or until wine is completely absorbed, then add 1½ cups of stock mixture and 1 teaspoon of salt.

❋ Black pepper

🥬 Beets

continued ⟶

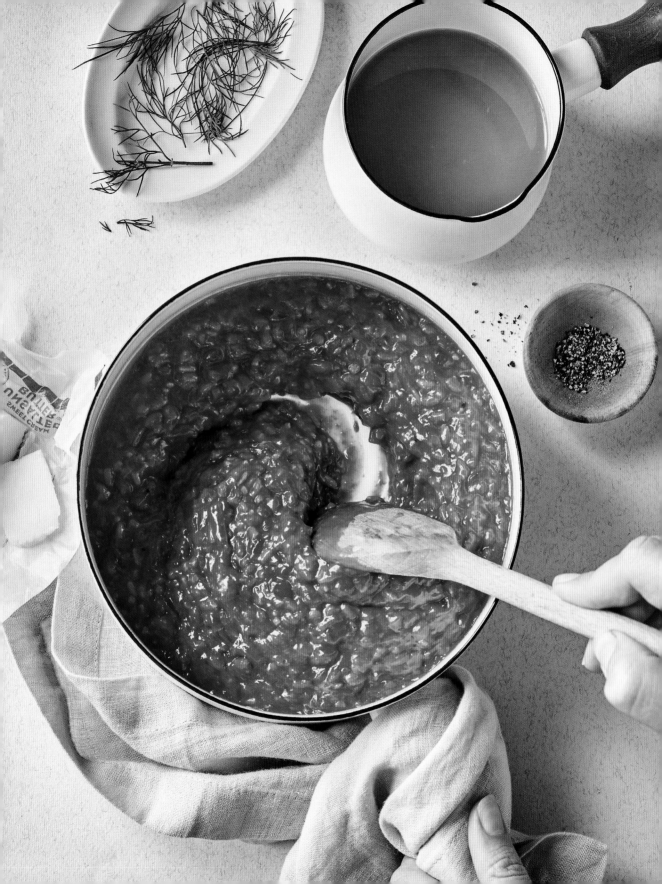

Lower heat to low and simmer, stirring constantly, until liquid has evaporated. Continue adding stock mixture, 1 cup at a time, stirring constantly and adding additional stock mixture after each addition is absorbed. Continue until rice is tender but still al dente, 30 to 40 minutes. (You might not use all of stock mixture, depending on how juicy your beets are. Stop adding when rice is al dente and you have a creamy sauce. Risotto should be *alla onde*, meaning that it can be jiggled like a wave, not solid and gloppy.)

To finish, turn off heat and stir in remaining 1½ teaspoons of butter until melted, then stir in chopped dill and lemon juice. Adjust salt and pepper to taste and garnish with additional dill.

8 ounces pasta, any shape (best if whole grain)

1 (4.4-ounce) can sardines (can be omitted if vegetarian/vegan; substitute 2 tablespoons capers, for brininess, and 2 tablespoons olive oil)

1 cup cherry or grape tomatoes, halved

1 (15-ounce) can white beans, such as cannellini, no-salt-added if possible, drained and rinsed

About 3 tablespoons chopped fresh mint, basil, or flat-leaf parsley

Pinch of salt

Freshly ground black pepper

Crushed red pepper flakes

ON A BUSY DAY, you might not cook if you haven't had a chance to get groceries. Or you might, if you have a well-stocked pantry. This is one of my back-pocket recipes for those busy days when having a stocked pantry is the difference between ordering takeout and being able to put together a delicious, balanced, and economical meal on the table. It may seem basic, but the flavors blend beautifully—and pack a nutritional punch (sardines are inexpensive, environmentally sustainable, low in mercury, and a great source of heart-healthy omega-3 fatty acids, among other nutrients).

PANTRY PASTA WITH CHERRY TOMATOES, WHITE BEANS, AND SARDINES

Serves 4 to 6

Cook pasta until al dente, then drain, reserving a cup of pasta cooking water.

In the same pot you used to cook pasta, combine cooked pasta with sardines, breaking up sardines with your spoon or spatula into bite-size chunks, and add sardine oil to pasta. Add some of the reserved pasta water to make a sauce with the sardine oil to coat pasta. Toss tomatoes, beans, mint, plus salt, black pepper, and red pepper flakes to taste and serve warm.

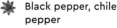

✳ Black pepper, chile pepper

Cannellini beans, sardines, tomatoes

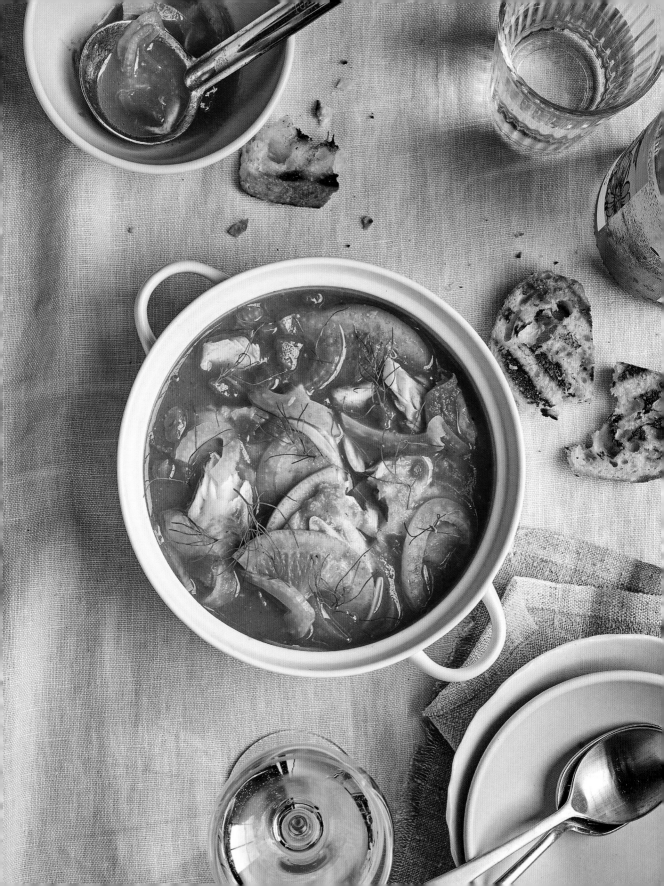

THIS IS A CLASSIC Mediterranean fish stew that tastes complex but comes together very quickly. It has fresh flavors from fennel, orange, and saffron. Saffron is expensive, but you don't need a lot and can buy it in bulk. It's worth it for this dish. You'll definitely want to have some crusty bread to sop up the fragrant broth.

SAFFRON-SCENTED MEDITERRANEAN FISH AND FENNEL STEW

Serves 2

Soak saffron in hot water for 20 minutes. This will bring out its flavor.

Meanwhile, prepare braising liquid: Heat olive oil in a Dutch oven or large skillet with a lid over medium-low heat and gently cook garlic until fragrant, less than a minute.

Add wine, water, tomato paste, diced tomatoes, and saffron in its liquid to skillet and stir well. Add fennel and orange slices and simmer over low heat, covered, for about 15 minutes, or until fennel is soft. Add additional water, if needed, to have about an inch of broth. Add salt to taste.

Season both sides of fish with salt and pepper and cut into 3-inch chunks (about four pieces per average-size fillet). Add fish pieces to braising liquid, partially submerging them.

Simmer, covered, over low heat for 7 to 10 minutes, checking for doneness after 5 minutes. When fish is opaque, it's done. Do not overcook.

To serve, first spoon some of braising liquid onto rimmed plate or shallow bowl, then top with a piece of fish. Garnish with reserved fennel fronds or other fresh herbs. Serve with olive oil–brushed grilled or toasted bread.

½ teaspoon saffron threads mixed with 2 tablespoons hot water

2 tablespoons extra-virgin olive oil

5 garlic cloves, thinly sliced

⅔ cup dry white wine

1 cup water

2 tablespoons tomato paste

1 (14.5-ounce) can no-salt-added diced tomatoes

1 fennel bulb, trimmed, cored, halved, then thinly sliced lengthwise, fronds reserved for later use

1 small navel orange, thinly sliced into 5 slices, rind on

Salt

1 pound skinless white fish fillet, such as cod, snapper, or halibut

Freshly ground black pepper to taste

Crusty bread, brushed with olive oil and grilled or toasted, for serving

Garlic, saffron

Fennel, fish, oranges, tomatoes

1 head cauliflower

1 tablespoon olive oil

A few pinches of salt

1 teaspoon garlic powder

1 teaspoon pimentón
(smoked paprika)

1 recipe Romesco (page 246)

Garnish: chopped fresh flat-
leaf parsley

CAULIFLOWER, though humble and pale in appearance, is a cruciferous vegetable with nutritional benefits comparable to kale's. And its architecture gives it another superpower: making a vegetable substitute for steaks. Its mild flavor is also a benefit, making it a best supporting actor for flavorful sauces, including romesco. This recipe seasons the cauliflower with garlic powder and smoked paprika, to mirror the flavors of the accompanying romesco.

SMOKY CAULIFLOWER STEAK WITH ROMESCO

Serves 2 to 4, depending on size of cauliflower

Preheat oven to 400°F. Line a baking sheet with parchment.

Cut cauliflower into steaks: Starting at the top center of the cauliflower head, cut 1-inch-thick slices, cutting down through stem end, so that each cross-section has the shape of cauliflower. An average-size cauliflower will yield two steaks. Reserve the rest of the cauliflower for another use.

Brush each side of cauliflower steaks with olive oil, then sprinkle with salt, garlic powder, and pimentón.

Place seasoned cauliflower steaks on prepared baking sheet and roast until tender, 8 to 10 minutes per each side. Check with a fork for doneness—should be tender, but not falling apart.

To serve, spoon some romesco onto the center of each of two dinner plates, then place a cauliflower steak on top and garnish with chopped parsley.

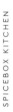

 Garlic, smoked paprika

Cauliflower

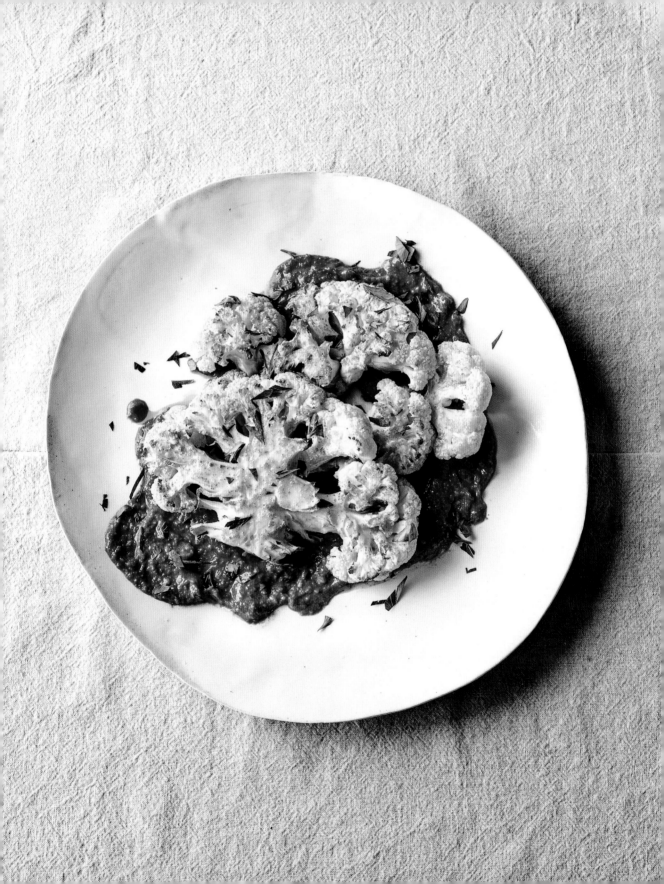

3 to 4 tablespoons extra-virgin olive oil, plus more for garnish (optional)

10 ounces fresh baby spinach

2 thick slices day-old bread, crusts removed, cubed

3 garlic cloves, chopped

1 teaspoon ground cumin

¼ to ½ teaspoon cayenne pepper

Freshly ground black pepper

2 tablespoons sherry vinegar or red wine vinegar

½ cup water

2 (15-ounce) cans no-salt-added chickpeas, drained and rinsed

¾ teaspoon kosher salt

1 teaspoon pimentón (smoked paprika), plus more for garnish (optional)

✳ Black pepper, cayenne, cumin, garlic, smoked paprika

🥬 Chickpeas, spinach

ANDALUCIA, in southern Spain, is known for flamenco and tapas. This classic tapas dish is a very satisfying vegan recipe with robust flavor from the garlic and spices. It can be served hot or warm, or make it an appetizer by serving on grilled toasts, if desired.

SPANISH SPINACH AND CHICKPEAS

Serves 4 as an entrée, 8 as an appetizer

Heat 2 tablespoons of olive oil in a large sauté pan over medium high heat.

Add spinach and sauté until just wilted. Transfer to a plate, straining off any liquid.

Add another 1 to 2 tablespoons of oil to pan and add cubed bread. Fry until bread is browned and crispy on each side. Lower heat to low, add garlic, cumin, cayenne, and black pepper, and sauté for a couple of minutes, until fragrant.

Transfer seasoned bread to a food processor and add vinegar and water. Process until you have a thick paste. Transfer paste to sauté pan and add chickpeas.

Stir gently until chickpeas are fully coated by sauce. Add additional water, if needed, to thin into a sauce.

Return spinach to pan and stir gently until evenly incorporated.

Season with salt, additional black pepper, and pimentón and stir to combine.

Serve hot or warm, and garnish, if desired, with a drizzle of additional olive oil and sprinkle of additional smoked paprika.

To enjoy as an appetizer, thickly slice rustic bread, brush with olive oil and grill on both sides, then top each toast with a few spoonfuls of this dish.

THIS IS ONE OF the simplest vegetable stews, and one of the first things I learned to make. It's a taste of summer; plus, eggplant's "meaty" texture makes it satisfying to nonvegetarians. The key to optimizing the flavors of this stew is to cook the vegetables separately so that they maintain their integrity, then simmer them together so their flavors can harmonize.

RATATOUILLE

Serves 6 to 8

Toss eggplant with several pinches of salt and allow to drain in a colander for 15 to 20 minutes, or until it begins to sweat. This is to reduce bitterness. Rinse with cold water and drain completely.

Heat 2 tablespoons of olive oil in a Dutch oven or other heavy pot over medium-high heat, then add eggplant with a pinch of salt. Cook until golden, about 10 minutes, stirring a few times, then transfer to a plate.

Add remaining 2 tablespoons of olive oil to the pot, add onion and garlic, and cook for a few minutes, until fragrant. Then, add zucchini and cook until slightly golden, 2 to 5 minutes, then tomatoes, cooking for another couple of minutes, then herbes de Provence, red pepper flakes, and black pepper. Stir, lower heat to medium-low, cover the pot, and cook for another 10 minutes, or until vegetables are tender but still maintain their shape. Return eggplant to the pot, cook for another 5 to 10 minutes, remove from heat, and stir in fresh basil. Adjust salt and pepper to taste before serving.

Serve with orzo or crusty bread.

1 pound eggplant, cut into ½-inch dice

Kosher salt

¼ cup olive oil

1 large onion, cut into ½-inch dice

6 garlic cloves, minced

1 pound zucchini, cut into ½-inch half-moons

1 pound Roma tomatoes (5 to 6 tomatoes), cut into ½-inch dice

1 teaspoon herbes de Provence or ½ teaspoon each dried oregano and dried thyme

¼ teaspoon red pepper flakes

Freshly ground black pepper

Garnish: ½ cup fresh basil, chiffonaded (cut into thin ribbons)

Cooked orzo or crusty bread, for serving

Black pepper, chile pepper, garlic

Eggplant, tomatoes, zucchini (summer squash)

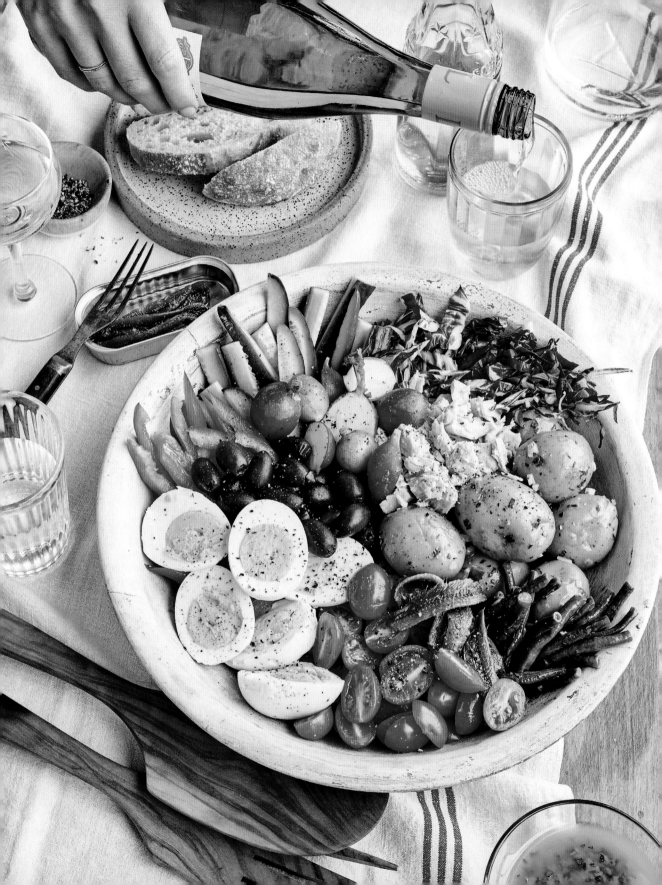

A FRENCH BISTRO STAPLE, this Provençale salad combines tuna, olives, cucumber, green beans, anchovies, and other spring vegetables for a filling and protein-rich meal—a way to take the simple nutrition advice to "eat the rainbow." It looks fancy but is very simple to make. Bring it on a picnic—pack each component separately, then plate on arrival.

SALADE NIÇOISE

Serves 6

Prepare dressing: First, make garlic paste by sprinkling minced garlic with salt, then using the edge of a chef's knife to mash into a paste. Place garlic paste in a jar, add remaining dressing ingredients, including pepper to taste, and shake until well combined.

Prepare salad: Boil the eggs. My foolproof method for cooking a hard-boiled egg that's easy to peel and has a perfectly yellow yolk: Place room-temperature eggs in a pot with enough cold water to cover them about an inch, bring water to a boil over high heat, then remove pot from heat, cover, and let stand for 10 minutes exactly. After 10 minutes, drain hot water and replace it with cold or ice water to stop cooking process, then let cool completely before peeling and slicing in half lengthwise.

Toss potatoes and haricots verts with enough vinaigrette to coat. Arrange them beautifully on a platter along with the other ingredients, including eggs, placing contrasting colors next to each other. Drizzle additional vinaigrette over entire salad and finish with a pinch of salt and a few grinds of pepper.

VINAIGRETTE

1 garlic clove, minced

Kosher salt

⅓ cup olive oil

Juice of 1 lemon

1 tablespoon Dijon mustard

1 shallot, minced

2 to 4 tablespoons minced fresh tarragon leaves

Freshly ground black pepper

SALAD

4 large eggs

1 pound small new potatoes, boiled until tender, 13 to 15 minutes

8 ounces haricots verts or green beans, trimmed and blanched

12 ounces cherry tomatoes, halved

1 red or yellow bell pepper, seeded and thinly sliced

½ cup black Niçoise or Kalamata olives

8 small radishes, trimmed and thinly sliced

8 salt-packed anchovies, rinsed and drained (from a 2-ounce can)

1 small cucumber, thinly sliced

2 (4-ounce) cans high-quality oil-packed tuna, drained

½ small head radicchio, sliced in bite-size pieces (about 1 cup)

✳ Black pepper

 Anchovies, bell pepper, cucumber, eggs, olives, potatoes, radicchio, tomatoes, tuna

FILLING

1 tablespoon olive oil, plus more for drizzling

1 medium-size onion, thinly sliced

1 to 2 pinches kosher salt, plus more for sprinkling

1½ cups mixed green and red grapes

1 cup feta cheese, coarsely crumbled by hand

1 teaspoon fresh minced rosemary

2 pinches freshly ground black pepper

GALETTE DOUGH

8 tablespoons (1 stick) cold, unsalted butter, cut into pea-size pieces

2 cups all-purpose flour, plus more for dusting

Pinch of salt

6 tablespoons ice water

THIS SAVORY TART takes inspiration from the flavors of the Mediterranean. The sweetness of mixed green and red grapes and caramelized onions contrasts with the brininess of feta. Roasting the grapes transforms their sweetness into a mellower taste not unlike roasted tomatoes. This galette makes a satisfying vegetarian meal; serve with a simple arugula salad, or cut into slices for an appetizer.

RUSTIC GRAPE, FETA, AND CARAMELIZED ONION GALETTE

Serves 4 as a main, 6 as an appetizer

Preheat oven to 350°F. Line a baking sheet with parchment paper.

Prepare filling: Heat a medium-size skillet over low-medium-low heat and add olive oil. Add onion and salt and cook, stirring every 5 minutes, until caramelized, about 30 minutes total. Add water, as needed, if onion begins to dry out. Remove from heat and cool slightly.

While onions are caramelizing, prepare galette dough: Cut together butter pieces and flour with a pastry cutter or food processor until you have a coarse meal. Add salt. Stir with fork/process continuously while slowly adding ice water, 1 tablespoon at a time, until dough sticks to itself. Form into a ball of dough, then roll out onto a flour-dusted surface into a 10-inch round. Transfer rolled-out dough to prepared baking sheet.

Assemble galette: First scatter cooled, caramelized onion in center of dough circle, leaving about a 1-inch rim of uncovered dough all around. Scatter grapes in a single layer over onion. Mix together crumbled feta and minced rosemary with your fingers or a spoon, then scatter among grapes.

Now, fold over uncovered rim of dough to encase filling, slightly overlapping each segment. Lightly brush rim of crust with a small amount of cold water. Sprinkle remaining salt and pepper onto water-glazed crust and over galette filling. Drizzle a small amount of olive oil over filling.

Bake for 40 to 45 minutes until grapes are roasted, crust is golden, and cheese starts to brown.

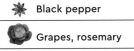

Black pepper

Grapes, rosemary

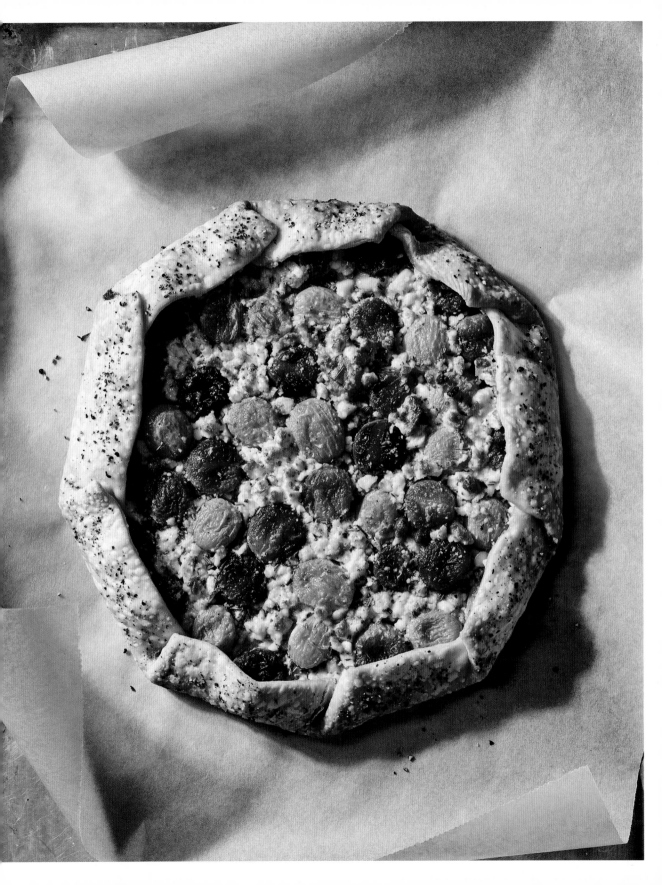

1 cup dried brown or green lentils

½ cup olive oil

1 teaspoon cumin seeds

3 medium-size onions, thinly sliced

Kosher salt

½ teaspoon ground cumin

¼ teaspoon ground allspice

¼ teaspoon ground cinnamon

¼ teaspoon cayenne pepper

¾ cup uncooked brown basmati rice

3 cups water

GARNISHES

2 tablespoons pine nuts

Chopped fresh flat-leaf parsley

Fresh lemon juice

Greek yogurt or labneh (see page 255 to make your own)

Allspice, cayenne, cinnamon, cumin

Brown rice (whole grains), lentils

THIS ONE-POT MEAL is a Middle Eastern version of a comforting dish enjoyed in many cultures—rice and beans, or in this case, rice and lentils. This recipe is a good example of three of my favorite tenets of cooking: simple is best, one ingredient can really elevate a dish, and spices can make it ethereal. Many versions of this dish are simply spiced with salt and pepper, with an essential topping of caramelized or crispy onions to enhance the flavor and texture of the dish. My version goes further to add sweet cinnamon, balanced with earthy cumin and allspice and a subtle kick of cayenne. Briefly toasting the spices to release their flavors is worth the extra step. Garnishing with Greek yogurt or labneh and toasted pine nuts adds even more flavor and textural contrast. *Mujadara* is a very simple dish that only tastes complex—*shh*, don't tell your dinner guests!

Adapted from Aarti Sequeira's recipe on www.FoodNetwork.com.

MUJADARA (RICE WITH LENTILS AND CARAMELIZED ONIONS)

Serves 6

Place lentils in a medium-size saucepan and add water to cover by an inch. Bring to a boil over medium-high heat, then lower heat to a simmer and cook, covered, until lentils are al dente, about 20 minutes. Drain and set aside.

While lentils cook, heat a large skillet with a lid over medium-high heat and add oil. When oil is shimmery, add cumin seeds and cook for up to a minute, until seeds are fragrant and slightly browned. Add onions and a pinch of kosher salt and cook over medium-low heat until onions caramelize, stirring often. This will take about 30 minutes. Check periodically and add a little water if onions begin to stick to the bottom of the pan. They're done when deep caramel in color and a little crisp around edges.

Once onions have caramelized, transfer half to a paper towel–lined plate and reserve for garnish.

To remaining onions in the skillet, add ground cumin, allspice, cinnamon, and cayenne and sauté for about 1 minute. Add rice and cook for 5 minutes, stirring thoroughly to coat rice with onions and spices. Then, add cooked lentils, 3 cups of water, and 1 teaspoon of salt and bring to a boil.

Lower heat to low and simmer, covered, for 30 minutes. Water should be completely evaporated and rice should be tender; if not, continue to cook for 5 to 10 minutes longer.

Once rice is done, turn off heat, fluff with a spoon, replace the lid, and allow to sit for another 5 minutes.

Meanwhile, prepare pine nuts to use for garnish: Toast pine nuts in a small, dry skillet over medium-low heat, shaking often, about 5 minutes. Be careful not to burn them, as they brown quickly.

To serve, mound mujadara on a large platter and top with reserved caramelized onions, toasted pine nuts, chopped parsley, and a squeeze of lemon juice. Garnish with Greek yogurt or labneh, if desired.

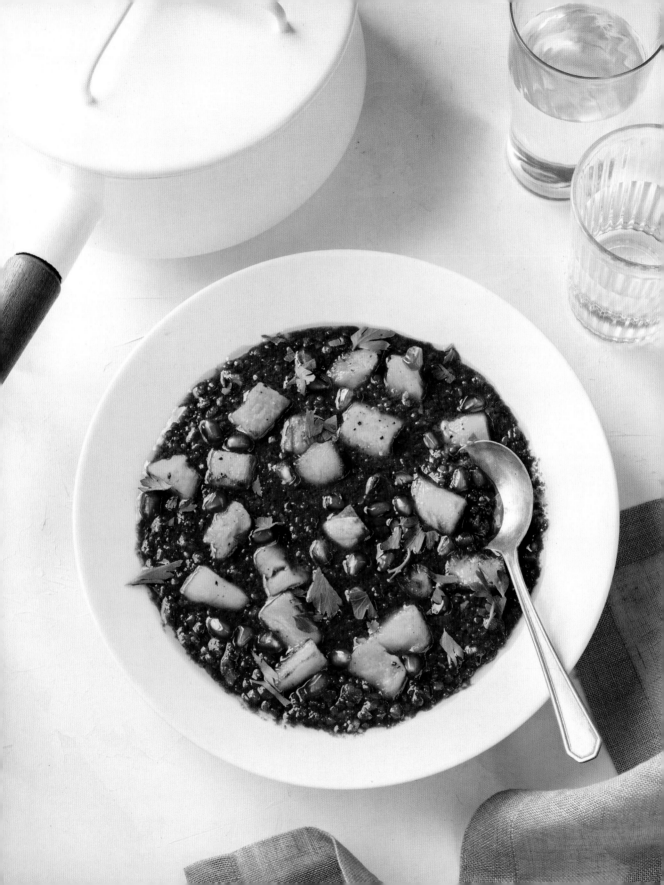

THIS STEW COMBINES the creamy richness of the slow-cooked ground walnut sauce with a sour-sweet undercurrent of pomegranate molasses. It's simple enough to make on a weeknight, but because of the luxuriousness of the ingredients, it can also be savored on special occasions. The dish is traditionally made with chicken or duck, but butternut squash makes a good substitute for a vegetarian/vegan version. Roasting the squash separately enhances its flavor and also prevents it from being overcooked. Slowly simmering the sauce will deepen the walnut flavor and allow its natural oils to be released, which makes for a smooth and rich sauce.

KHORESH FESENJAN (PERSIAN STEW WITH WALNUT AND POMEGRANATE SAUCE)

Serves 6 to 8

Heat oil in a large, heavy-bottomed pot, such as a Dutch oven, over medium heat. Add onion and sauté until translucent, about 5 minutes.

Stir in ground walnuts and stock. Bring to a boil, then lower heat to low, cover, and simmer for 20 minutes.

Stir in pomegranate molasses, cardamom, turmeric, cinnamon, and salt and pepper to taste. Simmer, stirring occasionally, for another 30 to 45 minutes, or until sauce is slightly thickened and walnuts begin to release their oil. Sauce should be dark brown. Adjust seasoning to taste, adding sugar if desired to balance tartness, and simmer for 10 more minutes.

While sauce is simmering, roast butternut squash: Preheat oven to 425°F. Toss butternut squash cubes on a baking sheet with a little olive oil, salt, and pepper, then roast in oven until tender, about 20 minutes, turning once. Set aside until sauce is at desired thickness and flavor, then add roasted squash just before serving.

Garnish finished stew with pomegranate seeds and chopped parsley. Serve over basmati rice.

---

2 tablespoons olive oil, plus more for roasting squash

1 large onion, thinly sliced

2 cups walnuts, finely ground with a mortar and pestle or in a food processor

1½ cups vegetable stock or water

⅔ cup pomegranate molasses (see page 251 to make your own)

½ teaspoon ground cardamom

½ teaspoon ground turmeric

¼ teaspoon ground cinnamon

1 tablespoon salt, or to taste, plus more for roasting squash

Freshly ground black pepper

Sugar (optional)

1 large butternut squash (about 2 pounds), peeled, seeded, and cut into 2-inch cubes

Garnishes: pomegranate seeds, chopped fresh flat-leaf parsley

Steamed basmati rice, for serving

✳ Black pepper, cardamom, cinnamon, turmeric

🥬 Butternut squash, walnuts

1 cup sugar

1 cup water

4 rosemary sprigs

1 tablespoon orange flower water

3 pounds oranges (about 8 navel oranges); for the prettiest presentation, use a mix of navel, Cara Cara, tangerines, and blood oranges

GARNISHES

2 tablespoons chopped pistachios

8 or more fresh mint leaves, torn

THIS LIGHT and elegant dessert brings together some iconic flavors of California—with a kiss of orange flower water, which is a distinctive taste from the Mediterranean. When you want to serve something a little more special, infusing the oranges in this syrup enhances and elevates their flavor. The brightness of the citrus contrasts with the floral, herbal syrup, accented nicely with the rich crunch of chopped pistachios. Orange flower water, also known as orange blossom water, is available from Middle Eastern groceries, stores specializing in cocktail ingredients, as well as online.

ORANGES IN ROSEMARY AND ORANGE FLOWER WATER SYRUP

Serves 8

Prepare syrup: Pour sugar and water into a saucepan and bring to a boil, whisking to dissolve sugar. Add rosemary sprigs and lower heat to a simmer. Simmer for 10 minutes, then remove from heat. Leave in rosemary sprigs to continue to infuse syrup as it cools. When cool, strain through a mesh strainer into a glass measuring cup or small bowl and stir in orange flower water.

While syrup is cooling, prepare oranges. Use a sharp knife to cut off top and bottom of each orange, so you have a stable base, then cut peel off orange, following along its curves. Trim off any remaining pith. Then, slice peeled oranges crosswise into 1/4-inch rounds and place in a shallow, wide bowl. (If using blood oranges, store those slices separately so their juice doesn't bleed into lighter-colored oranges.)

Pour syrup over orange slices, then cover with plastic wrap and refrigerate for at least 2 hours, turning occasionally so that orange slices get equally soaked.

To serve, arrange chilled marinated orange slices prettily on a large platter and drizzle with just enough syrup to moisten oranges; they shouldn't be swimming in syrup. Garnish with chopped pistachios and torn mint leaves.

🌼 Orange flower water

Oranges, mint, pistachio, rosemary

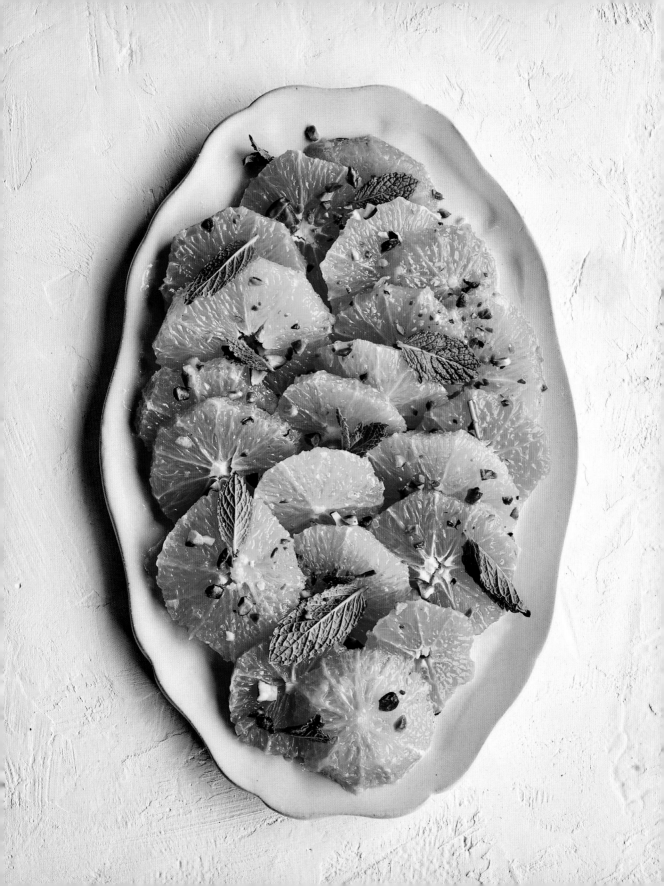

8 tablespoons (1 stick) unsalted butter, at room temperature, plus more for pan

¾ cup granulated sugar

4 large eggs

1 teaspoon orange flower water

2½ cups almond flour (make sure it's finely ground)

2 teaspoons baking powder

Garnish: confectioners' sugar

THIS IS A SIMPLE yet elegant gluten-free cake, with the enticing fragrance of orange flower water. It's light and elegant on its own or with a dusting of confectioners' sugar, but can also be frosted with a simple buttercream if the occasion calls for it.

ORANGE FLOWER WATER– SCENTED ALMOND CAKE

Serves 12

Preheat oven to 350°F. Butter an 8-inch round cake pan, line with parchment paper, and set aside.

In a large bowl, cream together butter and sugar with an electric mixer until light and fluffy. Mix in eggs, one at a time. Add orange flower water.

In another bowl, combine almond flour with baking powder.

Fold flour mixture into butter mixture until just combined. Pour batter into prepared pan.

Bake for 20 to 25 minutes, or until golden brown and a toothpick inserted into center comes out clean. Remove from oven and let cool in pan on a wire rack for at least 10 minutes before inverting and removing from pan. Sprinkle with sifted confectioners' sugar, if desired, before serving.

 Orange flower water

Almonds

2 lemons (for about ½ cup juice)

1½ cups water

2 tablespoons sugar, or to taste

1 tablespoon orange flower water

2 mint sprigs

Ice, for serving

I'VE MADE FRESH LEMONADE with herbs for years, with my favorites being thyme and mint. But I was inspired to make it even more special after a visit to Reem's in Oakland, California, where I had a memorable and refreshing glass of Syrian Lemonade. Whenever I serve this fragrant beverage, someone invariably asks what the subtle flavor is. Freshly squeezed lemonade on its own is delicious, muddled mint is refreshing, and the orange flower water is alluringly fragrant.

LEMONADE WITH ORANGE FLOWER WATER AND MINT

Serves 2

Squeeze lemon juice into a pitcher or jar, then add water and sugar and stir until dissolved. Stir in orange flower water. Keep cold until ready to serve.

To serve, pour into two ice-filled glasses. Add a mint sprig to each glass and muddle (gently crush mint leaves with a spoon).

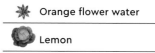

✳ Orange flower water

🥬 Lemon

1 tablespoon loose Chinese gunpowder green tea

6 cups boiling water

3 to 4 tablespoons sugar, or to taste (optional; traditionally, served almost syrupy sweet)

1 large bunch fresh mint (about 1 ounce)

FRESHLY BREWED mint tea is a part of daily life in Morocco. You can purchase preblended loose or bagged forms of this tea, but for optimal flavor, prepare it fresh using this traditional recipe with gunpowder green tea and loads of fresh mint. And ceremony. The ceremonial sharing of freshly brewed mint tea is symbolic of hospitality in Morocco. Traditionally, the tea is served three times. The amount of time it has been steeping gives each of the glasses of tea a unique flavor, described in this Maghrebi proverb:

Le premier verre est aussi doux que la vie,
le deuxième est aussi fort que l'amour,
le troisième est aussi amer que la mort.
The first glass is as gentle as life,
the second is as strong as love,
the third is as bitter as death.

MOROCCAN MINT TEA

Serves 4 to 6

Add loose tea to a teapot, pour in 1 cup of boiling water, and infuse for 30 seconds. Strain out and reserve this water, called the "spirit" of tea, keeping tea leaves in pot.

Add another cup of boiling water and allow tea leaves to steep for a minute, then swirl and discard infusion, reserving tea leaves in teapot. This is called "washing" tea leaves, and is meant to remove their bitterness.

Add remaining 4 cups of boiling water to washed tea leaves and let steep for 2 minutes. Add back reserved "spirit" of tea. Stir in sugar to taste (though untraditional to do so, leave out sugar to be added individually to taste, if desired) and mint sprigs and steep for 3 to 4 minutes more. Serve in small, heatproof glasses. Traditionally, this tea is poured from a great height back and forth between teapot and glasses, to aerate tea for optimal flavor.

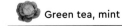 Green tea, mint

1 cup unsweetened
almond milk

¼ cup tahini

3 Medjool dates, pitted and
chopped

½ teaspoon ground
cardamom, plus more for
garnish

2 or 3 ice cubes

THIS TREAT combines two iconic flavors from the Middle East—tahini
and dates—into a rich drink perfect for a light dessert.

TAHINI DATE SHAKE

<u>Serves 4</u>

Combine all ingredients in a blender and blend until smooth. Serve in
four small glasses with a dusting of cardamom.

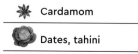

🌸 Cardamom

Dates, tahini

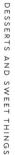

1 cup packed kale leaves, center rib removed, leaves chopped or torn

½ cup packed fresh basil leaves

2 tablespoons toasted, chopped walnuts

½ teaspoon salt, or to taste

1 garlic clove, chopped

2 to 4 tablespoons extra-virgin olive oil

OIL-FREE VERSION

1 cup packed kale leaves, center rib removed, leaves chopped or torn

½ cup packed fresh basil leaves

2 tablespoons toasted, chopped walnuts

½ teaspoon salt, or to taste

1 garlic clove, chopped

¼ cup vegetable stock

1 tablespoon nutritional yeast

THIS IS NOW my family's preferred version of pesto. Kale added to the traditional basil adds a nutrition and flavor boost, and the creaminess of the walnuts eliminates the need for cheese (although you could add some grated Parmesan, if desired). I've included an oil-free version for people who might prefer an even lighter recipe, or who are following a whole food, plant-based diet.

KALE-WALNUT PESTO

Makes 1 cup pesto

For olive oil version: Place all ingredients, except olive oil, in a small food processor and process until you have a coarse paste. Then, drizzle in olive oil until emulsified (it will look creamy). Add additional oil, if needed to loosen. Use immediately with pasta or grains, or keep refrigerated, covering with a thin layer of additional oil to prevent oxidation/discoloration.

For oil-free version: Place all ingredients in a small food processor and process until you have a coarse paste. Add additional stock, if needed to loosen. Use immediately with pasta or grains, or keep refrigerated, covering with a thin layer of additional stock to prevent oxidation/discoloration.

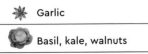

❋ Garlic

Basil, kale, walnuts

1 cup packed arugula

¾ cup packed fresh mint leaves (about ½ bunch)

2 tablespoons pistachios, toasted and chopped

½ teaspoon salt

1 garlic clove, minced

3 to 4 tablespoons extra-virgin olive oil

ALTHOUGH BASIL is traditional, any herbs can be made into pesto. I love the piquant brightness of this pesto, from both the mint and peppery arugula, and with pistachios, this version brings us a step closer to the Middle East. It pairs wonderfully with pita, pita chips, and crudités.

MINT-ARUGULA PESTO

Makes ¾ cup pesto

Place all ingredients, except oil, in a food processor and pulse until coarsely ground.

Slowly drizzle in olive oil while continuing to pulse, until you have a smooth paste. Adjust amount of oil to desired thickness.

Use immediately, or if refrigerating for later, pour a thin layer of olive oil on top to maintain color and freshness, before covering tightly.

✳ Garlic

Arugula, mint, pistachios

2 medium-size ancho chiles

1 large red bell pepper
(jarred already roasted,
seeded, peeled, and
chopped; or see directions)

1 cup blanched almonds

4 large garlic cloves, minced

1 cup canned, crushed
tomatoes

1 tablespoon pimentón
(smoked paprika)

½ teaspoon cayenne pepper

3 tablespoons red wine
vinegar or sherry vinegar

1 teaspoon salt

¾ cup extra-virgin olive oil

THIS CLASSIC Spanish sauce combines the flavors of roasted red peppers, garlic, tomatoes, and pimentón (smoked paprika) that will transport you immediately to a tapas bar in Spain. The flavors are complex, but this versatile recipe comes together very quickly. Enjoy it with Canary Island Wrinkled Potatoes (Papas Arrugadas) (page 217), roast vegetables, with cauliflower steaks (see page 226 for a recipe), or grilled meats, or as a dip with bread and crudités. Besides the fabulous flavor, this recipe is special to me because I first learned to make it at the Healthy Kitchens, Healthy Lives Conference, at the Culinary Institute of America at Greystone. It was at this fateful conference where I realized I could, should, and really wanted to combine my love of cooking with my practice of medicine. I taught my first cooking class one week after the conference (and the rest is history).

ROMESCO

Makes 4 cups sauce

Soak chiles in hot water to cover for 1 hour, or until softened. (*Tip*: Place a small plate on top of chiles to keep them submerged.) Drain, remove stems and seeds, and cut into small pieces.

Meanwhile, to roast bell pepper: Preheat oven to 450°F. Place whole bell pepper on a baking sheet and roast in oven for about 30 minutes, rotating a few times, until skin has blackened and pepper is soft to touch and limp when picked up with tongs. Remove from oven and transfer immediately to a small paper or resealable plastic bag and seal tightly, allowing cooked pepper to steam so skin can be peeled off easily. After about 5 to 10 minutes, remove from bag and quickly peel off skin by rubbing with your fingers (be careful, pepper will still be quite hot). Remove seeds, then slice pepper into long strips and set aside until ready to use. (Alternatively, place entire bell pepper directly over an open flame or on a grill/grill pan and roast until blackened on all sides and completely softened, about 20 minutes, turning every 5 minutes or so. Follow remaining steps as in first method.)

Place all ingredients, except olive oil, in a food processor and pulse a few times to make a chunky paste.

 Cayenne, chile peppers, garlic, smoked paprika

Almonds, bell peppers, olive oil, tomatoes

Add oil, 1 tablespoon at a time, to emulsify. You'll see sauce lighten in color and look creamier as oil emulsifies with rest of ingredients. Don't add oil all at once, or it won't combine properly.

Taste and adjust salt, vinegar, or cayenne, as desired.

GREMOLATA is a vibrant lemon peel and herb topping used traditionally in Italian cuisine to accompany osso buco but can also be used to add a bright and zesty flavor to any roasted proteins or vegetables, to swirl into soup, or sprinkle onto pasta. You can follow this recipe or just use a ratio of about 2:1:1 parsley:lemon peel:garlic. Make sure to peel the lemon lightly, to avoid adding too much of the bitter pith (the white part under the skin). A paring knife or vegetable peeler can be used for this purpose. (Note that because you'll be eating the lemon peel, it is best to use organic, unwaxed lemons, and make sure to wash thoroughly before using.) For a fun variation, feel free to experiment with other citrus zests (such as orange, lime, or grapefruit).

¼ cup finely chopped fresh flat-leaf parsley

2 teaspoons finely chopped lemon peel (from about 1 lemon)

2 garlic cloves, finely minced

GREMOLATA

Makes ¼ cup gremolata

Place chopped ingredients together on a cutting board and chop them again until well combined. Transfer to a bowl. Best used same day but can be stored in a paper towel–lined covered container in refrigerator for up to 3 days.

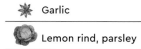

✳ Garlic

Lemon rind, parsley

1 cup tightly packed, chopped, fresh flat-leaf parsley

½ cup tightly packed fresh cilantro leaves

½ teaspoon capers, drained

1 teaspoon minced preserved lemon rind or lemon zest

½ teaspoon ground cumin

½ teaspoon hot paprika

1 garlic clove, chopped

¼ cup extra-virgin olive oil

Juice of 1 lemon

CHERMOULA is an assertively herbal marinade and relish used in Algerian, Libyan, Moroccan, and Tunisian cooking. It is traditionally used to flavor fish, seafood, or meat. Besides being used as a marinade, it adds intense flavor as a sauce for roasted vegetables or as a garnish swirled into pureed soup. Key ingredients include fresh cilantro, parsley, and lemon. For even zingier flavor, I use preserved lemon peel. If you can't get (or make) any, feel free to add some lemon zest instead.

CHERMOULA (NORTH AFRICAN HERB MARINADE)

Makes 1 cup chermoula

Combine all ingredients in a food processor and process until you have a fairly smooth, green sauce.

Keeps well in an airtight container in refrigerator for up to 5 days.

Cumin, paprika

Cilantro, lemon rind, parsley

½ teaspoon coriander seeds

½ teaspoon cumin seeds

½ teaspoon caraway seeds

1 teaspoon smoked hot paprika

1 teaspoon dried mint

½ teaspoon sugar

1 red bell pepper

3 garlic cloves, minced

2 teaspoons tomato paste

½ teaspoon minced preserved lemon rind

Juice of 1 lemon

2 tablespoons olive oil

HARISSA refers to a chile pepper paste or sauce first created in Tunisia but also popular in other parts of North Africa, including Morocco, where it is served alongside tagines and couscous. The key ingredients are roasted red peppers, hot chile peppers, garlic, and spices, such as coriander, caraway, and cumin, combined with olive oil. (Harissa is also available as a dried spice blend.) Don't skip the step of toasting the seeds, which is essential for bringing out their fragrance. Think of this as your new favorite chili sauce, and put it on anything that could use a touch of heat and spice.

HARISSA SAUCE

Makes ½ cup harissa

Toast coriander, cumin, and caraway seeds in a small, dry skillet over medium heat until fragrant, tossing often, about 30 seconds. Grind into a fine powder, using a spice grinder or mortar and pestle, then grind together with paprika, mint, and sugar.

To roast bell pepper: Preheat oven to 450°F. Place whole bell pepper on a baking sheet and roast for about 30 minutes, rotating a few times, until skin has blackened and pepper is soft to touch and limp when picked up with tongs. Remove from oven and transfer immediately to a small paper or resealable plastic bag and seal tightly, allowing cooked pepper to steam so skin can be peeled off easily. After 5 to 10 minutes, remove from bag and quickly peel off skin by rubbing with your fingers (be careful, pepper will still be quite hot). Remove seeds, then cut pepper into long strips and set aside until ready to use. (Alternatively, place entire bell pepper directly over an open flame or on a grill/grill pan, and roast until blackened on all sides and completely softened, about 20 minutes, turning every 5 minutes or so. Follow remaining steps as in first method.)

Combine all ingredients, except olive oil, in a food processor or blender until smooth, then slowly add olive oil until it is emulsified. You will notice that sauce lightens in color when this happens.

Keep tightly sealed in a jar, refrigerated, for up to 2 weeks.

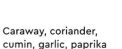

Caraway, coriander, cumin, garlic, paprika

Bell pepper, lemon rind, olive oil, tomato

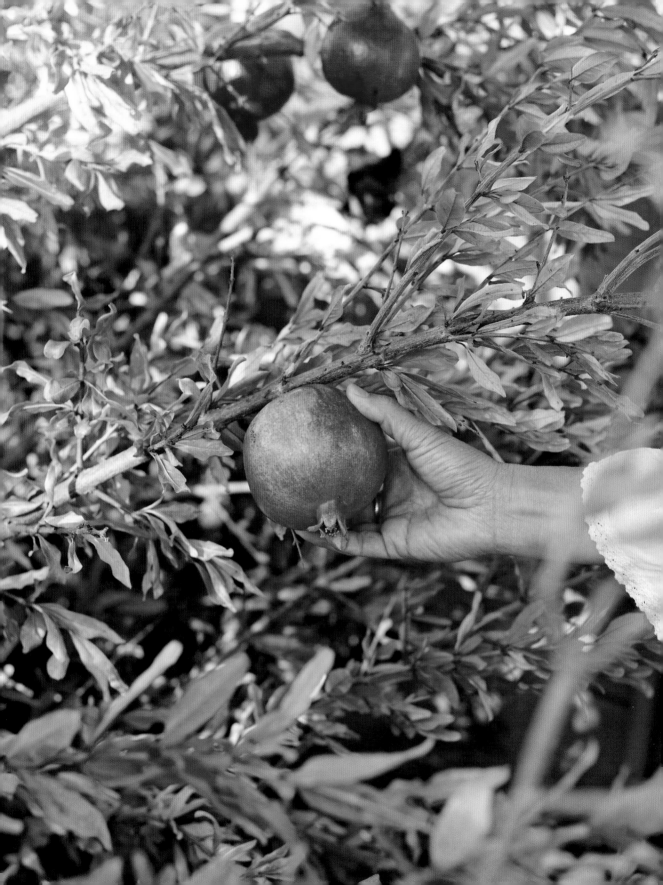

4 cups pomegranate juice

½ cup sugar

Juice of 1 lemon

THIS IS AN INGREDIENT in Muhammara (page 204), Khoresh Fesenjan (page 237), and Pomegranate Vinaigrette (page 256); it's also great to have on hand for glazing grilled vegetables.

HOMEMADE POMEGRANATE MOLASSES

Makes 1 cup pomegranate molasses

Place all ingredients in a medium-size saucepan. Bring to a low boil over medium-high heat and stir until sugar has dissolved.

Lower heat to a simmer and cook for about an hour, stirring occasionally, until mixture has reduced by three-quarters to a syrupy texture, thick enough to coat a spoon.

Remove from heat and let cool completely before storing in a glass jar in refrigerator for up to 6 months.

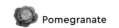 Pomegranate

¼ cup white sesame seeds

¼ cup pistachios

¼ cup roasted cashews

3 tablespoons ground coriander

1 tablespoon ground cumin

¼ teaspoon salt, or to taste

½ teaspoon dried mint

DUKKAH is an Egyptian spice and nut blend used with olive oil as a dip for bread and crudités. It's also excellent as a spice rub or crust for meat, fish, or roasted vegetables, and can be mixed into Greek yogurt for a savory dip. Use whatever nuts you like; pistachios and hazelnuts are common. Whatever nuts you use, make sure you toast them before using, for flavor and crunch. Key spices are cumin and coriander, but you can add others to your taste. A hint of dried mint is also a nice addition that brings freshness and sweetness to the mix.

DUKKAH

Makes 1 generous cup dukkah

Toast sesame seeds in a small, dry skillet over medium heat for 3 minutes, or until fragrant.

Toast shelled pistachios with cashews in a separate dry pan over medium heat for 3 to 5 minutes, or until lightly browned and fragrant.

Process pistachios and cashews in a spice grinder or small food processor until finely chopped, but not as fine as dust.

Transfer chopped nuts, toasted sesame seeds, coriander, cumin, salt, and mint to a bowl and stir until combined. After mixture has cooled, transfer to a sealed jar for up to 2 weeks at room temperature, or for 3 months refrigerated.

Coriander, cumin

Cashews, pistachios, sesame seeds

1 tablespoon sesame seeds

1½ tablespoons dried oregano

1½ tablespoons dried thyme

1 tablespoon sumac

2 teaspoons ground coriander

2 teaspoons kosher salt

THIS SPICE MIX from the Levant is traditionally made with fresh or dried oregano, thyme, and/or marjoram leaves, along with sumac, sesame seeds, salt, and sometimes other spices, such as cumin, coriander, or fennel seeds. Za'atar is closely tied to Palestinian cuisine but is popular throughout the Middle East. Its fragrant flavor makes a terrific topping for flatbreads and roasted root vegetables, which can be drizzled with olive oil before the za'atar is sprinkled on. It also makes a savory garnish for labneh, hummus, or other spreads. Feel free to experiment and use it anywhere you might use oregano. Sumac, a powdered dried berry that adds a tangy and lemony flavor, can be found in Middle Eastern groceries and online. If you can't find it, add some lemon zest for a similar taste.

ZA'ATAR

Makes ⅓ cup za'atar

Toast sesame seeds in a small, dry skillet over medium heat for 3 minutes, or until fragrant, and set aside to cool.

Meanwhile, grind together all remaining ingredients in a spice grinder, food processor, or mortar and pestle until you have a coarse powder. Stir in cooled, toasted sesame seeds. Store tightly sealed in refrigerator; za'atar will keep for 3 months.

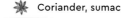

Coriander, sumac

Oregano, sesame seeds, thyme

12 lemons, preferably organic and unwaxed (may use any amount)

Fine sea salt or kosher salt

ONE OF THE FLAVOR THEMES, or perhaps the central flavor theme, of Moroccan cuisine is the preserved lemon. Preserved lemons are used as a condiment and seasoning to add brightness and depth of flavor— what I like to think of as citrusy umami. You can use preserved lemon peel countless ways; you'll find it in recipes throughout the book and can also use it to garnish a bowl of warmed olives; add to tagines or stews; puree with some olive oil and use as the base for a salad dressing; or add to recipes in place of lemon juice and salt.

This is one of the easiest pickles you'll ever make, using just salt and lemon juice to preserve. Try to get organic, unwaxed lemons because it is the peel that you will be eating.

PRESERVED LEMONS

Makes 6 preserved lemons

Scrub lemons vigorously with a brush under running water and then dry thoroughly. Have ready a wide-mouth glass jar that will fit half your lemons.

Prepare half your lemons: Slice each lemon into quarters, but not all the way, so that quarters are still attached and hold together at one end.

Cram as much salt as you can into exposed/cut areas of each lemon (up to a few tablespoons per lemon). As you finish each lemon, place it into your jar, cramming as many lemons as you can into the jar. When you can't fit any more, cut an equal number of lemons—the other half of your supply—and squeeze their juice over salted lemons until they are completely submerged (discard squeezed lemons after squeezing). Keeping the salted lemons covered is key to make sure that they are preserved rather than rotting. Now you can seal the jar, and keep in a dark cabinet at room temperature. Mark the date because you'll forget when you made them. For the first week, shake the sealed jar once daily to redistribute salt. Now here is the hard part: wait a minimum of one month but, if you can, perhaps 3 to 6 months for best flavor.

When they are ready, rinds will have softened, possibly changed color slightly. With very rare exceptions, you will only be using the rind (not pulp) of your lemons, and sometimes their brine.

 Lemons

To use, take a piece of lemon, rinse it to remove excess saltiness, and remove pulp with a knife or spoon. Scrape off as much of its pith (white part) as you can because, even preserved, it will be bitter.

Keep remaining lemons covered in liquid; you can also add some olive oil to top it off. After preserving, keeps indefinitely in refrigerator.

---

1 quart Greek yogurt

½ teaspoon fine kosher salt

Garnishes: a drizzle of olive oil, fresh herbs, dukkah or za'atar (see pages 252 and 253 to make your own), and/or pomegranate seeds

THIS STRAINED YOGURT, which is also known as "yogurt cheese," is a simple preparation of Greek yogurt strained through a cheesecloth until it has the consistency of cream cheese. This is enjoyed in many cuisines throughout the Mediterranean and Middle East. Serve with lavash, pita, or other flatbread on a meze platter, or as an accompaniment to grilled meat, vegetable, or grain dishes.

LABNEH

Makes 1 cup labneh

Stir salt into yogurt, then place yogurt in a cheesecloth-lined sieve.

Place sieve over a large bowl with a few inches of space at bottom. Cover top loosely with ends of cheesecloth or with a piece of plastic wrap. Place in refrigerator and allow to drain off whey for 12 to 24 hours.

Serve immediately or keep refrigerated. Before serving, garnish creatively for both aesthetics and flavor.

 Yogurt

¼ cup extra-virgin olive oil

2 tablespoons freshly squeezed lemon juice

1 tablespoon pomegranate molasses (see page 251 to make your own)

¼ teaspoon salt, or to taste

Freshly ground black pepper

USE THIS sweet and tart dressing for an herb salad to accompany any of the dishes in this section.

POMEGRANATE VINAIGRETTE

Makes ½ cup vinaigrette

Whisk all ingredients together, adding pepper to taste, in a small bowl or shake together in a lidded jar. Keeps for up to a week in refrigerator.

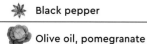 Black pepper

Olive oil, pomegranate

MEDITERRANEAN AND THE MIDDLE EAST MENUS

MEDITERRANEAN MENU

Classic Gazpacho

Spanish Orange and
Olive Salad

Saffron-Scented
Mediterranean Fish
and Fennel Stew

Spanish Spinach
and Chickpeas

Canary Island Wrinkled
Potatoes (Papas Arrugadas)
with Romesco

Orange Flower Water–
Scented Almond Cake

MIDDLE EASTERN MENU

Muhammara (Lebanese
Red Pepper, Walnut, and
Pomegranate Molasses Dip)
with Pita

Zaalouk (Moroccan
Roasted Eggplant Salad)

Salade Marocaine (Moroccan
Tomato Salad)

Mujadara (Rice with Lentils
and Caramelized Onions)

Oranges in Rosemary and
Orange Flower Water Syrup

Moroccan Mint Tea

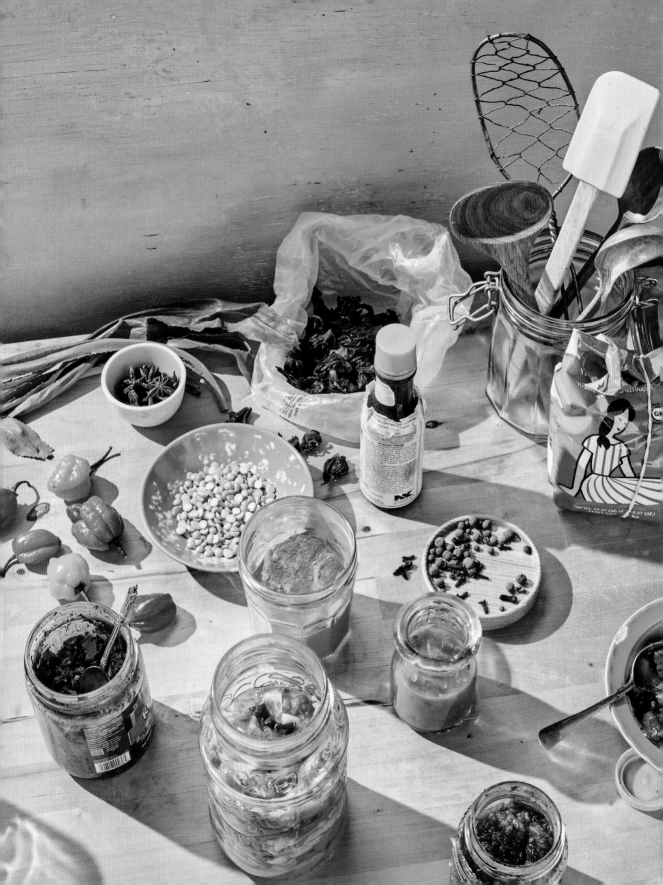

TRINIDAD

spices

allspice

amchar masala

cinnamon

cloves

cumin

Trinidad curry powder

turmeric

condiments and seasonings

Angostura bitters

green seasoning

kuchela

lime pepper

Scotch bonnet pepper sauce

tamarind sauce

herbs

bay leaf

cilantro

culantro (shado beni)

thyme

fats

canola or peanut oil

coconut oil

acid

lime

TRINIDAD

WHEN I FIRST HEARD PETER, the man who would become my husband, speak, I couldn't place his accent. When I learned he was from Trinidad, I knew embarrassingly little more about his homeland other than it is a Caribbean island and was the birthplace of limbo. When you fall in love with a person from another culture, you take a deep dive into learning about where they come from (and hopefully fall in love with their culture too). Over the past three decades, I have had the pleasure of learning about Trinidad and Tobago, as the former British colony is formally known. The island nation is populated by descendants of African slaves, Indian indentured laborers, Syrian and Chinese merchants, British and Scottish plantation owners and other Europeans from colonial times, native Arawaks and Caribs, and various combinations of these. Trinidad's culture and cuisine reflect this diversity. Trinidad's musical contributions are well known, from classic calypso to the infectious rhythms of modern-day soca. But for such a varied, unique, and flavorful cuisine, its food traditions are surprisingly less well known outside the Caribbean.

Everything I know about Trinidadian cuisine was taught to me by Peter's family and friends, along with the guidance of a decades-old classic community cookbook. *The Naparima Girls' High School Diamond Jubilee: Trinidad & Tobago Recipes*, originally published in 1988, is the best-known cookbook in Trinidad. Although the quality of the recipes vary, as should be expected with a community cookbook, the breadth of the recipes is reflective of what people eat in Trinidad. I used it as a guide for ideas on which recipes to include here and as a starting-off point for recipe development. I relied on my most trustworthy taste tester for Trinidadian cuisine to refine these recipes: Peter. I knew a recipe needed work when Peter would enjoy what I cooked, then ask what it was. But I also knew immediately when I got it right. When I made a recipe for a classic Trinidadian dish Peter hadn't had in years, there was pure joy on his face. When I got it right, one taste could bring back happy childhood memories, meals, and loved ones long forgotten.

This collection of recipes is a unique representation of Peter's Trinidad, which is largely reflected by his childhood in the south of Trinidad, with a large Indian population, and his own family history, which includes Chinese, Indian, and Scottish roots. In addition to learning Trinidadian recipes of Indian and African origin, you'll also see the influence of neighboring Latin America in such recipes as *sancoche* and *pastelles*. Vestiges of colonial influence hang on in the abundant use of nutmeg, rum, and Angostura bitters. You'll see a lot of Scotch bonnet pepper, which is really the only pepper locals refer to when they talk about "pepper" (not "chile").

Beyond the filter of Peter's personal upbringing, I have deliberately chosen more vegetable-forward recipes from a traditionally meat-loving cuisine, and in some cases made vegetarian versions. Also, somewhat controversially, I've snuck in a few recipes that come from neighboring Jamaica, a friendly rival, just because they are so good. For essential condiments and spice blends without which your Trinidadian meal will not taste authentic, I'll help you fill your pantry with *kuchela*, pepper sauce, tamarind sauce, green seasoning, Trinidad curry powder, and *amchar masala*. If you want to be truly authentic, you'll have to package these in repurposed containers, such as glass Nescafé jars, glass bottles from commercially made pepper sauce, and plastic liter-size soda bottles. If you're from the Caribbean, I see you nodding and laughing right now. Whether you're from the Caribbean or not, *veni mange* (come and eat)!

2 pounds salt fish, cleaned of skin and bones

2 tablespoons canola oil

1 onion, sliced

1 teaspoon minced fresh garlic

2 celery stalks, cut into ¼-inch dice

1 green bell pepper, seeded and cut into ¼-inch dice

1 tomato, cut into ¼-inch dice

3 pimientos, minced

Juice of 1 lime

Freshly ground black pepper

FOR SERVING

Sliced avocado

Provisions (see headnote), boiled until tender

Coconut Bake (page 266), or ciabatta or focaccia

Sliced Scotch bonnet or habanero peppers (optional)

BULJOL is a Trinidadian dish of prepared salt fish, usually cod. The most important part of the technique is to soak the salt fish in a large amount of water and squeeze out all the salt, or else the dish will be unpalatable, and also dangerously high in sodium. (This process can be done by soaking the fish overnight in cold water, but in Trinidad, the method consists of boiling the salt fish for a few minutes.) The rest of it is up to you. Trinis usually fry salt fish with onions, bell peppers, and tomatoes, and often serve it with a type of bread called bake (page 266), along with sliced avocado and boiled provisions (the Trinidadian term for boiled root vegetables—any combination of potatoes, sweet potatoes, and tropical root vegetables, including taro, cassava, and plantains, which you can find in Asian or Latin American markets).

I have found the best source of salt fish to be Italian specialty food stores. Pimientos are available fresh in Trinidad; leave them out of the recipe if you can only get a jarred version.

BULJOL (SALT FISH)

Serves 4 to 6

Prepare salt fish by placing in a pot with enough water to cover by an inch or so. Bring to a boil, drain cooking liquid, allow to cool, and squeeze out excess liquid. (You can taste it now, and if it is still too salty, repeat boiling and draining process again.) Allow to cool, and then carefully remove any remaining bones. Shred into flakes with your fingers.

Heat a large skillet, add oil, fry prepared salt fish for a few minutes, then add onion, garlic, celery, bell pepper, tomato, and pimientos, and sauté for another minute, or until vegetables are just slightly softened.

Squeeze lime juice and sprinkle black pepper onto prepared buljol just before serving.

Serve with sliced avocado, provisions, and bake and garnish with sliced Scotch bonnet or habanero, if you like heat.

Note: If you are concerned about the sodium in this, rest assured that you can soak and rinse the salt fish as many times as you desire to get rid of the excess salt.

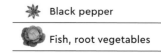

❋ Black pepper

Fish, root vegetables

2 tablespoons salted butter, melted, plus more for bowl and dough ball

1 tablespoon active dry yeast

2 teaspoons sugar

2½ cups warm water, about 110°F

8 cups all-purpose flour

1 tablespoon kosher salt

PETER WAS LUCKY to grow up surrounded by talented cooks. Granny would spy a lappe, agouti, or other wild animal, shoot it herself with a rifle, and curry it. Mommy was working in the shop all the time but would still cook the Cantonese comfort food that satisfied Daddy's soul. Auntie Doll was legendary for her Trinidadian Indian food. And then there was AhMoo, the matriarch of the family next door, literally the only other Chinese family in the village, and the family my sister-in-law married into. AhMoo, like Mommy, came from Toishan, but her culinary repertoire was far vaster and more adventurous than anyone could have imagined. She could make anything. And she made the best bread. On my first visit to Trinidad, we planned a weekend excursion; AhMoo roasted a ham and baked fresh hops bread to make sandwiches for our journey. These rolls look like hamburger buns, but the similarities stop there. Hops bread's popularity is attributed to an English immigrant, Jon Alfred Rapsey, who operated a bakery in Port of Spain in the late 1800s. He is credited with using an old technique he observed among the French Creole kitchens of Trinidad, which involved leavening dough with an extract of the male hop flower. At some point, the hops were replaced with yeast, but these rolls continue to hold a special place in the Trini heart. To get best results, allow time for three rises. You'll be rewarded with a flaky, moist interior and a slightly crisp exterior. (History source: www.izatrini.com)

HOPS BREAD

Makes 1 dozen rolls

Butter a large bowl and set aside.

Stir together yeast, sugar, and water in a small bowl until dissolved, and let sit for 10 minutes until bubbly and yeasty-smelling.

Mix together flour and salt in a separate, dry large bowl, make a well in its center, and drizzle in melted butter, then gradually add yeast mixture with a wooden spoon. Mix with your hands. Add additional water, if needed, to bring dough together.

Like all homemade bread, this recipe does wonders for your soul.

Knead until soft and smooth, 5 to 10 minutes. Then, place dough ball in prepared bowl, and butter top of dough. Cover with plastic wrap and let rest in a warm area for 45 minutes.

After first rise, punch down dough, form it back into a ball, cover, and allow it to rise for another 45 minutes.

Preheat oven to 400°F and line 2 baking sheets with parchment.

After second rise, punch down dough, divide into twelve balls, and place 2 inches apart on prepared baking sheets. Cover with a damp cloth and allow to rise a final time until doubled, another 15 minutes.

Remove cloth and bake rolls for 15 to 20 minutes, or until golden. Eat immediately with butter to experience hops bread in its ideal, crusty-topped form. Keeps best for 1 to 2 days.

2 cups all-purpose flour,
plus more for dusting

2 teaspoons baking powder

¼ teaspoon salt

4 tablespoons margarine
(salted butter may be
substituted but would not
be authentic)

¾ cup canned, full-fat
coconut milk, shaken
vigorously before using

THIS IS A BAKED VERSION of a Trinidadian flatbread that is usually deep-fried. Confusing, but delicious. This bake has the texture of your flakiest biscuit with the tropical flavor of coconut. Bake can be split in half to make a sandwich with buljol, or eaten for breakfast.

COCONUT BAKE

Makes 1 bake

Preheat oven to 350°F. Line a baking sheet with parchment.

Sift together dry ingredients in a medium-size bowl. Work in margarine with your fingertips until crumbly.

Add coconut milk, first stirring with a spoon and then with your hands to form dough into a smooth ball. Depending on your kitchen's humidity, you may need more coconut milk or more flour; add a tiny bit at a time. Allow dough to rest for 30 minutes, covered with a damp cloth.

After dough has rested, roll out onto a floured surface to form a 1-inch-thick circle. Transfer to prepared baking sheet and bake for about 30 minutes, until golden.

Bake can be eaten on its own, or split horizontally to make sandwiches with buljol, smoked herring, or for more familiar flavors, avocado, tomato and onion, ham, or eggs. Also consider rolling out and cutting with a biscuit cutter for an individual-size version.

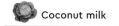 Coconut milk

1 large eggplant (about 2 pounds)

6 garlic cloves, peeled

¼ cup chopped onion

Hot pepper, sliced (e.g., Scotch bonnet, habanero; optional)

Salt and freshly ground black pepper

CHOKA REFERS TO a roasted vegetable dish, such as this eggplant version, which is similar to Middle Eastern baba ghanouj. It's served for breakfast with roti or buss up shut (see pages 275 and 270 to make your own), and sometimes as a side dish to curries.

EGGPLANT CHOKA (ROASTED EGGPLANT DIP)

Serves 4 to 6

Wash and dry eggplant. With a paring knife, slice an X into skin for each clove of garlic, then insert whole cloves into slits.

Roast eggplant: You'll get the best, smokiest flavor if you cook directly on a gas or charcoal grill. Cook until eggplant is completely tender (almost like a deflated balloon) and evenly charred on all sides, rotating occasionally with tongs. This will take 30 to 40 minutes. When done, wrap in foil and allow to rest for 15 minutes.

Alternatively, use the broiler. Preheat broiler to HIGH. Place eggplant on a foil-lined baking sheet and broil for about an hour, rotating occasionally with tongs, until it is completely tender and its skin is evenly charred, as above. Wrap, using same foil, and allow to rest for 15 minutes.

Scoop out flesh, remove garlic cloves, and transfer to a medium-size bowl. Discard skin.

Mash eggplant flesh together with garlic, and season with onion, sliced pepper (if using), and salt and pepper to taste.

Serve with your choice of accompaniments.

❋ Black pepper, garlic

🥬 Eggplant

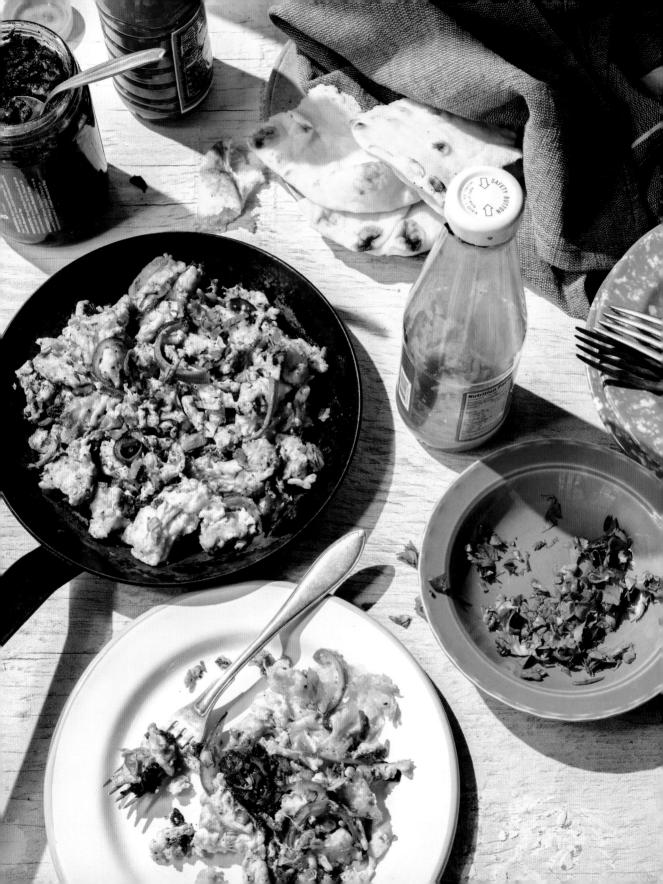

2 tablespoons oil

½ red onion, sliced

2 teaspoons cumin seeds

Pinch of salt

8 large eggs, beaten with a pinch or two of salt

¼ cup minced fresh cilantro

2 to 4 tablespoons kuchela (see page 319 to make your own)

CHUTNEYS, which originated in India, are condiments traditionally made with a variety of vegetables or fruits blended together with spices and chiles. *Kuchela*, a specific kind of mango chutney eaten in Trinidad, is very different from the mango chutney you'll find elsewhere. It's made of grated green mangoes and spiced with the unique taste of the spice blend amchar masala, garlic, and chile. The flavors are spicy, salty, and sour, without added sugar. It's used, like other chutneys, to enhance the flavor of curries, roti, rice dishes like pelau, and really just about everything. Here is one of my family's favorite ways to enjoy kuchela. This spin on scrambled eggs and toast is an easy, flavorful breakfast. To keep with the Indian theme, I recommend serving this with roti, buss up shut, or naan (see pages 275, 270, and 123 to make your own). Enjoy with spiced chai or other tea.

SCRAMBLED EGGS WITH KUCHELA

Serves 4 to 6

Heat oil in a skillet over medium heat. When shimmery, add sliced onion, cumin seeds, and a pinch of salt and cook for 1 minute, until just becoming translucent.

Lower heat to low, then add beaten eggs. When eggs are slightly set, after about 2 minutes, add minced cilantro.

Continue to scramble until eggs reach your desired firmness (1 more minute for softer, 2 to 3 minutes for firmer), then remove from heat and stir in kuchela. Serve immediately with your accompaniments of choice.

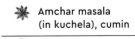

Amchar masala (in kuchela), cumin

Cilantro, eggs

2 cups all-purpose flour, plus more for dusting

1 cup whole wheat flour

1 teaspoon sugar

2 teaspoons baking powder

1½ teaspoons salt

1 tablespoon neutral oil, such as canola, plus more for pan

1¼ cups warm water, plus more if needed

6 tablespoons ghee or melted salted butter

ON MY FIRST VISIT to Trinidad, I had a little trouble understanding the accent, but I tried hard to figure out what people were telling me. I couldn't figure out what the *paratha*, the fluffy flatbread we were having with our curry, was—what was this "buss up shut"? Peter's nephews laughed hard and slowly enunciated for me, "It's *bursted up shirt*, Auntie Linda." That was almost three decades ago, and they just asked me about it again last month! Well, I had the last laugh—I've figured out how to make it at home, which no Trinidadian actually does. It's an interesting technique of laminating the dough and then literally beating up the just-cooked flatbread to lighten it up and create even more layers. In this version, I've substituted a bit of whole wheat flour to give a little bit more nutrition. If you want a more traditional version, use all-purpose flour only. Note that, dough-resting time included, this recipe takes 3 to 5 hours to complete.

BUSS UP SHUT (TRINIDADIAN PARATHA)

Makes 6 paratha

In a large bowl, sift together flours, sugar, baking powder, and salt.

Make a well in dry ingredients, then add oil and warm water and stir until dough begins to come together. Flour your hands and knead dough for about 30 seconds—dough will be very soft and sticky.

Divide dough into six equal pieces. Cover with a damp cloth and let it rest for 30 minutes.

After dough has rested, place each piece onto a floured surface and use a rolling pin to roll it into a circle. Then, brush each circle with some ghee or melted butter.

Use a knife to make a cut from center of circle to its edge. Then, pick up one cut edge and roll it clockwise onto rest of the dough circle, so that you have a cone.

continued ⟶

As a general rule in baking, replacing half the flour with *whole-grain flour*, in this case whole wheat, adds fiber and the other nutritional benefits of whole grains.

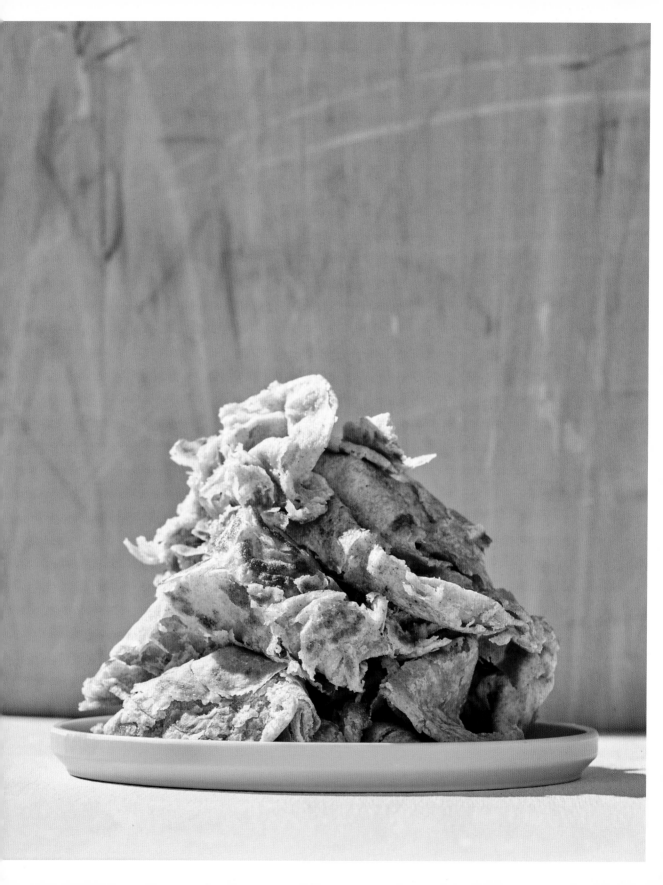

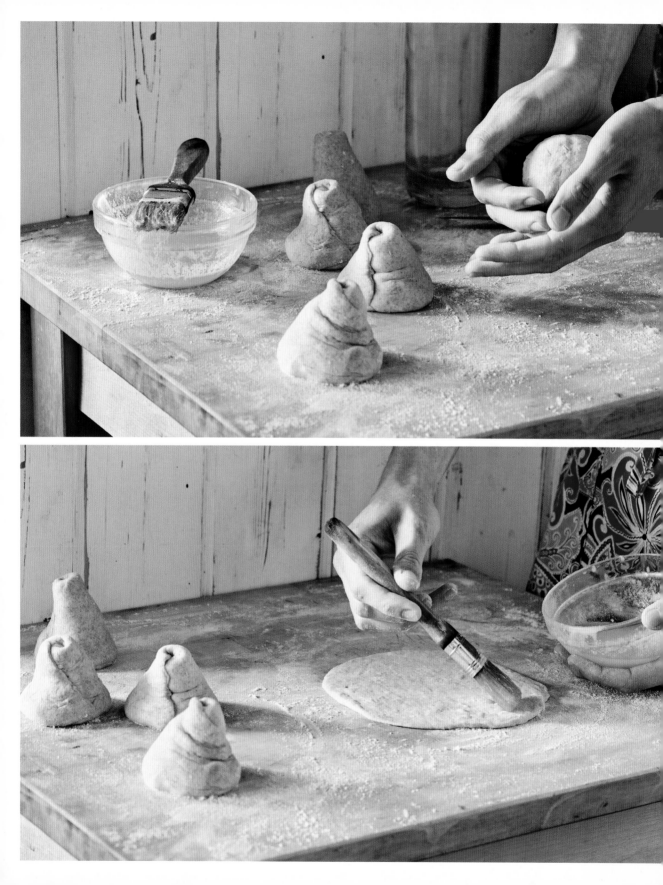

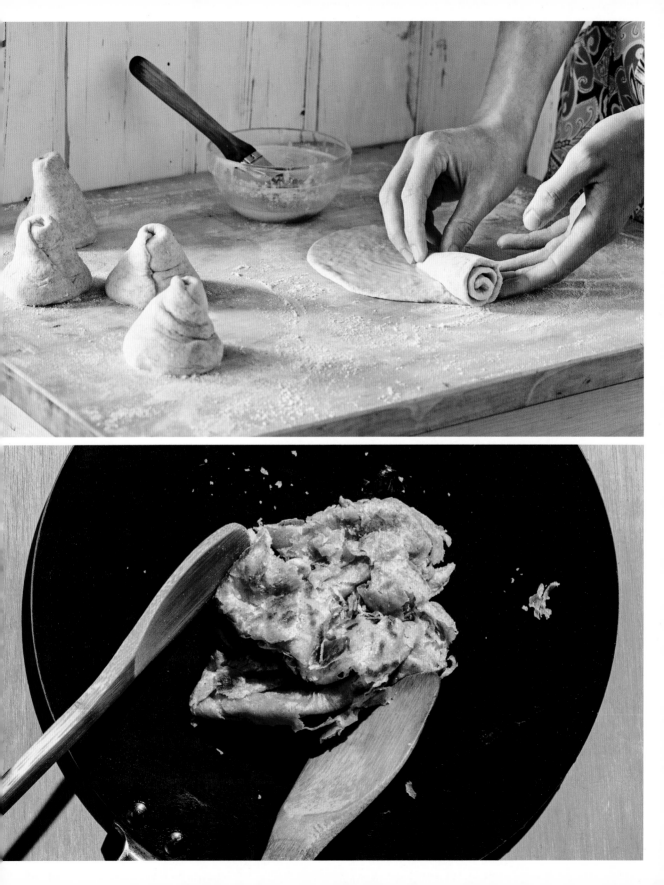

Next, tuck in the wide part of the cone so that you have a flat bottom, and then push in the tip of the cone. It will look like a little volcano. Repeat with remaining pieces of dough.

Place each rolled dough on an oiled baking sheet with a little space between, and cover with a damp cloth. Let rest for 2 to 4 hours.

When ready to cook, heat a nonstick or cast-iron griddle or skillet (traditionally, a *tawa*) over medium heat.

Using your rolling pin, roll each cone into a thin circle.

Gently place a rolled-out dough circle onto hot pan.

Brush the side that is facing up with ghee or melted butter while its bottom side is cooking. When dough begins to produce little air pockets, flip it over.

Allow the other side to cook for another 20 seconds, then make "buss up shut" by crushing paratha between two wooden spatulas (in Trinidad, long wooden spatulas called *dablas* are used). Pick up paratha with spatulas and bang spatulas together, smashing paratha between them. Repeat several times, beating, tearing, and folding paratha into fluffy, messy layers. Transfer to a platter and keep covered with a dry cloth. Repeat with remaining dough. Serve warm with a curry.

½ cup rolled oats

1 cup whole wheat flour

2 tablespoons ground flaxseeds

¼ teaspoon salt

About 1 cup warm water

Canola oil or coconut oil, for pan

PETER'S LATE GREAT-AUNT VICTORIA, known to all as Auntie Doll, was a talented cook and the one who taught me most of what I know about Trinidadian cooking. Even when her failing health required her to alter her recipes to be more heart and diabetes friendly, she had what Trinis call "sweet hands." Auntie Doll replaced the usual white flour in her roti (Indian flatbread) with a custom blend of oats, flaxseeds, and whole wheat. This just-right blend of flour is not only rich in fiber and nutrients but has a more interesting, nutty taste and remains tender and flaky. Enjoy this with the recipes in this section for eggplant or pumpkin choka (pages 267 and 286), dal (page 287), or other Indian food.

AUNTIE DOLL'S MULTIGRAIN ROTI

Makes 6 roti

Make oat flour by pulsing rolled oats in a food processor or high-speed blender until fine.

Transfer to a small bowl and add whole wheat flour, flaxseeds, and salt. Combine with a wooden spoon.

Gradually add just enough water to make a soft, pliable dough (depending on humidity and other conditions, you might not need all of it), stirring with spoon. Then, use your hands to roll dough into a ball, cover with a damp cloth, and allow to rest for 20 minutes.

After it has rested, divide dough into six small (golf ball–size) balls, then use a rolling pin to roll each ball into a thin, flat circle, with about a 5-inch diameter.

Heat a nonstick or cast-iron griddle or skillet and add a thin layer of oil. Add one dough circle at a time to pan. Cook until browned on one side, then flip over and cook until browned on the other side, about 1 minute per side. You'll see brown spots and roti will puff just a little. Repeat with remaining dough circles.

Serve warm.

 Flaxseeds, oats, whole wheat (whole grains)

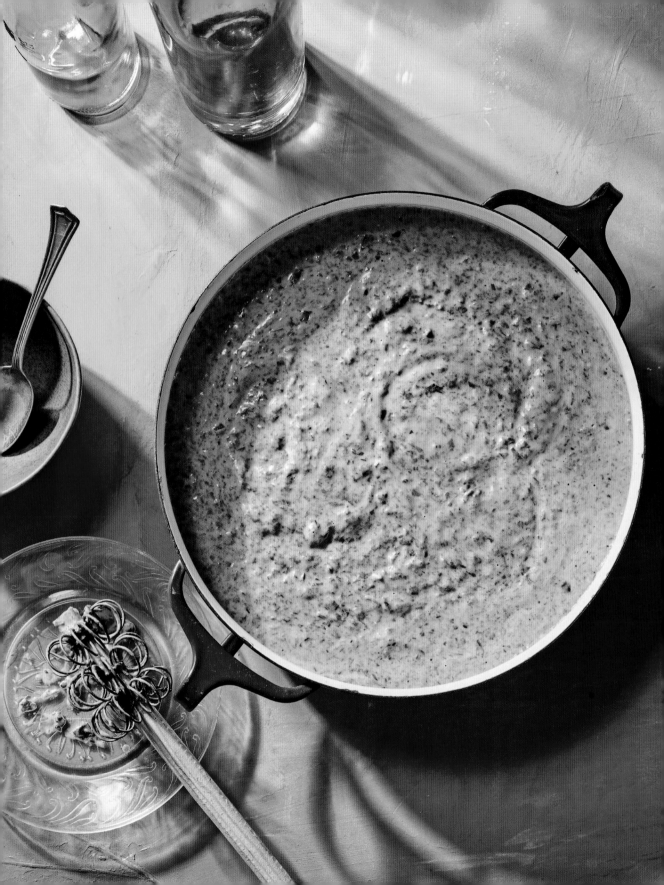

ON ONE OF HIS last visits before he passed away recently, Peter's childhood friend Heland, who made his living as an actor and independent filmmaker in New York, made us a delicious pot of callaloo. This green vegetable stew is hard to describe to outsiders; it's the kind of dish that you eat when your granny makes it for you, but can seem like too much work to make it yourself. But it is a taste of home, and worth the effort. The central ingredient is traditionally taro leaves, also called dasheen. Spinach is sometimes used and makes a fine substitute. The leafy greens are cooked with okra, coconut milk, peppers, a secret blend of spices, and sometimes salt pork and/or crab. This classic dish, which has humbler origins among Trinidad's African slaves, is part of what is known as Creole food in Trinidad. It's eaten alongside macaroni pie and *pelau* (rice with pigeon peas, see page 296) or simply served with rice.

HELAND'S CALLALOO

Serves 4 to 6

Melt butter in a stockpot over medium heat, then add onion and a pinch of salt. Sauté until onion is fragrant and translucent, about 5 minutes.

Add garlic and cook for 30 seconds.

Add taro, okra, green onions, minced pepper, thyme leaves, and another pinch of salt and stir. Cook for another 30 seconds. Stir in stock and coconut milk and bring to a boil. Lower heat, cover, and simmer for 30 minutes, until all vegetables are very soft.

Puree with an immersion blender or in a standard blender.

Return puree to pot. Add salt to taste.

If using crab, add to soup and bring to a boil. Cook for a few minutes until crabmeat is cooked.

Serve over hot rice or as a sauce or condiment for provisions or other starches.

2 tablespoons salted butter or coconut oil

1 onion, diced

Salt

3 garlic cloves, minced

1 pound taro leaves (about 12 leaves) stripped from central stem), roughly chopped, or whole leaf fresh spinach or frozen spinach

8 okra, diced

2 green onions, whites and greens, thinly sliced

1 Scotch bonnet or habanero pepper, minced

Leaves from 3 thyme sprigs

1 cup vegetable stock

4 cups canned unsweetened full-fat coconut milk

8 ounces lump crabmeat (optional)

Steamed rice (in the Caribbean, parboiled rice is typical) or roti, for serving

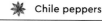

✳ Chile peppers

🥬 Okra, spinach, taro leaves, thyme

1 tablespoon vegetable oil

1 onion, chopped

2 garlic cloves, peeled and smashed

1 cup dried yellow split peas

2 tablespoons green seasoning (see page 324 to make your own)

1½ teaspoons pimentón (smoked paprika)

8 to 10 cups water

1 cup peeled, seeded, and diced pumpkin, or kabocha or butternut squash (1-inch dice); may use frozen

3 pounds mixed provisions: taro, sweet potato, green plantain, potatoes, peeled and cut into 1-inch dice

12 whole okra, trimmed and sliced in half crosswise

1 large carrot, peeled and cut into 1-inch chunks

1 tablespoon kosher salt

1 Scotch bonnet pepper

Trinidad Dumplings (page 324, optional)

PETER HAS FOND MEMORIES of Auntie Doll's sancoche, a hearty, comforting root vegetable stew with a base of salt beef or pigtail. When I said I was going to make a version without either of these preserved meats, both to make it more accessible to people outside the Caribbean and to offer a plant-based version, he was skeptical. But on tasting it, he was amazed, as I was able to re-create the smokiness with my pantry trick, smoked paprika. Sancoche, which has roots in the Spanish Caribbean, where it is known as *sancocho*, gets its Trinidadian flavor from the Scotch bonnet pepper and green seasoning.

SANCOCHE

Serves 12

Heat oil in a Dutch oven or stockpot, then sauté onion and garlic until onion is translucent, about 5 minutes. Add split peas, green seasoning, pimentón, and 4 cups of water, stir well, then simmer until split peas are soft, about 45 minutes.

Add remaining ingredients, except dumplings, with enough water to cover, and cook for another 30 to 45 minutes, or until root vegetables are completely soft and broth is thickened, with the consistency of stew. Adjust salt to taste.

If desired, prepare dumpling batter and cook on top of stew until done.

Chile pepper, smoked paprika

Okra, split peas, plantain, potatoes, pumpkin (winter squash), sweet potatoes, taro

THE INGREDIENTS used in this soup, which I've named after Trinidad's capital city, represent many of Trinidad's diverse cultures—corn from the indigenous Caribs, herbs from French settlers, split peas used for both dal and *dhalpourie roti* in local Indian cuisine, and root vegetables and dumplings from Creole cuisine. Another traditional Creole ingredient is salt-cured pigtail, but I'm substituting pimentón (smoked paprika) for smoky flavor. This is a hearty soup, suitable for a meal on its own. It's popular during Carnival, when it is traditionally sold by street vendors in Styrofoam cups as a thin broth, but you can serve it more like a stew, if desired. In Trinidad, most of the time all these ingredients would just be boiled together, but the flavor is much enhanced by these separate steps below, so I encourage you to do so.

PORT OF SPAIN CORN SOUP

Serves 8 to 12

Cut kernels off one ear of corn, place in a blender with ¼ cup of water, and blend until smooth. Set aside. Cut remaining ears of corn into 1½-inch lengths. Set aside.

Rinse split peas and bring to a boil in 6 cups of water for about 20 minutes, then drain and set aside.

Melt coconut oil in a stockpot over medium heat, then add onion, garlic, celery, and bell pepper with a pinch of salt and sauté for a few minutes, until onion is translucent. Add sweet potato, potatoes, pumpkin, and carrot with another pinch of salt and sauté for another minute.

Next, stir in split peas, corn puree, coconut milk, stock, and remaining 3 cups of water. Add thyme, parsley, chives, culantro, whole Scotch bonnet pepper, and pimentón, black pepper, and remaining salt, bring to a boil, then lower heat to a gentle simmer and cook, covered, for 30 to 45 minutes, stirring every 10 to 15 minutes.

continued ⟶

4 ears fresh corn

3¼ cups water

1 cup dried yellow split peas or orange lentils

2 tablespoons coconut oil

1 small onion, minced

3 garlic cloves, minced

1 celery stalk, minced

1 green bell pepper, seeded and minced

1½ teaspoons kosher salt, or to taste

1 large sweet potato, cut into ½-inch dice

2 medium-size Yukon Gold potatoes, cut into ½-inch dice

1 pound pumpkin or butternut squash, peeled, seeded, and cut into ½-inch dice (about 1½ cups)

1 large carrot, cut into ½-inch dice

1 (13.5-ounce) can coconut milk (about 1½ cups)

4 cups unsalted or low-sodium vegetable stock

3 thyme sprigs

2 tablespoons minced fresh parsley

5 fresh chives, minced

2 tablespoons minced fresh culantro (shado beni) or cilantro

1 Scotch bonnet or habanero pepper, left whole

1 teaspoon pimentón (smoked paprika)

A few grinds of black pepper

2 recipes Trinidad Dumplings batter (page 324)

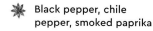

✳ Black pepper, chile pepper, smoked paprika

🌰 Corn, herbs, pumpkin, split peas

When all vegetables and split peas have cooked down so that they are starting to fall apart, remove thyme (and Scotch bonnet pepper if you don't want anyone to have a spicy surprise!) and add cut-up corn ears. Bring back to a boil and cook for another 15 to 20 minutes, adding additional water, if needed, to have a thin broth, and making sure to stir frequently, until kernels appear very soft. Lower heat to a simmer.

Adjust seasonings to taste, then drop in dumpling batter to make bite-size dumplings, about 2 tablespoons batter per dumpling. These will float at the top of the soup. Simmer for another 10 to 15 minutes, or until dumplings are cooked. Serve hot, garnishing individual servings with additional herbs, if desired. Enjoy soup as you normally would with a spoon, then finish off by eating corn off cobs with your hands.

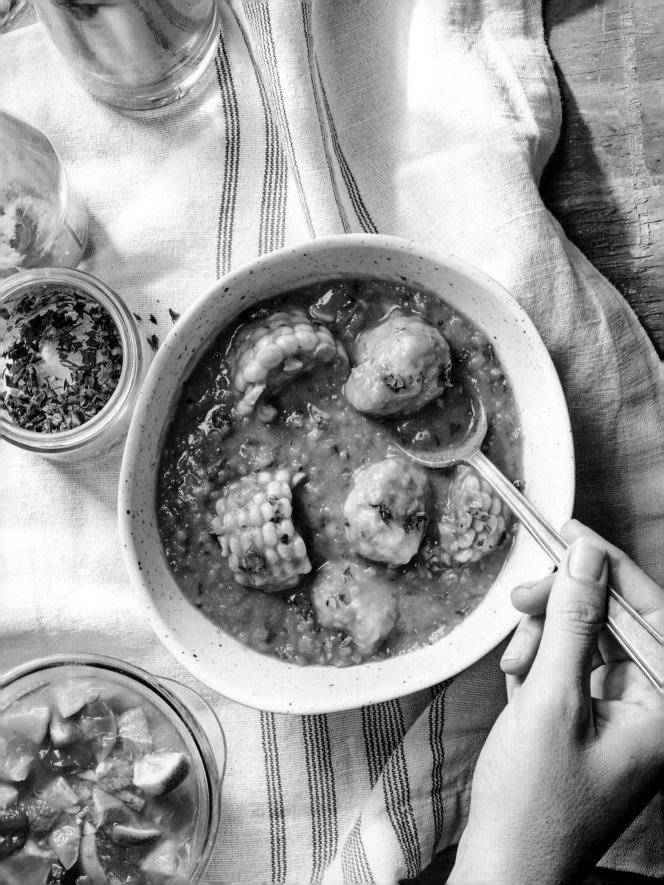

1½ pounds whole red snapper or similar firm, white-fleshed fish

Freshly squeezed lime juice, for soaking

Kosher salt

Freshly ground black pepper

3 tablespoons green seasoning (see page 324 to make your own)

1½ teaspoons canola or other neutral oil

1 small onion, peeled and thinly sliced

1 celery stalk, thinly sliced

8 ounces Yukon Gold potatoes, cut into bite-size chunks

1 pound sweet potatoes, peeled and cut into bite-size chunks

1 to 2 green (unripe) bananas, ideally small tropical variety, peeled and quartered

1 medium-size carrot, cut into bite-size chunks

4 to 6 okra, tops and ends removed

1 ripe Roma tomato, sliced

1 Scotch bonnet or habanero pepper, left whole

3 thyme sprigs

8 cups water

1 recipe Trinidad Dumplings batter (page 324)

Juice of 2 limes

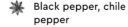 Black pepper, chile pepper

Fish, herbs, okra, tomato

<image name="SPICEBOX KITCHEN"></image>

DON'T BE FOOLED by the name; this recipe is a not a clear liquid, but more of a fish stew. Most notably, this Trinidadian favorite serves fish in a way that some may not be accustomed to—a cutup whole fish: head, skin, bones, and tail included—as opposed to deconstructed pieces of fillet. If you're not comfortable with cleaning your own fish, your fishmonger will be happy to cut and clean it for you. If that's not possible, fish steaks would be second best, but don't substitute fillet, as it won't be as flavorful. Make sure your guests are prepared to watch out for bones.

TRINIDAD FISH BROTH

Serves 6 to 8

Clean and descale fish, making sure to remove all scales. Then, use a traditional Trinidadian technique of "washing" fish in lime juice, by soaking in a bowl of lime juice and enough water to cover for a few minutes. After, remove fish from liquid (discard soaking liquid), then season inside and out with salt and black pepper and half of green seasoning. Cut seasoned fish into 2- to 3-inch chunks and marinate for at least an hour, refrigerated.

Heat oil in a stockpot over medium heat, then add onion and celery with a pinch of salt, and cook for 30 seconds to a minute, until fragrant. Add potatoes, sweet potatoes, bananas, carrot, okra, tomato, Scotch bonnet pepper, thyme, 1½ teaspoons of salt, black pepper to taste, water, and remaining green seasoning, stir well, and bring to a boil.

Lower heat to a simmer, cover, and cook, stirring once or twice, until vegetables are fork-tender but not falling apart, 20 to 30 minutes.

Once vegetables are done, add seasoned fish and cook, covered, for about 5 minutes.

Remove thyme and Scotch bonnet pepper, if desired. Adjust salt and black pepper to taste.

Bring soup back to a gentle boil and drop in dumpling batter by the spoonful to make bite-size dumplings (about 2 tablespoons batter). Once all dumplings have been added, lower heat back to a simmer and cook, covered, for another 10 minutes, or until dumplings are done. Stir in lime juice and serve.

1 tablespoon coconut oil

1 onion, sliced

Salt

3 garlic cloves, chopped

2 dozen okra, sliced, or
1 pound frozen sliced okra

2 cups parboiled (converted)
rice

1½ cups water

1½ cups canned full-fat
coconut milk

1 Scotch bonnet pepper

Freshly ground black pepper

THIS CREOLE DISH, with African roots, is a delicate tasting combination of naturally sweet coconut milk with mild, grassy tasting okra. Because the okra is simmered with the rice, its potentially gummy interior gets absorbed into the rice grains. Enjoy this with Pumpkin Choka (page 286), Trinidadian Black-Eyed Peas for Old Year's and New Beginnings (page 289), or Stew Pigeon Peas and Pumpkin (page 303).

OKRA RICE

Serves 8

Melt coconut oil in a Dutch oven or deep sauté pan with a lid over medium heat. Add onion and a pinch of salt and cook until translucent, a few minutes. Then, add garlic and cook for another 30 seconds.

Add okra and a pinch of salt, and stir to combine with onions and garlic, about a minute.

Add rice, water, coconut milk, Scotch bonnet pepper, and ½ teaspoon of salt and bring to a boil.

Lower heat and simmer, covered, until rice is tender, about 30 minutes. Check after 20 minutes to add additional water, if needed.

When done, adjust salt and black pepper to taste.

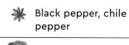

Black pepper, chile pepper

Okra, rice

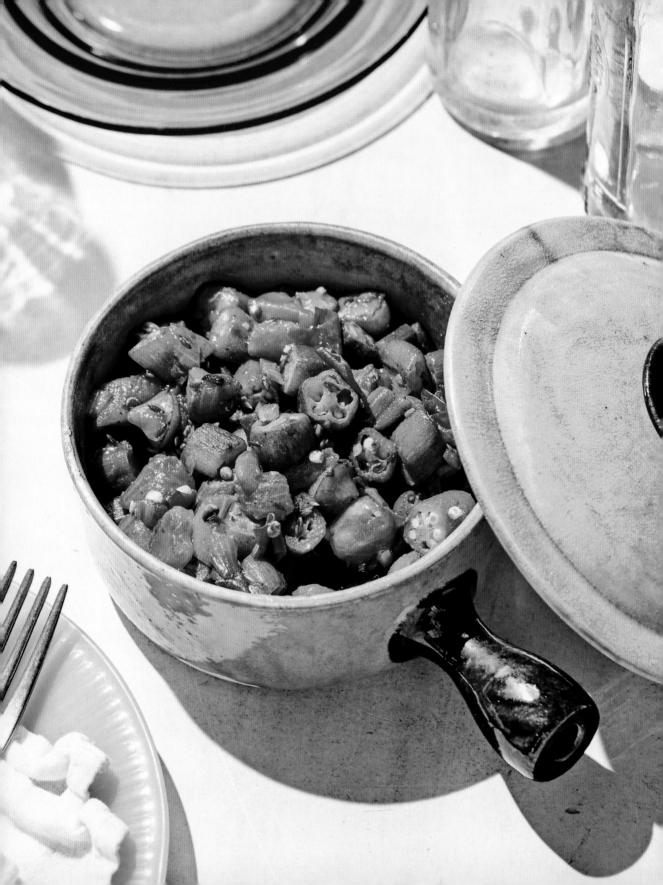

1 tablespoon coconut oil

½ cup diced onion

Salt and freshly ground black pepper

2 garlic cloves, chopped

1 teaspoon cumin seeds

8 ounces fresh okra, top and tail trimmed, sliced into ½-inch pieces, or frozen, sliced okra

1 Roma tomato, cut into ½-inch dice

TRINIDAD

THIS DISH IS BASED ON an African recipe of stewed okra and tomatoes. It also has a hint of Indian influence with the addition of cumin and the cooking method, which, rather than stewing, involves searing the okra over very high heat until slightly charred. For people who may not enjoy okra due to its gummy starches, this demonstrates two pro tips for reducing that characteristic—cooking okra with something acidic, in this case tomatoes, and cooking at high heat.

OKRA AND TOMATOES

Serves 4 as a side dish

Heat a medium-size skillet, ideally cast iron, over medium heat, then melt coconut oil in skillet.

Add onion with a pinch of salt and cook for about 30 seconds, then add garlic and cumin seeds and cook for another 30 seconds.

Increase heat to high, add okra, and cook, stirring, for 30 to 60 seconds, or until slightly charred.

Add tomato plus salt and pepper to taste, stir to combine, and cook for another 3 minutes, until tender but not mushy. Adjust seasonings to taste.

SIDES

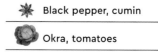

Black pepper, cumin

Okra, tomatoes

1 tablespoon canola oil

1 small onion, diced

Salt and freshly ground black pepper

2 garlic cloves, minced

½ teaspoon cumin seeds

2 cups peeled and cubed calabaza pumpkin, or kabocha or butternut squash, (1-inch cubes)

½ cup water

Garnish: fresh cilantro

Cooked rice or roti, for serving

UNLIKE OTHER CHOKAS, such as eggplant (page 267), which involve roasting and are typically served at breakfast, pumpkin choka involves boiling or steaming. Chokas are a popular breakfast, and pumpkin choka is also commonly eaten as a side dish with curries. The pumpkin used in Trinidad is usually the calabaza pumpkin. Kabocha or butternut squash, which are more readily available in North America, make very good substitutes. In a pinch, or out of season, you can also use prepared, frozen winter squash, commonly stocked in supermarket freezers.

PUMPKIN CHOKA

Serves 4

Heat a sauté pan over medium heat and add oil, add onion with a pinch of salt and cook until translucent, then add garlic and cumin seeds and cook until fragrant, about 30 seconds.

Add calabaza and coat in oil and aromatics, then add water and bring to a low boil.

Cover, lower heat to low, and simmer for about 20 minutes, until mashable. Add more water, if needed, to cook completely.

Mash cooked pumpkin with a wooden spoon or spatula. This should have texture of a chunky puree. Add salt and pepper to taste and cook for another minute.

Garnish with cilantro. Serve with rice or roti.

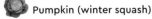 Black pepper, cumin, garlic

Pumpkin (winter squash)

1½ tablespoons canola oil

½ onion, sliced

2 garlic cloves, roughly chopped

2 teaspoons Trinidad curry powder (see page 325 to make your own), or other curry powder, combined with 2 teaspoons water to make a paste

Salt

1 cup dried yellow split peas

4½ cups water

Freshly ground black pepper

½ teaspoon cumin seeds

DAL, which can be made with pretty much any legume, can be enjoyed as a soup or a side dish, depending on how thick or thin you make it. In Trinidad, it is made with yellow split peas and made on the watery side, served as a sauce alongside roti and curry. In most versions, everything is just boiled together. In my version, I prefer to cook the aromatics and curry powder first, to bring out their flavor. The last step, of toasting whole spices in hot oil, is an Indian technique known as *tadka*, or tempering in English, and adds intense flavor.

DAL

Serves 4 to 6

Heat about 1½ teaspoons of oil in a medium-size saucepan with a lid over medium heat, then add onion, garlic, curry powder paste, and a pinch of salt. Stir and cook for a minute, until onion is translucent and softened. Stir in split peas and water and bring to boil over high heat.

Lower heat and simmer, covered, stirring occasionally, for 45 to 60 minutes, or until split peas are soft and starting to break apart. (Time will depend on age of split peas.)

When split peas are very soft, use an immersion blender or swizzle stick (a type of whisk used in Trinidad) to thicken dal slightly in the pot, or transfer about one-third of the dal to a blender, blend till smooth, then add back to the pot. If you desire a thicker dal, bring back to a rolling boil and boil, uncovered, until reduced to desired thickness. Add salt and pepper to taste.

In a small skillet, heat remaining tablespoon of oil over medium heat, then add cumin seeds and cook in oil until fragrant and slightly toasted, up to 30 seconds. Pour spiced oil on top of dal before serving.

Black pepper, cumin, curry powder

Split peas

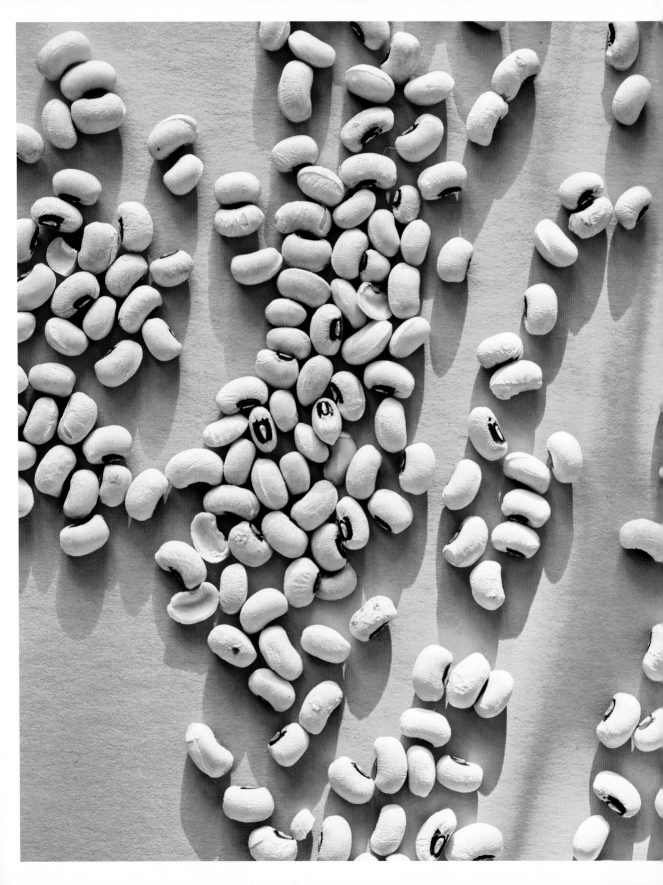

1 tablespoon oil

½ large onion, diced

2 garlic cloves, smashed

Kosher salt and freshly ground black pepper

1 teaspoon pimentón (smoked paprika), or to taste

1 pound dried black-eyed peas, soaked in enough water to cover by a few inches for 8 hours or overnight, then rinsed and drained

6 cups water

1 bay leaf

1 to 2 tablespoons green seasoning (see page 324 to make your own)

1 Scotch bonnet pepper, left whole

Cooked rice (parboiled rice is most common in Trinidad), for serving

WHAT MOST OF THE WORLD celebrates as New Year's Eve is known as Old Year's in Trinidad. The name suggests that you review and reflect upon the old year before it's gone. Similar to the tradition of eating Hoppin' John in the American South, Trinidadians also believe that eating black-eyed peas on Old Year's will bring good luck in the New Year. For my plant-based version, I've left out the traditional ham hock or pigtail and swapped in smoked paprika for smokiness. With the distinctive flavors of green seasoning and Scotch bonnet pepper, it's one of the dishes that I make for Peter to keep him feeling connected to his childhood home.

TRINIDADIAN BLACK-EYED PEAS FOR OLD YEAR'S AND NEW BEGINNINGS

Serves 8 to 12

Heat oil in a stockpot over medium heat and cook onion and garlic with a pinch of salt and pimentón until onion is translucent, about 3 minutes.

Add drained peas, water, bay leaf, green seasoning, and whole Scotch bonnet pepper and bring to a boil. Simmer, covered, for about 45 minutes, or until peas have reached your desired tenderness. Add more water, if desired, or bring to a boil to reduce water if it's too soupy. Add salt and black pepper and adjust other seasonings as desired, and simmer for another 5 minutes.

Remove bay leaf and whole pepper before serving. Serve over rice.

✳ Black pepper, chile pepper, smoked paprika

 Black eyed peas, green seasoning (herbs)

2 large partially ripe mangoes (about 2½ pounds), skin on, cut into 2-inch chunks and pit reserved (mangoes should be firm, mainly green with a slight orange blush in a few areas)

2 tablespoons kosher salt

3 tablespoons Trinidad curry powder (see page 325 to make your own)

1 teaspoon ground turmeric

1 teaspoon ground cumin

1 tablespoon oil

1 onion, chopped

2 garlic cloves, chopped

1 Scotch bonnet or habanero pepper, sliced

1 tablespoon chopped fresh culantro (shado beni) leaves or cilantro

Freshly ground black pepper

THIS VEGETARIAN CURRY is served as a savory and fruity side dish with other curries and can also be enjoyed as a main dish. Make sure you use only partially ripened mangoes, or it will be too sweet.

CURRY MANGO

Serves 4

Place mangoes, pit included, in a medium-size saucepan. Add water to cover, along with salt. Bring to a boil and cook until softened, 5 to 10 minutes. Drain and set aside, reserving water.

Mix curry powder, turmeric, and cumin together in a small bowl with an equal amount of cold water, until you have a pourable slurry.

Heat a sauté pan over medium heat and add oil. When oil is shimmery, add onion and sauté until translucent, about a minute, then add garlic and sliced Scotch bonnet pepper and cook for another 30 seconds. Add spice mixture and cook for 2 minutes, or until slightly reduced, then transfer cooked, drained mangoes to curry mixture. Stir to coat.

Add about ½ cup of reserved mango cooking water and culantro. Stir and simmer, uncovered, for another 10 to 15 minutes, until mangoes are tender and curry sauce has reduced. Add pepper and adjust seasonings to taste.

Serve with rice or roti. (Pit is included for flavor and is not meant to be chewed and swallowed, but can be savored by sucking off flesh by someone who knows their way around mangoes.)

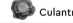 Black pepper, cumin, curry powder, turmeric

Culantro, mangoes

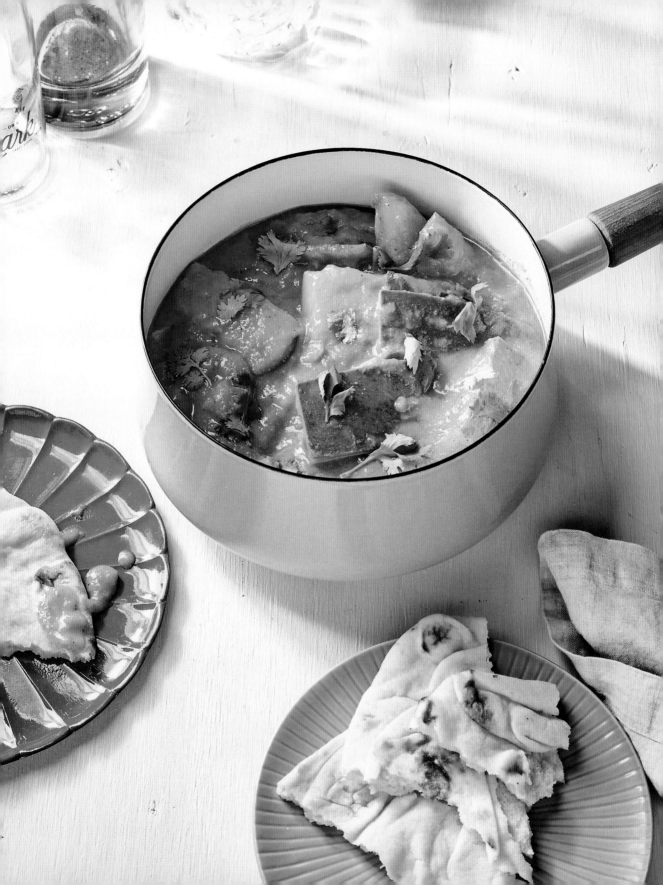

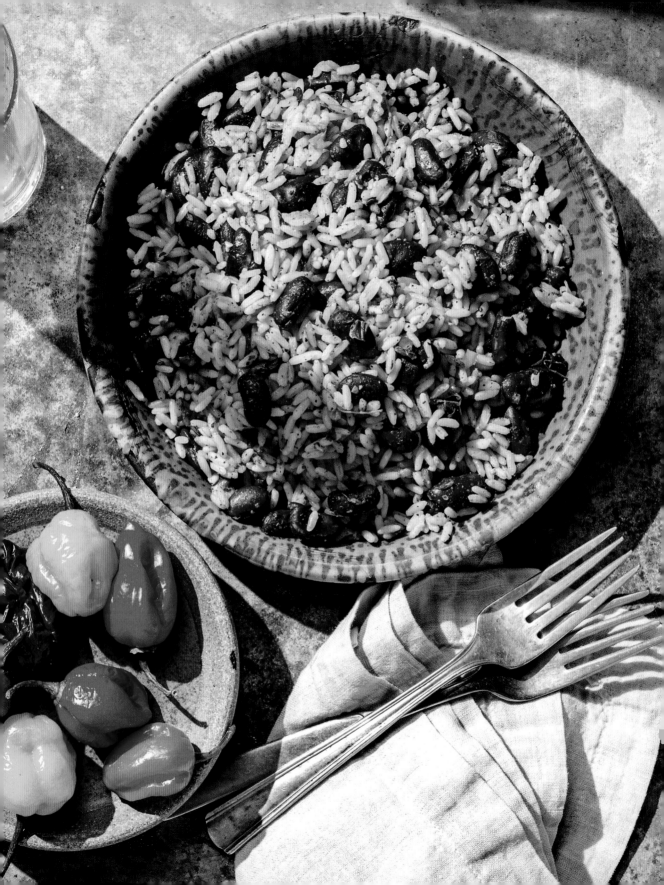

TRINIDAD

1 cup parboiled (converted) rice

1 cup canned, full-fat coconut milk

2 scallions, chopped

2 garlic cloves, chopped

2 tablespoons fresh thyme leaves

1¼ cups canned no-salt-added red kidney beans, drained and rinsed

½ Scotch bonnet or habanero pepper, seeded and diced

¾ teaspoon salt

½ teaspoon freshly ground black pepper

½ teaspoon ground allspice

1¼ cups water

THIS WEEKNIGHT ADAPTATION of the classic Jamaican dish rice and peas (which are not green peas, but small red beans similar to kidney beans) uses the convenience of a rice cooker to make a hands-off, one-pot meal. If you don't have a rice cooker, you can certainly make this on the stove, using any pot with a lid, including a Dutch oven. Parboiled rice holds up better than white rice to the cooking liquid, so it can absorb all of the flavor while maintaining its texture. It's also more nutritious than white rice. This dish pairs well with Jamaican Jerk Tempeh Kebabs (page 294).

RICE COOKER JAMAICAN RICE AND PEAS

Serves 8

Place all ingredients in a 3-cup or larger rice cooker and stir well. Set to cook. Alternatively, if cooking on stovetop, place all ingredients in a medium-size pot with a lid or a small Dutch oven, stir well, bring to a boil over high heat, then lower heat to a simmer and cook, covered, until all liquid has been absorbed, 20 to 30 minutes.

After rice has finished cooking, stir again and allow to sit, covered, for another 5 to 10 minutes. Fluff with a fork before serving.

MAINS

✳ Allspice, black pepper

 Kidney beans, parboiled (converted) rice, thyme

2 (8-ounce) packages
tempeh (original, not
seasoned)

½ cup jerk marinade
(see page 323 to make
your own)

JERK IS A SPICE RUB or marinade that is synonymous with Jamaican,
not Trinidadian, cuisine. Historically, the two islands have been rivals
for cultural dominance, though Trinidadians will insist that their
cuisine is indisputably the finest in the Caribbean. All that aside, I did
notice on a recent trip back to Trinidad that there were a couple of
jerk sheds on the roadsides. Perhaps a détente? This allspice-heavy
marinade brings concentrated, deep flavor to anything you put it on.
It can be used to marinate any protein; here I've chosen to use tempeh,
which is a fermented soy product with a nutty taste and hearty texture.
It has enough heft to take the place of meat, takes up marinade nicely,
and can stand up to the grill. As a vegan option, it also is a nod to the
plant-based Ital diet followed by Rastafarians in Jamaica.

JAMAICAN JERK TEMPEH KEBABS

4 to 6

Cut tempeh into bite-size pieces (about 2 inches) and submerge in
marinade in a resealable plastic bag or a covered container. Marinate,
refrigerated, for at least 4 hours or overnight.

If using bamboo skewers, soak in water for at least 30 minutes
before using.

When ready to cook: preheat oven to 400°F and line a sheet pan
with foil.

Remove tempeh from marinade and thread onto skewers, then transfer
to prepared sheet pan, leaving some space around each kebab. If you
aren't using skewers, just place cubes on sheet pan.

Roast until edges start to crisp, 15 to 20 minutes total, turning over after
10 minutes. Alternatively, these kebabs can be cooked on a grill.

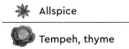

✳ Allspice

Tempeh, thyme

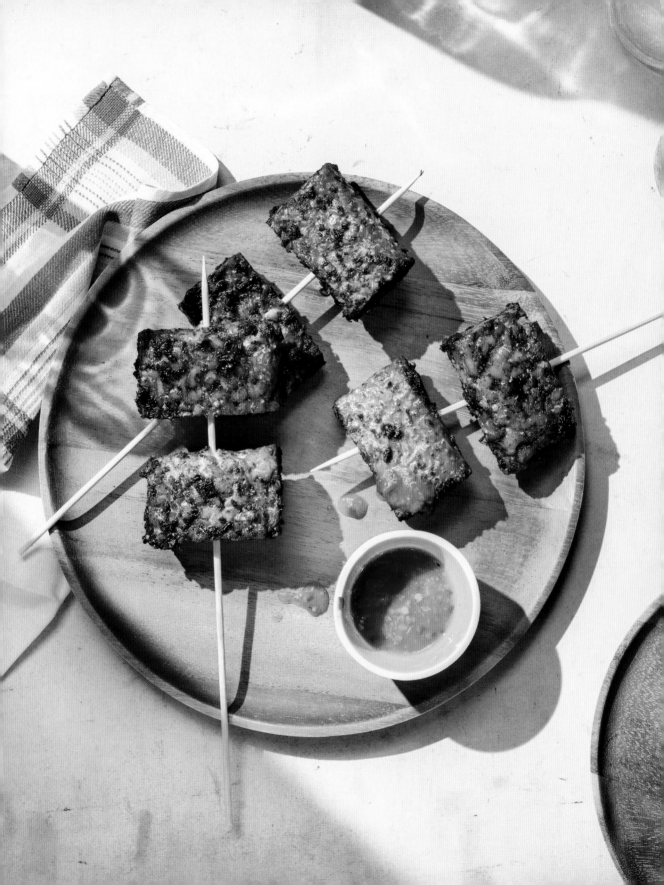

1 teaspoon freshly ground black pepper

1 small onion, diced

1 teaspoon ketchup

1 teaspoon soy sauce

1 teaspoon Worcestershire sauce

1 tablespoon dark rum

1 teaspoon Trinidadian Scotch bonnet pepper sauce (see page 320 to make your own, or purchase online from Matouk's); habanero sauce can substitute in a pinch but is not ideal

2 tablespoons green seasoning (see page 324 to make your own)

2 teaspoons canola oil

¼ cup sugar

4 cups parboiled rice

1 bell pepper, seeded and diced

1 (15-ounce) can green pigeon peas (about 2 cups), drained and rinsed (available from Goya), or frozen black-eyed peas

1 (13.5-ounce) can full-fat coconut milk

3 cups water

2 teaspoons salt

2 pounds kabocha or butternut squash, peeled, seeded, and cut into 2-inch chunks

2 tablespoons olive oil

✴ Black pepper

 Parboiled rice, pigeon peas, pumpkin

PELAU, a rice, bean, and often meat (usually chicken) dish, is thought of as an Afro-Trinidadian dish. However, you may note the remarkable similarity of its name to the Indian rice dish known as *pulao*, or in other derivations, *pilaf*. The basic ingredients of rice, beans, vegetables, and meat are indeed similar throughout the various cultures. But the flavorings used in pelau are distinctly Trinidadian. The coconut milk is a common Caribbean ingredient, and the type of beans used, pigeon peas, are also a hallmark of Caribbean cooking, as are the flavors of green seasoning, rum, and a little bit of Scotch bonnet pepper sauce. I've adapted this recipe from *The Naparima Girls' High School Diamond Jubilee: Trinidad & Tobago Recipes*, a community cookbook that was originally published in 1988. For this vegetarian version, I've added chunks of roasted kabocha or butternut squash, which are similar to what would be called "pumpkin" in Trinidad.

PELAU WITH ROASTED PUMPKIN

Serves 8

In a small bowl, stir together black pepper, onion, ketchup, soy sauce, Worcestershire sauce, rum, pepper sauce, and green seasoning. Set aside.

Make "browning" when you're ready to cook: Heat canola oil in a heavy pot with a lid over medium heat. Then, add sugar and allow to cook, stirring occasionally, until almost black.

When browning has liquefied and is almost black, add rice to pot and stir for a few minutes to coat.

Add bell pepper, pigeon peas, and seasoning mixture, stir, and cook until onion is translucent, about 3 minutes.

Add coconut milk, water, and salt and stir until all ingredients in pot are well combined. Cover pot and bring to a low boil, then lower heat to low and allow to cook for 20 to 30 minutes, stirring about every

continued ⟼

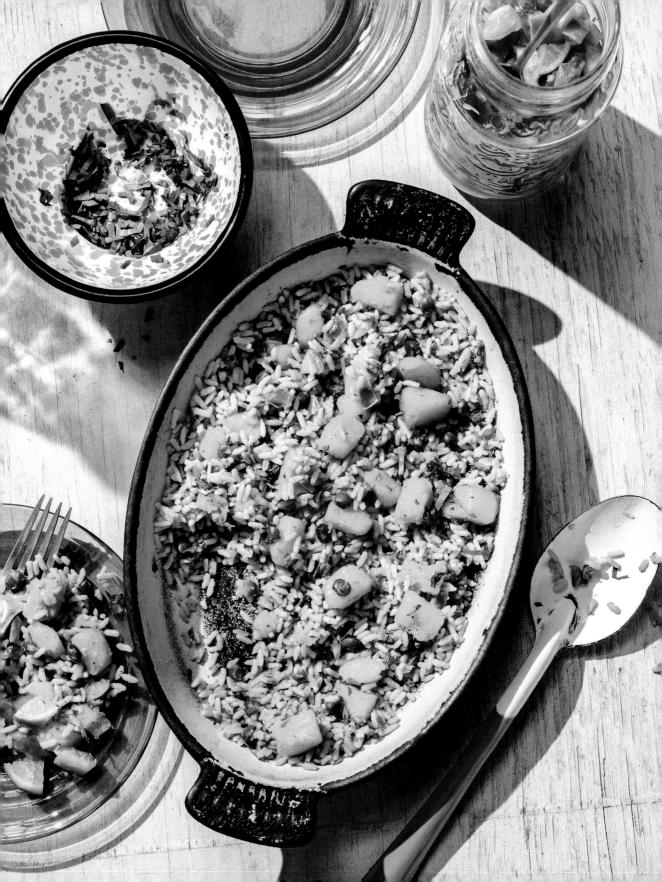

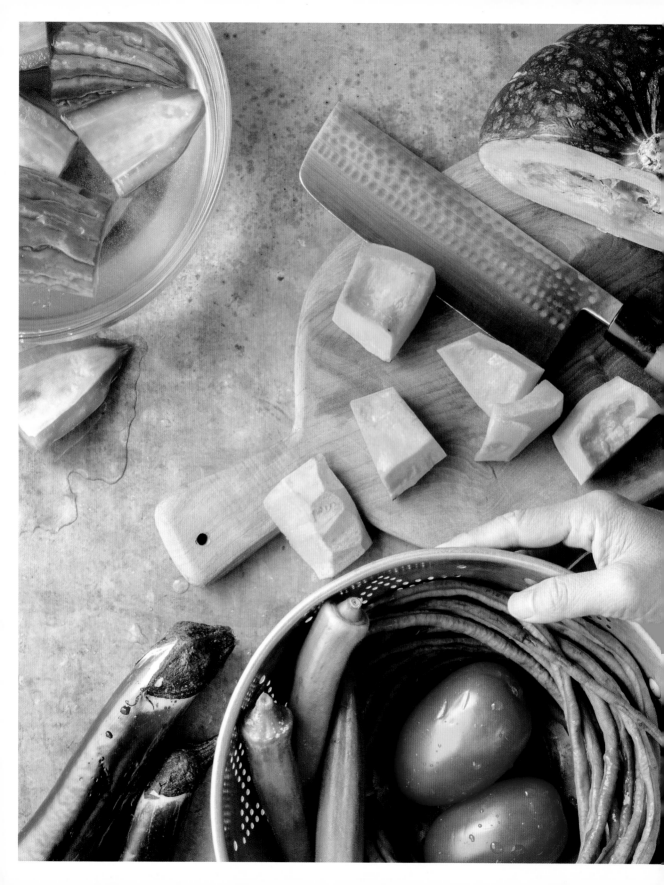

10 minutes to prevent rice from sticking to bottom. Dish is ready when
all liquid has been absorbed and rice is fully cooked. If needed, stir
in additional water and continue to cook to achieve desired level of
softness. Remove from heat, adjust salt and pepper to taste, stir to fluff,
and keep covered for at least 10 minutes before serving.

While rice is cooking, roast squash. Preheat oven to 425°F and line a
baking sheet with parchment. Toss squash cubes in olive oil and salt,
arrange in a single layer on prepared baking sheet, then roast in oven
for about 20 minutes, turning over at the 10-minute point, until lightly
caramelized. Add to pelau when ready to serve.

MARINADE

1½ teaspoons kosher salt

½ teaspoon freshly ground black pepper

1 Scotch bonnet or habanero pepper, seeded and minced, or ½ teaspoon Scotch bonnet pepper sauce or habanero chili sauce

2 tablespoons green seasoning (see page 324 to make your own)

——

2 pounds shrimp, peeled and deveined

2 tablespoons Trinidad curry powder (see headnote)

1 tablespoon ground cumin

1 tablespoon ground turmeric

1½ teaspoons garam masala

1½ cups water

3 tablespoons canola or other neutral oil

½ teaspoon cumin seeds

4 garlic cloves, minced

½ onion, thinly sliced

2 Roma tomatoes, diced

1 tablespoon tamarind sauce (see headnote)

2 tablespoons minced fresh culantro or cilantro

Salt and freshly ground black pepper

❋ Black pepper, coriander, cumin, curry powder, garam masala, turmeric

🥬 Shrimp

THE FIRST TIME I met my future mother-in-law, my welcome meal was a curry, which was not unexpected. What was curried was a complete surprise, however: armadillo, locally known as *tatu*. Despite having been a recently lapsed vegetarian, and despite the still visible impressions on the flesh from the armadillo's bony plates, I tasted it, under my mother-in-law's watchful gaze. More common proteins used in Trinidadian curries are chicken, duck, or goat. Shrimp is served on special occasions, and it's the protein base here. The flavor base is Trinidadian curry powder, which is a distinctive blend of spices, including cumin, coriander, turmeric, fenugreek, fennel, and chile pepper. You can make your own (page 325) or buy Trini favorite Chief brand online. Tamarind sauce (see page 321 to make your own) lends a sweet-and-sour flavor. If you can't find tamarind pulp or sauce, you can substitute a dash of Worcestershire sauce (which contains tamarind), or blend together some dates, raisins, and/or prunes with lime juice. Aside from this particular blend of spices and seasonings, the preparation of Trini-style curry, without coconut milk, gives it a more intense curry flavor and a thinner sauce than Indian or Malaysian-style curries. Curries in Trinidad are served with either dhalpourie roti, which is distinctively filled with spiced, ground split peas, or paratha, a multilayered, buttery flatbread. Both are difficult to obtain outside Trinidad. You can substitute naan (page 123), Buss Up Shut (page 270), Auntie Doll's Multigrain Roti (page 275), or rice. Wash it down with sorrel or Carib beer, play some calypso, soca, or steel band, and enjoy your fete.

TRINIDADIAN CURRY SHRIMP

Serves 6 to 8

Prepare marinade: Stir together marinade ingredients in a medium-size bowl, then add shrimp. Stir well, then marinate for 30 minutes in refrigerator. In a small bowl, combine curry powder, cumin, turmeric, and garam masala with ¾ cup of water to make a slurry.

Heat a Dutch oven or sauté pan over medium heat, add oil, and heat until shimmering.

Add cumin seeds and cook for 10 seconds, or until fragrant, then add garlic and onion to hot oil and sauté for another 2 minutes.

Add spice slurry to onion mixture and cook for another 2 minutes, or until slightly reduced.

Increase heat to high, then add marinated shrimp, stir to evenly coat with curry mixture, and cook for 2 minutes, uncovered. Add tomatoes, tamarind sauce, and culantro and fry for another 30 seconds, then add remaining ¾ cup water.

Mix well and cook for about 5 minutes, or until water has reduced by half and sauce is slightly thickened. Adjust salt to taste.

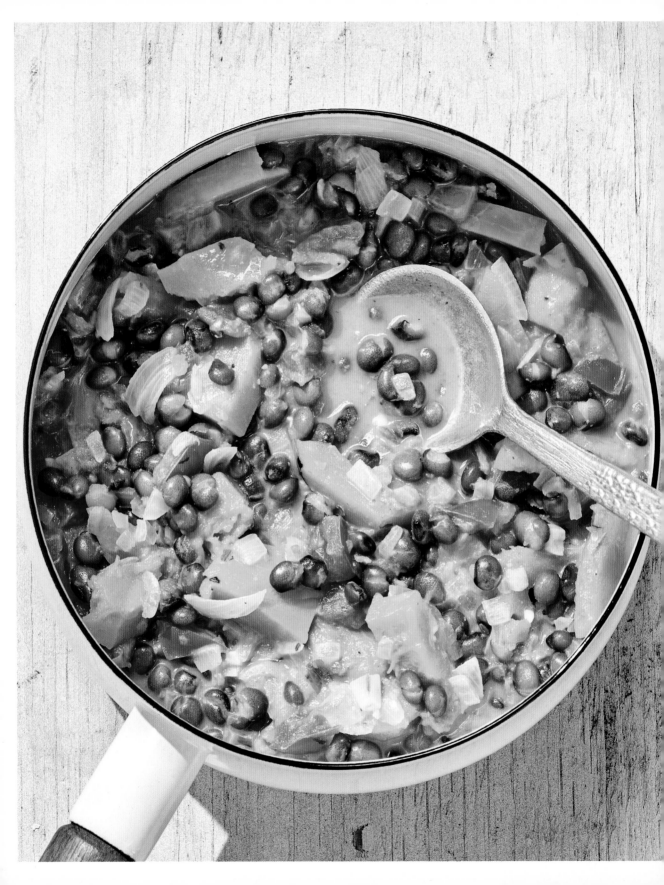

ONE OF THE MAIN TYPES of recipes in the Caribbean is "stew," which most commonly involves chicken cooked in browning, with additional flavors of green seasoning and Scotch bonnet pepper, and often with pigeon peas. This is an equally satisfying plant-based version, naturally sweet from the pumpkin, and with the added fragrant richness of coconut milk. Serve with plain parboiled rice or with Okra Rice (page 283).

STEW PIGEON PEAS AND PUMPKIN

Serves 4 to 6

1 tablespoon coconut oil

½ medium-size onion, diced

½ teaspoon kosher salt, or to taste

2 garlic cloves

1 Roma tomato, diced

1 Scotch bonnet pepper, left whole

1 (15.5-ounce) canned brown or green pigeon peas, drained and rinsed

1 pound pumpkin or butternut squash, peeled, seeded, and cut in 2-inch chunks

1 teaspoon green seasoning (see page 324 to make your own)

1 cup canned, light coconut milk

Freshly ground black pepper

Garnish: chopped fresh cilantro

Melt coconut oil in a Dutch oven or large sauté pan with a lid over medium heat. Add onion and a pinch of salt and sauté until onion is soft and translucent, about a minute. Add garlic and stir for another 30 seconds. Add tomato and cook for another 30 seconds.

Add whole pepper, pigeon peas, pumpkin, green seasoning, and coconut milk and stir to combine. Add additional water, if needed, to cover all ingredients, then simmer, covered, 10 to 15 minutes, or until pumpkin is just tender. Add salt and black pepper to taste.

Garnish with cilantro.

 Black pepper

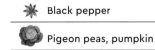 Pigeon peas, pumpkin

12 dried black or shiitake mushrooms

12 ounces dried Chinese egg noodles (chow mein noodles)

½ small onion, sliced

1 cup shredded green cabbage

1 large carrot, peeled and julienned

1 chayote squash, peeled and cut into thin, bite-size slices

½ green bell pepper, cut in half at the equator, then seeded and thinly sliced

2 celery stalks, cut thinly on the diagonal

2 scallions, whites and greens, thinly sliced

¼ cup canola or other neutral oil

6 garlic cloves, peeled and chopped

Salt

1 tablespoon oyster sauce or vegetarian stir-fry sauce

1 tablespoon low-sodium soy sauce

1 tablespoon char siew sauce

1 teaspoon rum, or ½ teaspoon sugar

A few coarse grinds of black pepper

Scotch bonnet pepper sauce and kuchela (see pages 320 and 319 to make your own), for serving

✳ Black pepper

🥬 Bell pepper, cabbage, carrots, celery, chayote, mushrooms

MY MOTHER-IN-LAW, Sue, whom we call Mommy, was born and raised in wartime rural Toishan, Guangdong Province, China. When she moved to Trinidad, she brought her resilience and the tastes of home. Chow mein is one of her signature dishes. This stir-fried noodle dish will be familiar to anyone who has eaten Cantonese food. The elements that bridge this recipe's Cantonese roots with its new home in the Caribbean are the inclusion of chayote squash, and the condiments that are served with it, including Scotch bonnet pepper sauce and kuchela. I've made Mommy's recipe vegetarian, added a little rum to bring in more Caribbean flavor, used less oil, and cooked the noodles al dente, but it is otherwise faithful to her exacting specifications, down to how the vegetables should be sliced ("Not like that, like this!"). Extra mushrooms take the place of the pork that Mommy uses. As with all stir-fry dishes, mise en place is essential for success, as the cooking time is literally a flash in the pan.

MOMMY'S TOISHAN-TO-TRINIDAD CHOW MEIN

Serves 6 to 8

Soak mushrooms in hot water for 5 minutes to soften and remove any grit, then drain, and remove and discard stem. Place in a bowl and cover with fresh hot water to soften completely, about 15 minutes.

Bring a large pot of water to a rolling boil, then add noodles and cook, using chopsticks or tongs to submerge and help loosen bundles of noodles. Cook until just softened, just a few minutes, as they will continue to cook in remaining steps. Drain and rinse in cold water. Set aside.

Ensure all vegetables have been prepped and set aside.

Heat a few tablespoons of oil in a wok or large sauté pan over high heat. Add half of garlic along with a few pinches of salt, and cook for

continued ⟼

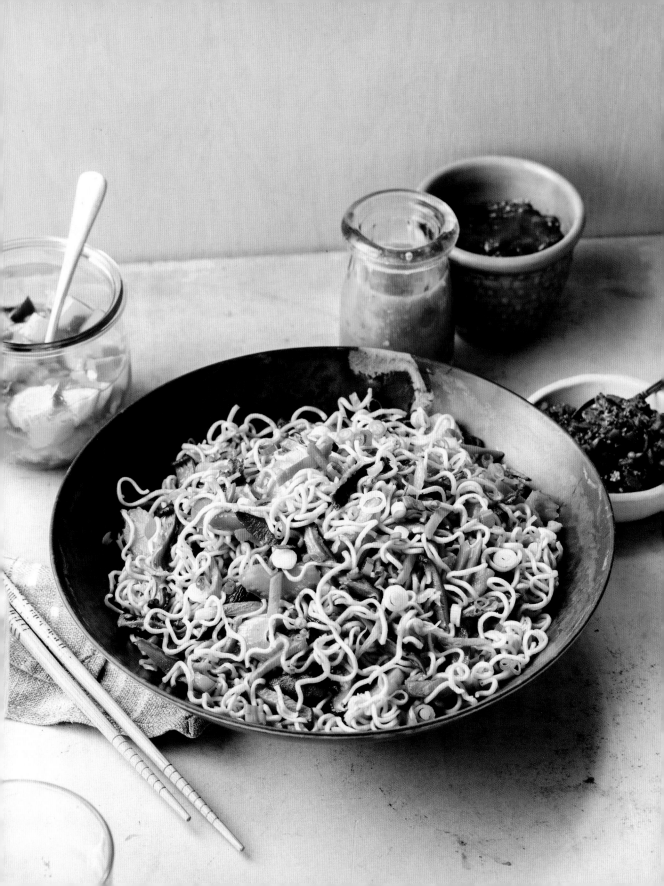

a few seconds, or until garlic is fragrant. Add noodles and cook until any residual liquid is cooked off. Transfer to a plate and set aside. Use a metal spatula to scrape off any residue from pan.

Add a few more tablespoons of oil to pan, then add sliced, soaked mushrooms and their liquid and cook until all liquid is evaporated, using spatula to deglaze pan.

Meanwhile, stir together oyster, soy, and char siew sauces with rum and black pepper in a small bowl and set aside.

When liquid in wok has evaporated, add all vegetables except scallions. Stir-fry for a few minutes, until vegetables are just tender. Add sauce mixture and stir to coat.

Add prepared noodles and gently combine with stir-fry mixture in same pan, to coat noodles evenly. Adjust sauces or salt to taste. Remove from heat and garnish with scallions.

Serve straight from wok. Season to taste with Scotch bonnet pepper sauce and kuchela on the side.

AUNTIE DOLL, Peter's great-aunt, was a gentle soul whose Trinidadian Indian and Creole cooking are legendary. Much of what I know about Trinidadian cooking comes from her. When we were last able to bring Auntie Doll over for the long journey to visit us in San Francisco, I hoped she would share some of her cooking pearls with me (along with dirt from Peter's childhood, of course). I needed to learn some basic techniques of Caribbean cooking, plus there were a few recipes I was desperate to learn: pelau, pastelles, sorrel, and her version of Trinidadian curry. Luckily, she shared a few secrets, including her coveted recipe for pastelles. These are the Trinidadian equivalent of Latin American tamales, filled with a slightly sweet minced filling studded with raisins, and are normally wrapped in banana leaves. Trinidadian pastelles are a treat served on special occasions, traditionally during Christmas celebrations. Auntie Doll didn't want me to go through the trouble of wrapping the filling in banana leaves, so she invented a casserole version, "baked pastelles." If true pastelles are like tamales, these baked pastelles are like tamale pie, or even shepherd's pie. Connoisseurs of true pastelles might not be satisfied, but should keep an open mind and take a bite—this is pure comfort food, Caribbean style.

AUNTIE DOLL'S BAKED PASTELLES

Serves 8 as an entrée; makes 20 to 25 bite-size appetizers

Preheat oven to 350°F and grease a 9 x 13 x 2-inch casserole or cake pan with margarine or butter.

Place cooked lentils in a bowl, then season with salt, pepper, pepper sauce, Worcestershire sauce, and green seasoning. Stir well and allow to sit for at least 10 minutes.

Melt margarine in a large sauté pan over medium-high heat, then add corn flour slowly, stirring constantly so it doesn't clump. Add seasoned lentils, onions, raisins, capers, olives, bell pepper, and celery and continue to stir and fry.

continued ⟶

Margarine or salted butter, for pan

1½ cups cooked green lentils

A few pinches of salt and black pepper

¼ to ½ teaspoon Scotch bonnet pepper sauce

A few splashes of Worcestershire sauce

1 teaspoon green seasoning (see page 324 to make your own)

½ pound (2 sticks) margarine (not butter, if you want to be authentic)

1½ cups corn flour (in Trinidad, this is Promasa brand, which can be purchased online; otherwise, substitute arepa flour or masa—what's used for tamales—but not standard cornmeal)

2 small onions, finely chopped

2 tablespoons raisins

2 tablespoons capers

2 tablespoons minced green olives

2 tablespoons seeded and minced red bell pepper

2 tablespoons minced celery,

1 (14.75-ounce) can creamed-style corn

2 large eggs

1½ cups evaporated milk

✳ Black pepper, chile pepper

🥬 Cornmeal, lentils

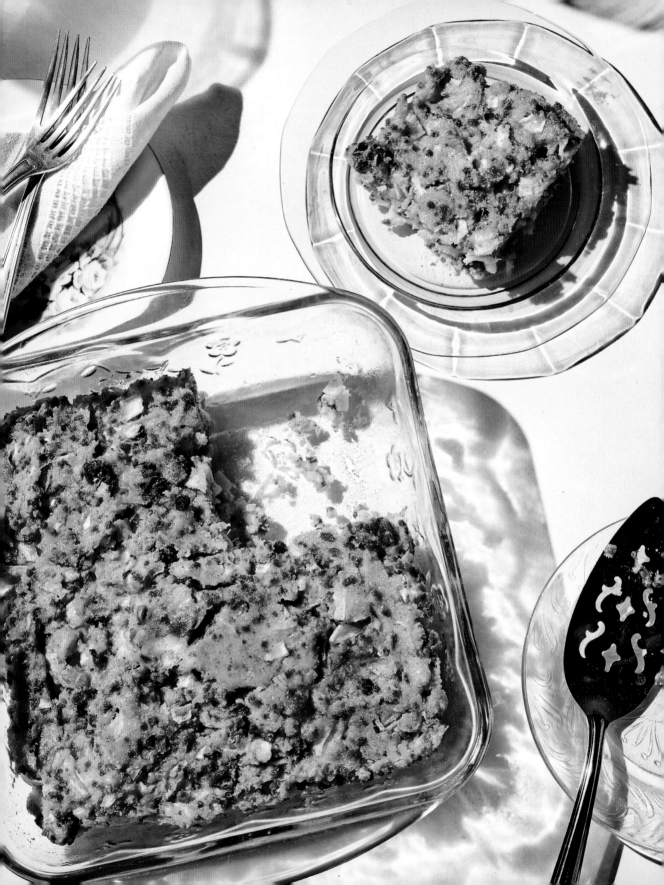

Auntie Doll's Baked Pastelles,
continued

Once onions are slightly translucent, pour in creamed corn and stir to combine. Remove pot from heat.

In a small bowl, beat eggs with evaporated milk. Stir into lentil mixture.

Transfer contents of pot to prepared pan, then bake for 30 to 35 minutes, or until top is slightly golden. Test for doneness with a knife inserted into center, which should come out clean. Remove from oven and allow to cool slightly before slicing and serving.

Tip: You can also make this into appetizers by baking in mini muffin pans. Check after 10 minutes for doneness. (Auntie Doll would have loved this innovation!)

1 cup dried chickpeas
(will make about 2½ cups
cooked)

2 tablespoons canola oil

1 small onion, diced

3 garlic cloves, chopped

2 tablespoons Trinidad curry
powder (see page 325 to
make your own) mixed with
3 tablespoons water, to make
a pourable slurry

1 pound Yukon Gold
potatoes, skin on, quartered

1 Scotch bonnet or habanero
pepper, stemmed, seeded,
and minced

Salt and freshly ground black
pepper

1 tablespoon green
seasoning (see page 324 to
make your own)

VEGETARIANISM is not very popular in Trinidad. Most curries have meat, and if you go to a roti shop, you'll always find chicken and goat, sometimes duck. Vegetables are the side dishes. But carnivorous Trinis all seem to adore this very simple, but surprisingly flavorful dish of curried chickpeas (chana) with potatoes (aloo). The potatoes used most commonly in Trinidad are russet, but I prefer to use Yukon Gold potatoes, skin on, for added nutrition and fiber. The potatoes are typically cut in large chunks. For authentic flavor and texture, I do not recommend canned chickpeas, but they can be used in a pinch. Serve with rice, roti (page 275), or on hops bread (page 264), as a sandwich. Bring out all of your Trini condiments to go with this—kuchela, pepper sauce, and tamarind sauce (see pages 319, 320, and 321 to make your own).

CHANA AND ALOO (CURRIED CHICKPEAS AND POTATO)

Serves 4 to 6

First, soak chickpeas (overnight, if you have the time). Place them in a large bowl and cover with several inches of cold water, to allow for expansion. (If you don't have time to soak overnight, you can use "quick soak" method, which will take 1 hour. Soak as above, then bring to a boil for 5 minutes. Remove from heat. Let chickpeas soak in hot water, covered, for at least 1 hour.) After soaking with either technique, drain water and rinse chickpeas before cooking.

Place soaked chickpeas in a large pot and cover with several inches of water, about 4 cups. Bring to a boil, then lower heat to a simmer. Cook for 60 to 90 minutes, or until they reach your desired tenderness. This will depend on age of your chickpeas. When chickpeas are fully cooked, drain in a colander and allow to cool.

In a Dutch oven or similar heavy pot, heat oil until shimmering, then add onion and stir-fry until translucent, about 5 minutes. Then, add garlic and stir-fry for a few seconds, until fragrant.

✳ Black pepper, curry
powder

Chickpeas, potatoes

Add curry mixture to pot and cook until slightly thickened, 1 to 2 minutes.

Add potatoes and stir to coat in curry mixture.

Add water to cover by 1 inch, along with Scotch bonnet pepper and 1 teaspoon of salt, and boil until potatoes are tender, 10 to 15 minutes, adding more water, if needed, to fully cook potatoes.

Add cooked chickpeas, bring back to a boil, then lower heat and simmer, uncovered, stirring often, until curry sauce is thickened, like a thin gravy. When sauce is at your desired texture, adjust salt and add black pepper and green seasoning.

2 cups sorrel (a.k.a. hibiscus); available at Latin American and Caribbean markets as *flor de Jamaica*

1 cinnamon stick

2 to 3 star anise

6 cloves

1 slice fresh ginger

3 quarts water

Sugar (preferably demerara), start with ½ cup plus 2 tablespoons, or to taste

Auntie Doll's secret ingredient: brandy (optional)

IN TRINIDAD, Christmas is much less commercialized, and celebrated by people of all faiths—it is not unusual to see a Christmas tree in a Hindu or Muslim home. As a time to connect with family and friends, the season is celebrated with local traditions and foods that illustrate the multicultural influences that shaped Trinidad's Creole culture— Amerindian, African, Indian, and British colonial. You'll still find a Christmas ham, but it will be flanked by such treats as pastelles, curry, and roti (see page 307, 290, and 275 to make your own), and serious home cooks are baking traditional Trinidad black cakes with fruit that's been soaking in rum since the year before. Instead of Christmas tree–shaped sugar cookies you're more likely to find *barfi*, the Indian milk sweet. You'll need a drink to wash down this feast. It would likely be ginger beer, Trinidad's Carib beer, or *ponche de creme*, the local version of eggnog that's spiked with tropical flavors of lime, Angostura bitters, and local rum. Or my favorite, sorrel, which is brewed from dried hibiscus flowers, sweetened with sugar, and steeped with sweet spices. Peter's Auntie Doll makes a mean sorrel. Her secret? Brandy "to taste." If you leave out Auntie Doll's brandy, you can also think of this as a nonalcoholic alternative to mulled wine. Cheers!

SORREL

Makes 12 (8-ounce) servings

Place hibiscus flowers, spices, and water into a large pot and bring to a boil. Add sugar to taste.

Turn off heat and steep until you have a beverage that is the color of cranberry juice, at least 1 hour, up to 4 hours. The longer you steep it, the stronger the flavor.

Strain and add brandy to taste, if you like.

Serve over ice.

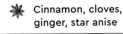

Cinnamon, cloves, ginger, star anise

Sorrel

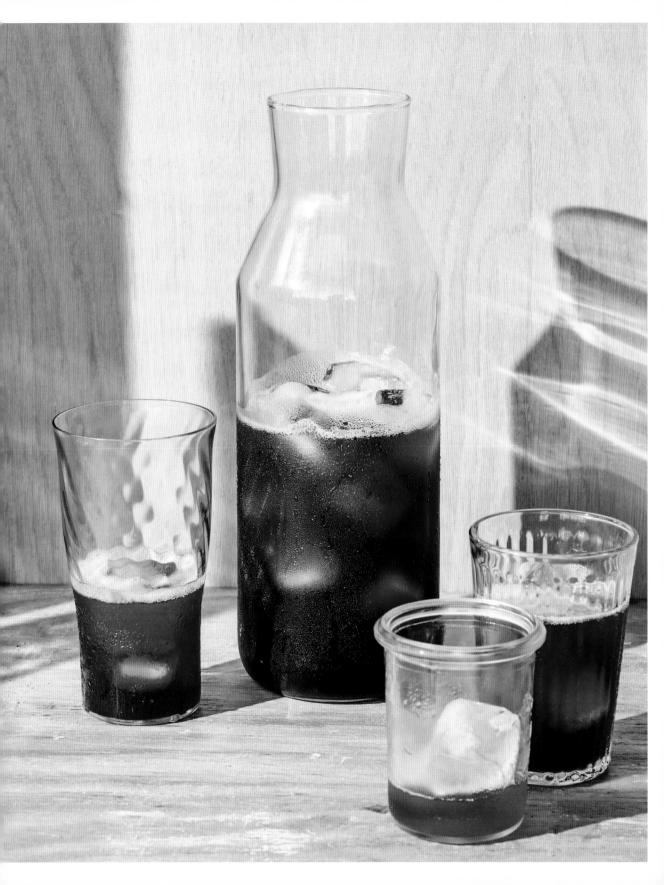

1 pound fresh ginger

2 cups water

Juice of 1 lime

Demerara sugar, about 1 to 2 cups, to taste

5 cloves

Angostura bitters

Still or sparkling water, for serving (optional)

I DAYDREAM of those lazy summers of my youth, where bicycle trips to the local library would reward me with global adventures. I was in fifth grade when I stumbled upon a tattered paperback copy of *Five Fall into Adventure*, one of the volumes in the expansive Famous Five series by British children's author Enid Blyton. I may have been a shy and bookish girly girl, but when I opened *Five Fall into Adventure*, I was Georgina, the brave tomboy heroine my age, always on a quest for adventure. It's been decades since I read the book, but I haven't forgotten the images of her taking rather civilized breaks to have a proper picnic of homemade sandwiches washed down with ginger beer. It took me many years and a trip to the Caribbean to understand that ginger beer can be a strong brew, but a nonalcoholic one. Trinidadian ginger beer is not carbonated, so if you want fizz, add some sparkling water for serving. This is a popular drink at Christmas.

FAMOUS FIVE GINGER BEER

Makes 3 quarts ginger beer

Peel ginger and coarsely chop. Place in a blender with 2 cups of water and blend.

Transfer to one or more large jars or bottles.

Juice lime, and place lime juice and rind in jar along with sugar to taste and cloves. Stir well (sugar doesn't need to completely dissolve; it will as it sits) and screw on lid.

Place jar in sun for an entire hot summer day. If you live in San Francisco as I do and don't have hot sun, allow it to sit at room temperature for 2 to 3 days, checking daily to release any air and to see whether it has a spicy bite.

Strain out solids. Stir in a few splashes of bitters.

Serve over ice, and dilute with still or sparkling water to taste. Keep remainder refrigerated for up to 2 weeks.

❋ Cloves, ginger

PONE IS A RICH, dense pudding made with sweet cassava, pumpkin, and coconut. If you're a fan of Hawaiian butter mochi, you'll find the gooey, bouncy texture of pone familiarly appealing.

Pone is thought to have originated from Trinidad and Tobago, an adaptation of a recipe from a local Amerindian tribe. This dessert is a little labor-intensive to make, particularly if you choose to grate all your ingredients by hand. I recommend using a few prepared ingredients to make this much easier. Traditional recipes include grated coconut, but you can use just coconut milk for a smoother texture. Most traditional recipes also call for evaporated milk, but I think it's rich enough with the coconut milk and I wanted to keep this vegan. I've added much less sugar than usual as well.

PONE

Serves 24

Preheat oven to 350°F, or 325°F if using a glass pan (which I recommend, for easier surveillance). Grease a 9 x 13-inch cake pan with baking spray. A round, ceramic dish that you'd usually use for pies also works well for this. Set aside.

Place all ingredients in a large bowl and stir with a whisk or wooden spoon until combined, a minute or two.

Pour batter into prepared pan and set in middle of oven. Bake for 40 to 45 minutes, or until a knife inserted in center comes out clean and top is very light golden brown. It will not be jiggly and will bounce back if gently touched with a finger.

Remove from oven and allow to cool for 15 minutes before slicing. This pone recipe is great served up on its own, or with a side of fresh coconut ice cream, if you prefer.

Baking spray, butter, or oil, for pan

3 cups grated fresh or frozen cassava (equivalent to two 1-pound packages frozen, available in Asian markets)

¾ cup unsweetened shredded coconut

½ cup canned pure pumpkin puree

1 cup demerara or light brown sugar

½ teaspoon ground cinnamon

½ teaspoon ground ginger

1 teaspoon freshly grated nutmeg

¼ teaspoon ground cloves

2 tablespoons melted vegan butter or coconut oil

1 cup canned full-fat coconut milk

1 teaspoon baking powder

1 teaspoon pure vanilla extract

1 teaspoon Angostura bitters

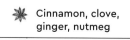

✳ Cinnamon, clove, ginger, nutmeg

Cassava, pumpkin

2 cups milk, any type
(traditionally evaporated
milk)

½ cup natural creamy peanut
butter

1 tablespoon light brown
sugar (traditionally,
condensed milk), or to taste

2 ice cubes

A few dashes of Angostura
bitters

½ teaspoon freshly grated
nutmeg

IVY, PETER'S GRANDMOTHER, knew how to handle a rifle. Granny was equally famous for making a British-style Sunday lunch as she was for her sharpshooting skills, shooting wild game that made their way into the shop with her rifle, to later curry for dinner. She had a sweet tooth, too, and peanut punch was one of her favorites. Peanut punch is an old-fashioned peanut milk shake, made more interesting and less rich with nutmeg and bitters, that is sold in roadside stands but popular enough to also be mass produced and sold in single-serve cartons. The last time I saw Granny, she was in her early nineties and in the last stages of dementia. The last time we came to visit her, though, she brightened at the sight of the peanut punch we brought her, sat up, and guzzled it down with gusto.

GRANNY'S PEANUT PUNCH

Serves 2

Place all ingredients in a blender in order listed, with ¼ teaspoon of nutmeg. Blend until smooth. Adjust sweetness to taste.

Pour into two 8-ounce glasses and dust with remaining nutmeg.

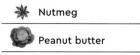

✳ Nutmeg

🌰 Peanut butter

3 ounces freshly squeezed lime juice (from about 5 small limes)

3 cups cold water

2 tablespoons sugar

A few splashes of Angostura bitters (⅛ teaspoon)

ALTHOUGH MOST AMERICAN CHILDREN grow up drinking lemonade, my children were raised on lime juice, with a splash of Angostura bitters, which come from Trinidad. They have a pretty interesting history, involving three continents, indigenous herbs, and a secret recipe. Why not add a little intrigue (and color) to your limeade with a splash of Angostura, the way people do in Trinidad? For authenticity, sweeten with either granulated or demerara sugar, not superfine sugar or simple syrup. Trinidadians have a sweet tooth, so would probably sweeten this much more than I've called for. Feel free to adjust to taste!

PETER'S LIME JUICE WITH ANGOSTURA BITTERS

Makes almost 1 quart juice, with ice

Juice limes into a pitcher and add water and sugar.

Stir with a chopstick (or other stirrer, but I'm giving you the authentic recipe here!)

Add Angostura.

Serve over "plenty" ice.

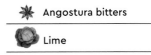

| ✴ | Angostura bitters |
| 🥬 | Lime |

1 barely ripe mango (slightly yielding, not rock hard) or other tart fruits (pommecythere, plums, Granny Smith apples, pineapple)

1 to 2 garlic cloves, minced

1 to 2 tablespoons minced fresh culantro, or cilantro

Trinidadian or habanero pepper sauce

Juice of 1 lime

Salt and freshly ground black pepper to taste

THIS IS A VERY SIMPLE RECIPE but one of the most beloved for Trinidadians. Three ingredients—mango, garlic, and culantro (known in Trinidad as shado beni)—are the soul of this zesty snack, to which you can add other seasonings to taste—pepper sauce, lime juice, salt, and pepper, sometimes soy sauce. It's basically a garlicky, spicy fruit salad. I didn't understand what was so great about chow until a trip to Trinidad to visit my in-laws, when I had a chow revelation during a nature outing. Ever since my first trip to Trinidad two decades ago, I had longed to see Trinidad's national bird, the scarlet ibis, in its natural habitat, Caroni Swamp. But after a long drive along the winding, bumpy roads, I started the two-hour boat tour of Caroni Swamp nauseated, and afraid I wouldn't be able to enjoy the long-anticipated tour. It didn't help that we were surrounded by a lively and loud family that talked, laughed, and snacked nonstop. I didn't mind helping pass their snacks back and forth to various members of their group, and was excited to accept an offer of their homemade chow made of mango and pommecythere (a tart, plumlike fruit). One bite of the tart, garlicky, and spicy snack, and my nausea disappeared. I was rejuvenated just in time to appreciate the wildlife of Caroni, and the finale—the astonishing and memorable flock of scarlet ibis flying in to roost for the night in the mangrove trees, looking like dozens of red poinsettia blooms.

CARONI MANGO CHOW

Serves 2 as a snack; make more, make new friends!

Peel mango, then slice into strips or slices and place in a bowl. Include pit—it's the lucky one who gets to suck on that.

Add garlic, culantro, and pepper sauce to taste, and squeeze lime juice over mixture. Add salt and black pepper to taste, if desired.

Stir it up, and eat up!

SPICEBOX KITCHEN

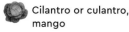
Black pepper, chile pepper, garlic

Cilantro or culantro, mango

1 green (unripe) mango

2 garlic cloves, minced

½ Scotch bonnet pepper, stemmed and minced

1 tablespoon amchar masala (see page 325 to make your own, or look for Chief brand, available online)

¾ teaspoon salt

¼ cup neutral oil, such as canola

THIS IS MY FAVORITE of the condiments that make up the Trinidadian Indian cupboard. Don't confuse amchar masala (page 325), a spice mixture used for pickling that is unique to Trinidad's Indian community, with amchur, which in India refers to a powder made *from* green mangoes, used to add sour flavor to savory dishes. In place of the traditional mustard oil, I have substituted more available vegetable oil, without a discernable change in flavor. This condiment is most often made with green mango but also popular with a tart plumlike fruit called pommecythere. An overabundance of plums on my backyard tree led me to experiment with making another version of this recipe with shredded just short-of-ripe plum, and the results were divine. Kuchela is eaten as a condiment for roti, curries, pretty much anything.

KUCHELA (MANGO PICKLE)

Makes about 1 cup kuchela

Peel and grate mango, place in a clean towel, and squeeze out any liquid, then spread out on a sheet pan to dry in the sun for a day, or in a low oven (250°F) for a few hours.

Combine all ingredients, except oil, in a bowl and then blend in oil. Allow to sit for 30 minutes before consuming.

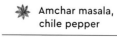 Amchar masala, chile pepper

 Mango

12 Scotch bonnet peppers (different colors, if available), stemmed and chopped

6 garlic cloves, peeled and chopped

1½ cups freshly squeezed lime juice (from 3 to 4 medium-size limes)

2 tablespoons chopped fresh cilantro or culantro (shado beni)

¾ cup peeled and chopped mango

Salt

THE MORUGA scorpion pepper might have put Peter's hometown on the map, but the pepper that Trinidadians and other people of the Caribbean use in all their cooking is the still fiery but more edible Scotch bonnet pepper (over 1.2 million vs. 80,000 to 400,000 Scoville units). This chile is not only spicy but fruity. To bring out the fruitiness and tame the spice a little, some recipes add a little shredded carrot or fruit. I like the addition of a little mango, which contains pectin to naturally thicken this sauce. You could also try papaya or pineapple, or if you're going for thickening only, a little dry or prepared mustard. Scotch bonnet peppers can be hard to source, so if needed, substitute habaneros, which are similar in heat but less fruity.

MORUGA ROAD PEPPER SAUCE

Makes about 2 cups sauce

Combine all ingredients in a food processor or blender and process until finely minced. Adjust flavors to taste. Keep refrigerated.

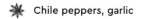 Chile peppers, garlic

Lime, mango

1 (14-ounce) package "wet tamarind" (pulp with seeds, available in Asian markets)

3 cups water, plus more if needed

2 garlic cloves, minced

1 Scotch bonnet pepper, minced

2 tablespoons minced fresh culantro (shado beni) or cilantro

3 tablespoons dark brown sugar, or to taste

1½ teaspoons salt

THE BACKYARD of my in-laws' former home in Fifth Company Village, in the south of Trinidad, is overrun with all the tropical fruit of your dreams. Pineapple, papaya, sorrel, tamarind, and other fruits all grow profusely. My sister-in-law, Jean, picks tamarind pods to make into spicy, sweet and sour tamarind balls, a far cry from the one-dimensionally sweet candy bars we can pick up in the grocery aisle stateside. I also love the flavor of tamarind but prefer it in condiment form, to go with roti and all types of Trini food. Unlike my sister-in-law, tamarind pods are not dropping from the sky for me. So I've made this recipe using tamarind pulp, easily found in Asian markets. Use it like ketchup.

TAMARIND SAUCE

Makes 2 cups sauce

Place tamarind pulp in a medium-size saucepan, cover with water, and bring to a boil over medium heat. Continue to simmer for 10 minutes or so, breaking apart, mashing and stirring with a wooden spoon, until tamarind begins to dissolve. Your goal is to have as much pulp as possible separate from seeds and fibrous membrane. Add more water, as needed.

When pulp has mainly come off seeds, pour mixture through a sieve into a bowl or another saucepan. Pass through additional water to get as much pulp as you can, pressing down with a wooden spoon. Return strained pulp to saucepan.

Add remaining ingredients and bring sauce to a simmer to marry flavors and thicken. Sauce will thicken and darken, and garlic and pepper will cook down. Once sauce is at the consistency you want, in 15 to 30 minutes (longer if you've added a lot of water), adjust salt and sugar to taste, remove from heat, and allow sauce to cool before transferring to a jar. Keep refrigerated; it will last for up to 6 months.

 Tamarind

½ small bitter melon
(optional)

12 Scotch bonnet peppers,
various colors

1 carrot

2 limes, plus juice of 4 limes

3 garlic cloves

1½ teaspoons salt

About 1 cup white vinegar

AUNTIE DOLL kept her small house immaculate. It was decorated from another time, with lace doilies covering armrests and lace curtains blowing in the wind. Her kitchen was cleverly outfitted with pegboard cabinet doors painted white, with S-hooks inserted to hold kitchen towels and small utensils, à la Julia Child's kitchen. On top of the cabinets in her sunny kitchen were jars of colorful pickles, mainly lime pickle, which is similar to Scotch bonnet pepper sauce, but chunky and coarse, and including tart pieces of lime peel, bitter melon, and carrots. Note that many people do not like the bitterness of bitter melon, so omit if you are one of those people. However, the pickling process definitely balances out a lot of the bitterness. Use this as a condiment, as you would pepper/chile sauce. If you can't tolerate that much heat, use just the liquid. If you can tolerate heat, eat the solids like a pickle.

AUNTIE DOLL'S LIME PEPPER

Makes about 3 cups lime pepper

Slice bitter melon in half lengthwise, then scoop out flesh and seeds. Slice crosswise into half-moons. If desired, soak for 15 minutes in salt water to decrease bitterness, then rinse. Reserve half for another use.

Stem peppers and slice thinly crosswise.

Cut carrots on the diagonal into thin coins, then cut each of those into thick sticks.

Wash limes thoroughly, then dry and cut into 1-inch chunks or small wedges.

Place all cut produce in a 24-ounce mason jar, alternating colors to make it pretty.

Add garlic, salt, and lime juice. Top off with white vinegar, adding enough to cover all vegetables.

Seal tightly with lid, then shake thoroughly. Place in a sunny spot for at least 3 days, up to 2 weeks, until all vegetables are slightly softened. Adjust salt to taste.

Keeps refrigerated for up to 6 months.

🌟 Chile peppers, garlic

🥬 Bitter melon, carrot, lime

JERK IS A SPICE RUB or marinade that is synonymous with Jamaican, not Trinidadian, cuisine but too good not to include in this book! This allspice-heavy marinade brings concentrated, deep flavor to anything you put it on. Use it to marinate any protein, such as tempeh (page 294), tofu, or fish.

JERK MARINADE

Makes about 2 cups marinade, enough for 4 to 5 pounds of protein

Blend all ingredients together in a food processor or blender until smooth. Adjust salt to taste.

Place your protein in a nonreactive, lidded container or resealable plastic bag and cover it with enough jerk sauce to coat on all sides. Cover/seal and marinate for at least 4 hours, or overnight, refrigerated.

To cook, remove protein from marinade (discard marinade), then grill or roast in oven.

1 small onion, chopped

4 scallions, chopped

4 garlic cloves, chopped

2 teaspoons minced fresh ginger

2 Scotch bonnet peppers, stemmed, seeded, and coarsely chopped

Leaves from 5 thyme sprigs

1 tablespoon ground allspice

½ teaspoon ground cinnamon

½ teaspoon freshly grated nutmeg

1 tablespoon demerara sugar or dark brown sugar

1 tablespoon kosher salt, or to taste

1 teaspoon freshly ground black pepper, or to taste

2 tablespoons white vinegar

Juice of 1 lime

¼ cup soy sauce

¼ cup canola oil

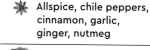 Allspice, chile peppers, cinnamon, garlic, ginger, nutmeg

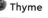 Thyme

½ cup chopped fresh chives

1 cup fresh thyme leaves

½ cup fresh parsley, chopped

½ cup culantro (shado beni), chopped

½ cup diced onion

4 garlic cloves, chopped

1 teaspoon salt

2 to 4 tablespoons water, for blending

Freshly ground black pepper

1 tablespoon white vinegar

THIS IS THE FRESH HERB MIXTURE that is one of the characteristic flavors of Trinidadian cooking. The herbs, which are grown in Paramin, in the north of Trinidad, reflect both Trinidad's colonial history, with the chives, thyme, and parsley coming from the French, and the culantro (shado beni) native to Trinidad, which was originally part of South America. If you can't get culantro, substitute cilantro. A batch of green seasoning can be refrigerated for up to 5 days, but for longer use, try freezing it in ice cube trays, and storing those small amounts for ready use in freezer bags.

GREEN SEASONING

Makes 1 cup seasoning

 Garlic

Culantro, parsley, thyme

Puree all ingredients together in a blender or food processor until you have a slightly chunky paste.

CREOLE SOUPS are often adorned with boiled flour dumplings that are similar to those served in the American South. Experiment with the amount of liquid to get a denser or softer dumpling, depending on your preference.

1 cup all-purpose flour

½ teaspoon salt

2 teaspoons baking powder

½ cup water

TRINIDAD DUMPLINGS

Serves 6

Stir dry ingredients together in a small bowl.

Stir in water, beginning with ¼ cup, adding spoon by spoon until dough reaches your desired texture. These can either be made firm enough to be rolled and shaped, or soft enough to be dropped from a spoon.

Drop into hot broth or soup, cover, and simmer for 15 minutes, or until done.

THE **SIGNATURE FLAVOR** of Trinidad curry is the local brand Chief's particular blend, which is easy to procure on the internet. If you want to make your own, this recipe comes close.

TRINIDAD CURRY POWDER

Makes ⅔ cup curry powder

¼ cup cumin seed

2 tablespoons coriander seeds

1 tablespoon fenugreek seeds

1 teaspoon fennel seeds

¼ cup ground turmeric

½ teaspoon ground cayenne pepper

½ teaspoon salt

Toast cumin, coriander, fenugreek, and fennel seeds in a dry sauté pan over medium heat until fragrant, shaking pan constantly, just a few minutes. Remove from heat and allow to cool.

Grind together cooled, roasted spices in a spice grinder. Once ground, add remaining ingredients and grind together.

Place in an airtight container and store in a cool, dry place for up to several months.

 Cayenne, cumin, coriander, fennel, fenugreek, turmeric

AMCHAR MASALA is the earthy, pungent spice blend that is necessary to making kuchela (page 319), an essential Trinidadian condiment. Since this is not easily available outside the Caribbean, try making your own.

3 tablespoons cumin seeds

¼ cup whole coriander seeds

4 teaspoons black mustard seeds

1 tablespoon fenugreek seeds

2 teaspoons fennel seeds

AMCHAR MASALA

Makes a generous ½ cup amchar masala

Place cumin seeds in a small, heavy, dry skillet over medium heat and toast for 2 minutes or more, until fragrant and deep brown.

Add remaining spices to pan and toast for another minute until all are fragrant. Remove from pan, allow to cool, and then grind as finely as possible in a spice grinder.

Coriander, cumin, fennel, fenugreek, mustard seeds

TRINIDAD MENUS

SOCA SUNDAY LUNCH

Caroni Mango Chow

Coconut Bake

Heland's Callaloo

Auntie Doll's Baked Pastelles

Pelau with Roasted Pumpkin

Sorrel

VEGETARIAN LIME

Lime (noun or verb) is the word used in Trinidad to mean "hang out, have a good time." More specifically, it refers to the art of doing nothing while sharing food, drink, conversation, and laughter.

Dal

Buss Up Shut

Curry Mango

Okra and Tomatoes

Chana and Aloo

Peter's Lime Juice with Angostura Bitters

resources

WHERE TO FIND ME

Blog: Spiceboxtravels.com

FB: www.Facebook.com/
TheDoctorsSpicebox

Twitter and Instagram:
@spiceboxtravels

YouTube: Linda Shiue, MD, Chef.
The Doctor's Spicebox

NUTRITION

https://www.choosemyplate.gov/
eathealthy/WhatIsMyPlate/

www.NutritionFacts.org/

SUSTAINABLE
GROCERY SHOPPING

PRODUCE

www.ewg.org/

**To find local farmers' markets,
search by zip code**: https://
www.ams.usda.gov/services/
local-regional/food-directories/

To find a CSA: https://www.ams
.usda.gov/local-food-directories/
csas

**To find out what's in season
in your area**: https://www
.seasonalfoodguide.org

SEAFOOD

www.seafoodwatch.org

https://www.epa.gov/fish-tech/

GUIDES TO
PREPARING PRODUCE

Anthony, Michael. *V Is for
Vegetables.* New York: Little,
Brown and Company, 2015.

Lipe, Mi Ae. *Bounty from the Box:
The CSA Farm Cookbook.* Bothell,
WA: Twisted Carrot, 2015.

Mangini, Cara. *The Vegetable
Butcher.* New York: Workman
Publishing, 2016.

SPICES

Lakshmi, Padma. *The Encyclopedia
of Spices and Herbs: An Essential
Guide to the Flavors of the World.*
New York: Ecco, 2016.

MacAller, Natasha. *Spice Health
Heroes.* London: Jacqui Small LLP,
2016.

Sercarz, Lior Lev. *The Spice
Companion: A Guide to the World
of Spices: A Cookbook.* New York:
Clarkson Potter, 2016.

WHOLE GRAINS

Speck, Maria. *Ancient Grains
for Modern Meals.* New York:
Ten Speed Press, 2011.

Wholegrainscouncil.org

LEARNING TO
COOK INTUITIVELY

Nosrat, Samin. *Salt, Fat, Acid, Heat.*
New York: Simon & Schuster,
2017.

REDUCING
FOOD WASTE

James Beard Foundation. *Waste
Not.* New York: Rizzoli, 2018.

INGREDIENTS
SOURCES

Beans: Rancho Gordo

Grains: Bob's Red Mill

Spices: Burlap & Barrel,
Diaspora Co., Oaktown Spice
Shop, Penzey's, Spicely

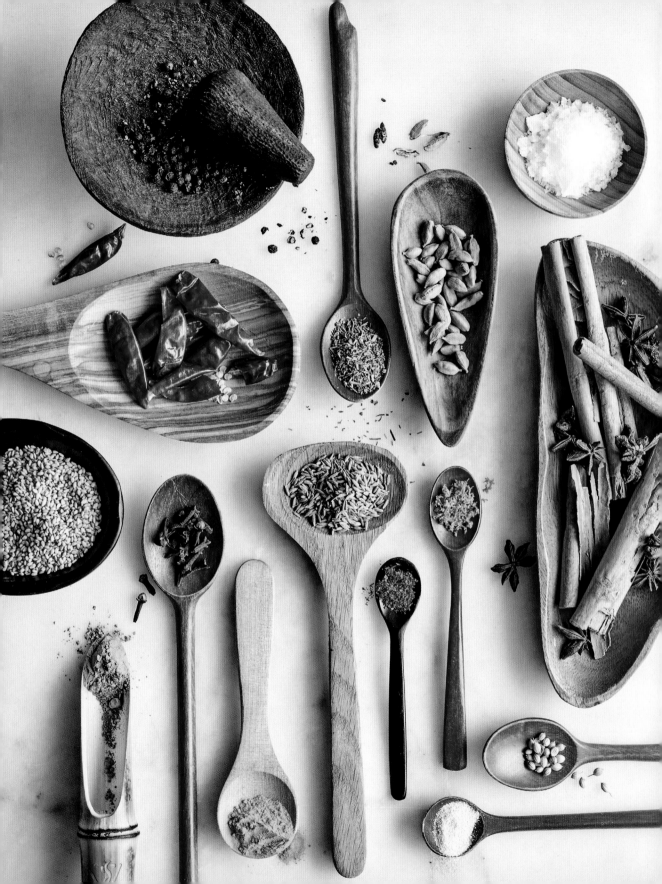

acknowledgments

THIS BOOK has been a long and delightful journey, one that began with taste memories from the kitchens of my family, friends, and people I've met along the way. When I made the leap into imagining that I could make food a part of my career, after writing my first recipes for Francis Lam's Salon Kitchen Challenge, I found myself surrounded by tremendous supporters who encouraged this crazy idea.

My first inspiration was David Eisenberg's Healthy Kitchens, Healthy Lives conference. I taught my first classes in Palo Alto with support from Tony Marzoni, Albert Chan, Martin Entwistle, Shauna Hyde, Shaun McElrath, Linda Klieman, and Martha Simmons. Aside from the kitchen, my other happy place is the public library, so it was a thrill to teach in the stacks—thanks, Chris Gray and Alex Perez! Thanks, Kara Rosenberg at Palo Alto Adult School and Kathleen Taggart and Abigail Crayne at Draeger's Cooking School, for taking a chance on me to teach my first hands-on classes. Fellow doctor-chefs Julia Nordgren, Michelle Hauser, Drew Ramsey, and John La Puma inspired and encouraged me.

Thank you, Jodi Liano, Catherine Pantsios, and Kirsten Salazar at San Francisco Cooking School, for honing my skills, expanding my palate, and modeling how to be a good cooking teacher. Thank you, Mourad Lahlou and everyone who taught me during my externship at Mourad.

My San Francisco cooking classes couldn't have happened without the support of Maria Ansari, Gene Lau, James Lawrence, Ray Liu, Dawn Ogawa, Connie Bonilla, Yvonne Gallot, Lisa Pecache, Rudolph Allen, Kelly Lam, and Erick Orozco. And huge thanks to the many volunteers who have helped out in my classes over the years, especially Dan Santiago, and to my students—you're the reason I do this.

I also thank three generous cookbook authors who got my feet wet in cookbook writing: Mi Ae Lipe, Natasha MacAller, and Pat Tanumihardja.

I am eternally grateful to my incredible food styling and photography team for your talent, attention to detail, and hard work. Haley Hazell, you always find just the right prop for every dish and make everything so beautiful. Michelle K. Min, people would be lucky if they were as photogenic as you made my food look. Thanks for capturing the light. Sara Remington, thanks for so generously sharing your beautiful photo studio. I also had a tremendous team of photo shoot volunteers, who as a group represented both the culinary and medical worlds: Antonia Diodate, Siobhan McDonnell, Marcus Olivares-Peres, Dana Quinn, Jessica Tien, and Adrienne Yang.

Much gratitude to the amazing publishing team that patiently and enthusiastically shepherded me through this process: Amanda Annis, my literary agent at Trident Media Group; and the entire crew at Hachette: editor Renée Sedliar, Alison Dalafave, Cisca Schreefel, creative director Amanda Kain, designer Toni Tajima, copyeditor Iris Bass, and proofreaders Katie McHugh Malm and Lori Lewis. Chef Bryant Terry, thank you for taking time to write the foreword. You're a wonderful collaborator and I look forward to planning more community programs with you.

Without the support of my family, this book would not have happened. I don't think my parents, Grace and Chyng Yann Shiue, ever expected me to write a cookbook. Thank you, Mama, for your unconditional love, support, and encouragement; allowing me to make many messes in the kitchen; and for chhá bí-hún and beef noodle soup. Thank you, Dad, for breaking with tradition to try, and sometimes like, my "weird food." Thank you to my brother, Peter Shiue, who ate many of my kitchen experiments growing up and is the best uncle my kids could wish for. I spent a lot of time away from my daughters to create this book. Thank you, Emmy and Coco, for that sacrifice; I hope it inspires you to follow your dreams. Peter, I am grateful for your support, encouragement, and taste testing, and for being my partner in adventure for so many years.

index

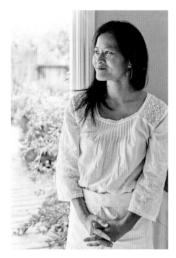

ASIDE FROM DURIAN AND BITTER MELON, **Linda Shiue** hasn't met a fruit or vegetable she doesn't like. Her openness to new flavors has led others to challenge her with armadillo and bunny ears, and white lies about her ethnicity in an attempt to access the secret menu at a local Cambodian restaurant. After she took her first French cooking class at age seven, it took almost forty more years before she finally went to culinary school at San Francisco Cooking School. In between, she studied anthropology and medicine at Brown University, with fieldwork in rural Sichuan, China, and in über-urban Singapore; continued her medical training at the University of California, San Francisco; and learned about plant-based nutrition at Cornell University. She has been known to play spin-the-globe to choose travel destinations. An enthusiastic eater, she inspires strangers to copy her order and restaurant chefs to send her a little something special. Linda is a practicing physician in San Francisco, where she also founded a popular vegetable-forward teaching kitchen to inspire people to cook for health. Follow her on Twitter and Instagram @spiceboxtravels, on Facebook and YouTube at The Doctors Spicebox, and on her blog, SpiceboxTravels.com.